due for return on or before the last date shown below.

2011

Mental
HEALTH
FROM POLICY TO PRACTICE

BROOKER, CH...

Mental Health: From Policy To Practice

0443103836   -

Churchill Livingstone   2009

Dedication

This book is dedicated to our mothers, Margaret and Pat, who both died in 2007

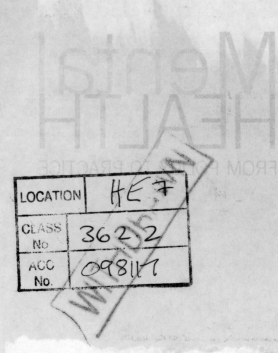

For Elsevier:
Commissioning Editor: Steven Black
Development Editor: Janice Urquhart
Project Manager: Kerrie-Anne Jarvis
Designer: Stewart Larking
Illustrator: Merlyn Harvey

Mental
HEALTH
FROM POLICY TO PRACTICE

Edited by

Charlie Brooker BA MSs PhD
Professor of Criminal Justice and Mental Health,
Centre for Clinical and Academic Workforce Innovation
(CCAWI), University of Lincoln,
Lincoln, UK

Julie Repper RGN RMN BA MPhil PhD
Associate Professor and Reader in Mental Health Nursing
and Social Care, University of Nottingham,
Nottingham, UK

Foreword by

Martin Brown
Interim Chief Executive, Barnet,
Enfield and Haringey Mental Health NHS Trust;
Head of Mental Health Policy, Department of Health (1995–2001)

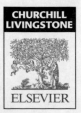

CHURCHILL
LIVINGSTONE

ELSEVIER

Edinburgh   London   New York   Oxford   Philadelphia   St Louis   Sydney   Toronto 2009

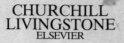

CHURCHILL
LIVINGSTONE
ELSEVIER

First published 2009

ISBN: 9780443103834

British Library Cataloguing in Publication Data
A catalogue record for this book is available from the British Library

Library of Congress Cataloging in Publication Data
A catalog record for this book is available from the Library of Congress

Notice
Knowledge and best practice in this field are constantly changing. As new research and experience broaden our knowledge, changes in practice, treatment and drug therapy may become necessary or appropriate. Readers are advised to check the most current information provided (i) on procedures featured or (ii) by the manufacturer of each product to be administered, to verify the recommended dose or formula, the method and duration of administration, and contraindications. It is the responsibility of the practitioner, relying on their own experience and knowledge of the patient, to make diagnoses, to determine dosages and the best treatment for each individual patient, and to take all appropriate safety precautions. To the fullest extent of the law, neither the Publisher nor the Editors assume any liability for any injury and/or damage to persons or property arising out or related to any use of the material contained in this book.

The Publisher

Printed in China

Contents

Contributors

Ian Baguley MPhil RMN DipPSI CPNCert
Co-Director, Centre for Clinical and
Academic Workforce Innovation
(CCAWI); Professor of Mental Health,
University of Lincoln; Associate Director
Education and Training National Institute
of Mental Health England (NIMHE), UK

Peter Bartlett BA MA LLB PhD
Barrister and Solicitor (Ontario);
Nottinghamshire Healthcare NHS
Trust Professor of Mental Health Law,
University of Nottingham, Nottingham, UK

Joanna Bennett PhD BA RN RM
Senior Lecturer in Nursing (Mental
Health), University of the West Indies,
Mona Campus, Jamaica; Breaking the
Circles of Fear Project, Sainsbury Centre
for Mental Health, London, UK

Max Birchwood BSc MSc PhD DSc FBPsS
Professor of Mental Health, School of
Psychology, University of Birmingham
and Birmingham and Solihul Mental
Health NHS Trust, Birmingham, UK

Jed Boardman MBBS BSc PhD FRCPsych
Consultant Psychiatrist and Senior
Lecturer in Social Psychiatry, South
London and Maudsley NHS Foundation
Trust and Health Services and Population
Research Department, Institute of
Psychiatry, London, UK

Charlie Brooker BA MSs PhD
Professor of Criminal Justice and Mental
Health, Centre for Clinical and Academic
Workforce Innovation (CCAWI),
University of Lincoln, Lincoln, UK

Jenny Bywaters MA BM BCh FFPH CCCert
Consultant in Public Health, Care Services
Improvement Partnership and North East
Public Health Observatory, UK

Julie Carlisle BA MPhil PhD
Postdoctoral Research Associate,
University of Liverpool, Liverpool, UK

Clair Chilvers BSc MSc DSc
Chair, Nottinghamshire Healthcare NHS
Trust and formerly Director of Research,
National Institute for Mental Health in
England, UK

Michael Clark BA MPhil PhD
Research Manager, Care Services
Improvement Partnership, UK

Kim Dent-Brown DipCOT BSc
AdvDipDramatherapy PG Cert(Psychotherapy) PhD
Research Fellow, Centre for
Psychological Services Research,
University of Sheffield, Sheffield, UK

David Ekers MSc DipCBT RMN
Nurse Consultant, Tees, Esk & Wear
Valleys NHS Trust, UK

Alison Faulkner BSc MSc
Independent Service User and
Researcher, London

John Freeman RMN MA
Faculty of Health & Wellbeing, Sheffield
Hallam University, Assertive Community
Treatment Association, Sheffield, UK

Kevin Gournay CBE FRCPsych FMedSci FRCN
PhD CPsychol AFBPsS CSci
CertBehaviouralPsychotherapy RN
Emeritus Professor, Institute of Psychiatry,
King's College London, London, UK

Richard Gray RN DipHE BSc MSc DLSHTM
FEANS PhD
Professor of Nursing, University of East
Anglia, Norwich, UK

Hilary Guite MSc FFPH MRCGP DCH
Consultant in Public Health, Greenwich
TPCT and Associate London
Development Centre for Mental Health,
London, UK

Guy Howland BSc
Public Affairs Consultant to the Mental
Health Foundation, London, UK

Naomi Humber BSc
Research Assistant, Department of Psychiatry, University of Manchester, Manchester, UK

Zaffer Iqbal BSc DClinPsy PhD CPsychol AFBPsS
Consultant Clinical Psychologist and Director of Research Training, Clinical Psychology Unit, The University of Sheffield, Sheffield, UK

Ian Kerr BSc MD MRCPsych MemACAT AssMemBAP
Consultant Psychiatrist and Psychotherapist, Sheffield Care Trust; Honorary Senior Lecturer, School of Health and Related Research (ScHaRR), University of Sheffield, Sheffield, UK

Karen Linde PhD
Senior Development Consultant, Strategy and Development/Research Fellow, Rotherham NHS Primary Care Trust, Rotherham, UK

Andrew McCulloch MA PhD
Chief Executive, Mental Health Foundation, London, UK

Stephen McGowan RMHN
Early Intervention in Psychosis Lead, National Institute for Mental Health in England (North East Yorkshire and the Humber) and Bradford and Airedale Teaching PCT, UK

Steve Onyett PhD MSc CClinPsychol AFBPsS
Senior Development Consultant, Care Service Improvement Partnership SW (Incorporating NIMHE), Visiting Professor, School of Health and Social Care, University of the West of England, Bristol, UK

Glenys Parry BA DipClinPsych PHD CPsychol FBPsS
Professor of Applied Psychological Therapies, Centre for Psychological Services Research, ScHARR, The University of Sheffield, Sheffield, UK

Michael Parsonage BA
Senior Policy Advisor, The Sainsbury Centre for Mental Health, London, UK

Rachel Perkins BA PhD MPhil(Clinical Psychology)
Director of Quality Assurance and User/Carer Experience, South West London and St George's Mental Health NHS Trust, London, UK

Julie Repper RGN RMN BA MPhil PhD
Associate Professor and Reader in Mental Health Nursing and Social Care, University of Nottingham, Nottingham, UK

Tom Ricketts RMN BSc CertAdultBehaviouralPsychotherapy PhD
Nurse Consultant in Psychotherapy & Research, Specialist Psychotherapy Service, Sheffield Care NHS Trust, Sheffield, UK

David Rushforth MPhil BA RN(MH) RNT
Principal Lecturer, National Project Lead, Centre for Clinical and Academic Workforce Innovation (CCAWI), University of Lincoln, Lincoln, UK

Elizabeth Sayce BA MSc
Chief Executive Officer, RADAR (Royal Association for Disability and Rehabilitation), London, UK

Jane Senior BA MA RMN PhD
Research Project Manager, Department of Psychiatry, University of Manchester, Manchester, UK

Jenny Shaw MB ChB FRCPsych PhD
Consultant Forensic Psychiatrist, Lancashire Care NHS Trust; Professor of Forensic Psychiatry, University of Manchester, Manchester, UK

Alan Simpson PhD PGDip(Couns) BA RMN
Senior Research Fellow, City University, London, UK

Harvey Wells BSc MSc PGCAP
Lecturer, Institute of Psychiatry, London, UK

Foreword

The Mental Health National Service Framework (MHNSF) was a key component in the policy approach to mental health implemented by the new Labour administration in 1997. Their analysis of the state of mental health care was informed by specialist advice pre election, constituency experiences and media opinion; and a post election realisation that much of mental health policy had been reactive and piecemeal.

Their judgement (soon arrived at) was that mental health services were resistant to change and modernisation (by which they primarily meant the ability of the service to incorporate new and effective approaches to care); were of variable quality both within and between organisations; that there was no overall strategy on what mental health services were supposed to be delivering, and that services were not focussed on preventing harm to users and the public at large. Clarity of expectation became a key driver for ministers: 'if we are not clear what the service is supposed to do, it is difficult to hold them to account for performance'. In judging policy made then, we must remember how things were then.

They were clear that mental health services were under-funded, and that mental health should be a major component of the first comprehensive spending review. In order to make a winnable case to the Treasury, it was agreed that two things must be in place. Firstly, an overarching strategic statement that clarified the purpose and role of mental health services. This strategy was published as Safe, Sound and Supportive in January 1998. The ordering of the words within the title is not random, and was the subject of much debate with ministers and others. It is important to recognise that there was just as much focus on public safety from the new administration as the one it replaced. Secondly, the production of a National Service Framework for mental health (the subject of this book). At that time, National Service Frameworks were seen as a way of delivering equity of national service provision, and equality of service delivery.

The NSF for mental health was therefore a structural device to drive system conformity. It also acted as a template against which service investment could be made. Any assessment of policy implementation must focus on what was expected, and the extent to which this has been delivered. As with most policy implementation, things are never quite as good as people hoped, but not quite as bad as they feared. A mixed picture is the standard.

But another consequence of the MHNSF is also important: it has acted as a defence against changing NHS priorities and financial imperatives. However far short implementation falls, not to have had it at all would have been be far worse. New imperatives have arisen. We need to complete the delivery of structures and systems, but also focus more on the individual processes that deliver high quality care. The National Service User Surveys clearly highlight where we need to be putting our energy. This book reports on progress in implementing the MHNSF. The key question is: are mental health services safer, sounder and more supportive now than they were in 1997? If the answer is no, then we have failed. If the answer is a yes, albeit a qualified yes, then we are on the right track.

Martin Brown

Preface

The origin of this book lies in our perception that mental health policy has been in almost constant and dynamic flux over the past ten years. The broad provenance of such system change might be attributed to the National Service Framework but this does not reflect the complexity or range of developments.

In this book we have attempted to examine the multi-faceted process of mental health service development from a wide variety of perspectives. The primacy of recovery-orientated approaches is emphasised. The functional service models of the NSF are dissected, not by us, but by experts in the relevant fields. We have also invited expert commentary on key support functions such as education and training, evidence-based practice and research, alongside other important changes, for example, disability rights and mental health legislation. The conclusion we reach does not chime wholeheartedly with the policy-makers. This is neither perhaps surprising nor overly pessimistic. Meaningful change has occurred, and given the costs involved, this is perhaps the least that should have been expected. There is still, however, a great deal more that needs to be done both in challenging the culture of services and addressing the needs of particular groups. For example, involving carers more effectively; establishing the fidelity of service models; identifying the funds for education and training; developing primary care mental health services; and ensuring that user led values underpin practice in all levels and types of services. This is not an exhaustive list by any means.

Our final concern is that the impetus for mental health service development is on the wane. This text serves to demonstrate that a new, more radical, policy push is required now that the NSF is stumbling into the final phase of its timetable.

Charlie Brooker and *Julie Repper*

Abbreviations

A&E	Accident and Emergency
AO	Assertive Outreach
BME	Black and Minority Ethnic
CAMHS	Child and Adolescent Mental Health Services
CBT	Cognitive Behaviour Therapy
CCBT	Computerised Cognitive Behaviour Therapy
CDWs	Community Development Workers
CHI	Commission for Healthcare Improvement
CMHT	Community Mental Health Team
CPA	Care Programme Approach
CRE	Commission for Racial Equality
CSIP	Care Service Improvement Partnerships
DH/DoH	Department of Health
DRE	Delivering Race Equality
DSPD	Dangerous and Severe Personality Disorder
ECT	Electro-convulsive Therapy
FISs	Focused Implementation Sites
GP	General Practitioner
HCHS	Hospital and Community Health Services
IWL	Improving Working Lives
LDP	Local Delivery Plan
LIT	Local Implementation Team
MDO	Mentally Disordered Offenders
MHMDS	Mental Health Minimum Data Set
MHP	Mental Health Promotion
NAPIU	National Association of Psychiatric In-patient Care Units
NCMH	Northern Centre for Mental Health
NHS	National Health Service
NICE	National Institute for Clinical Excellence
NIMHE	National Institute for Mental Health (England)
NSF	National Service Framework
NVQ	National Vocational Qualification
NWP	National Workforce Programme
ONS	Office for National Statistics
PCTs	Primary Care Trusts
PICU	Psychiatric Intensive Care Unit
PSS	Local Authority Personal Social Services

RELs	Race Equality Leads
RES	Race Equality Scheme
R&D	Research and Development
RRAA	Race Relations Amendment Act
SDO	NHS Service Delivery Organisation
SEU	Social Exclusion Unit
SHA	Strategic Health Authority
SSRI	Selective Serotonin Re-uptake Inhibitor
STORM	Skills based Training On Risk Management
STR	Support Time and Recovery (Worker)
WAT	Workforce Action Team

Recovery and social inclusion:
the changing mental health agenda

J. Repper • R. Perkins

Published in 2000, the Department of Health's NHS Plan, and its associated national service frameworks and implementation guidance, heralded major changes in the NHS. It is easy to think only of the structural changes that have occurred: like the major reorganisation of provider organisations and commissioning arrangements and the creation of new teams: 'Home Treatment', 'Early Intervention', 'Assertive Outreach'. However, the more profound changes lay in a fundamental redefinition of the vision and purpose of services proclaimed in the Plan. A move away from a 'sickness service' whose sole function is to treat illnesses towards one designed to promote health and well-being. A move away from a system that considers only symptoms and dysfunctions to one that recognises the intimate inter-relationship between the health and social facets of people's lives. A move away from an over-centralised service where patients have to 'fit in' – where 'the convenience of the patient can come a poor second to the convenience of the system' (p15) – to one designed around the concerns, convenience and needs of those who it serves. A move away from a service that disempowers those who use it – a service where people feel 'talked at' rather than 'listened to' – to one in which patients have a genuine say at all levels, from decisions about their individual care to decisions about the operation and development of services as a whole.

This vision has been elaborated in subsequent policy and guidance. The Department of Health 'NHS Improvement Plan' of 2004 – 'Putting people at the heart of public services' (DH 2004a) – signalled three big shifts:

- putting patients and service users first through more personalised care
- a focus on the whole of health and well-being, not only illness
- further devolution of decision making.

It was these priorities that formed the basis of the health and social care standards and planning framework for 2005–2008 'National Standards, Local Action' (DH 2004b). In relation to mental health, this framework again emphasised the interconnections between health and social concerns: the importance of social isolation and unemployment as risk factors in deteriorating mental health and suicide, and the need for mental health services to help people to gain and retain work and engage in community life more generally. Most importantly services must decrease health inequalities and ensure equality of access, experience and outcome irrespective of race/ethnicity, disability, gender, age, faith or belief and sexuality.

The imperative of moving away from a centrally directed system to one which is patient led was further elaborated in 'Creating a Patient-led NHS: Delivering the NHS Improvement Plan' (DH 2005a). The policy direction in relation to social care was further signalled in 'Independence, Well-being and Choice' (DH 2005b). This describes a vision of social care in which people using services have more control via the wider use of direct payments and the piloting of the 'individual budgets'. It also places a greater focus on preventative services, early intervention, social inclusion and the promotion of well-being.

The white paper describing new directions for community services – 'Our Health, Our Care, Our Say' (DH 2006a) – identified five key areas for change:

- more personalised care driven by better access and more funding following the patient
- services brought closer to people's homes and away from centralised hospitals
- better co-ordination between local councils and the NHS
- increased choice underpinned by systems for enabling people to pay for their own care and support and regular patient surveys
- prevention of illness.

The need for people to have greater control over decisions about their care and support is a theme running through the whole NHS reform agenda and is emphasised in the Cabinet Office Strategy Unit 2005 report 'Improving the Life Chances of Disabled People' which explicitly includes people with mental health problems. Such control is epitomised by the extension of direct payments to groups that have historically been excluded – including people with mental health problems – and most especially the cross government initiative to pilot 'individualised budgets' (see DH 2006b). The aim of individualised budgets is to give people the power to decide the nature of services that they need. In 13 pilot areas the Department of Health, Department for Communities and Local Government and the Department of Work and Pensions have worked together to bring together historically separate funding streams (council provided social care services, independent living fund, supporting people, disabled facilities grant, integrated community equipment services and access to work) to provide people with their own budgets for purchasing the care and support they need. Decisions about whether these will be rolled out more generally will be taken in 2008 when the results of the pilots are known, but the direction of travel is clear: greater control and choice for those on the receiving end of services to determine the type of services that they receive.

Within this policy context mental health services face three major challenges:

- A move away from a sole focus on symptoms, deficits and dysfunctions and the treatment of problems (whether via psychological, pharmacological or systemic means) towards a focus of individuals' strengths and possibilities and enabling them to live the lives they wish to lead and do the things they want to do (see Repper & Perkins 2003).
- A move away from the altruism of former years in which decisions about what people need are the exclusive preserve of expert professionals and people are expected to be grateful for what they are given, to a consumer culture in which individuals have choice and control over the support they receive.
- A move away from a focus on care and looking after people to a focus on opportunity and providing the support that people need to look after themselves: enabling those with mental health problems to access the opportunities that other citizens take for granted.

To be a mental patient

In mental health services we are very used to thinking about service users' needs and experience in terms of the supports and services that mental health workers provide: inpatient facilities, community teams, medication, occupational therapy, art therapy, 'psychosocial interventions'. People are deemed to need 'assertive outreach' or a 'day centre' or 'nursing input'. We monitor the effectiveness of these services and interventions in terms of indicators like symptom reduction, decrease in the duration of inpatient stays, progress in moving from higher to lower levels of support (from a hostel to a flat or from a sheltered workshop to open employment) and progression towards 'independence': decreases in the amount of support they receive.

If we are to develop the 'patient-led' services envisioned in national policy and genuinely place service users at the heart of services, we can no longer think about where people fit into our services but how our services fit into people's lives and the impact they have on them – for good or ill. But people do not exist in a vacuum – they live in a social context. Mental health problems affect not only the individual but those around them: the impact of what we do on others in the person's life is also critical (parents, siblings, partners, close friends and confidantes, neighbours, employers, workmates, teachers, people in the local faith community, or at the gym) so the impact of our services on wider social networks is critical.

It is difficult to describe what it is like to be diagnosed as having mental health problems – particularly more serious ones. The bottom falls out of your world. You have to cope with strange and often frightening symptoms ... symptoms that may stop you being able to think properly, stop you doing the ordinary everyday things that everyone takes for granted, may cause you to have experiences that no-one around you believes. Your confidence and belief in yourself hit rock bottom. You feel very alone ... very frightened – not only about what is happening to you, but also of using psychiatric services. Unthinkable things may happen to you – you may be picked up by the police and taken to hospital, detained against your will ...

And on top of all of this you experience all the prejudice and discrimination that go hand in hand with mental health problems in our society. People start treating you differently – as if you are dangerous, or stupid, or both – behave as if they are walking on egg-shells fearful that at the slightest provocation you may either explode with anger or dissolve into tears. You risk losing everything you hold dear: your job, your college place, your friends, even your home … Too many who use mental health services have lost everything that they value in life (Sayce 2000, Repper & Perkins 2003, Thornicroft 2006). People with mental health problems are among the most excluded in our communities (Dunn 1999, Social Exclusion Unit 2004) and frequently have difficulty in accessing those ordinary services that every citizen expects like justice and physical health care. A person who has serious mental health problems is more likely to get major killer diseases like strokes, respiratory or heart disease, diabetes, bowel cancer, and breast cancer, but they are also more likely to get them at a younger age and die from them more quickly (Disability Rights Commission 2006).

In the face of all this, is it any wonder that many people either deny that there is anything wrong with them (the idea of being 'mentally ill' being just to horrible to contemplate) or give up on themselves and their lives in the face of what seem to be insurmountable odds? Too many choose to end their lives completely (DH 2001a).

But it doesn't have to be like this. Recovery is possible.

The concept of 'recovery' in mental health

The concept of 'recovery' in mental health captures the key elements outlined in government health policy: a focus on the individual and their wants, wishes and concerns; the inter-relationship between health and social facets of people's lives; the importance of choice and control; the importance of promoting well-being and social inclusion and helping people to live the lives they want to lead. Ideas about recovery are genuinely user-centred having emerged not from the work of learned professionals but from the lived experience of people with mental health problems (see, for example, Deegan 1989, 1996, Leete 1989, Anthony 1996, Reeves 1998, Coleman 1999, Repper & Perkins 2003).

'Recovery refers to the lived or real life experience of people as they accept and overcome the challenge of the disability … they experience themselves as recovering a new sense of self and of purpose within and beyond the limits of the disability.'

(Deegan 1988)

'… a deeply personal, unique process of changing one's attitudes, values, feelings, goals, skills, and/or roles. It is a way of living a satisfying, hopeful, and contributing life even with limitations caused by illness. Recovery involves the development of new meaning and purpose in one's life as one grows beyond the catastrophic effects of mental illness.'

(Anthony 1996)

Every one of the people who experiences mental health problems faces the task of recovery: the task of living with and growing beyond what has happened to them in order to retain or rebuild a meaningful, valued and satisfying life. Relatives, friends and others who are important in the person's life face a parallel challenge of accepting and living with what has happened to the person they care about and accommodating it into their relationships with the person so that both the individual, and their relationships with him/her, can flourish and grow.

The first elaboration of the centrality of a recovery perspective in UK national mental policy can be found in the Department of Health publication 'The Journey to Recovery' (DH 2001b). This publication emphasises the need to replace the hopelessness and pessimism that pervade mental health services with a positive and optimistic approach. Recovery is possible if people are:

'supported by appropriate services, driven by the right values and attitudes. The mental health system must support people in settings of their own choosing, enable access to community resources including housing, education, work, friendships – or whatever they think is critical to their own recovery – and enable and empower people with mental health difficulties to take their full place in society.'

(DH 2001b, p24)

The centrality of a recovery perspective has been reinforced in 'From Values to Action' (DH 2006e) which states that 'Mental health nursing should incorporate the broad principles of the Recovery Approach into every aspect of their practice.'

It is important, however, to be clear about what is, and what is not, meant by 'recovery'. It is a term that tends to mean different things to different people. Following from the work of Deegan (1989, 1996) and Anthony (1996):

- *Recovery is not a professional intervention like medication or psychotherapy.* It is the journey of people who have mental health problems, not a characteristic of a specific service or therapy. Recovery is not a set of techniques: 'Once recovery becomes systematised, you've got it wrong. Once it is reduced to a set of principles it is wrong. It is a unique and individualised process.' (Deegan 1989)
- *Recovery is not the same as cure.* It does not mean that all suffering has disappeared, or that all symptoms have been removed, or that functioning has been completely restored. Rather that remaining symptoms and problems interfere less with a person's life.
- *Recovery is about growth.* Growing within and beyond the limits imposed by ongoing symptoms and difficulties. It is all too easy for a person to become nothing other than their 'illness' – 'a schizophrenic', 'a manic depressive'. Recovery involves redefining identity in a way which includes, but moves beyond, the limitations of 'illness'. People can and do develop a new sense of self, value, meaning and purpose in their lives in the face of continuing mental health problems.

- *Recovery does not refer to an end product or a result.* Recovery is not an outcome or end state but a continuing journey.
- *Recovery can and does occur without professional intervention.* Mental health workers do not hold the key to recovery. A person's own resources and those available to them outside the mental health system are central. There is no formula for recovery … there are many, many paths … including choosing not to be involved in the mental health system.
- *A recovery vision is not limited to a particular theory about the nature and causes of mental health problems.* It does not commit one to a social, or a psychological, or a spiritual, or an organic understanding of distress and disability, nor to the use or non-use of medical interventions. Whatever understanding of their situation a person chooses, recovery is an equally important process.
- *Recovery is not specific to mental health problems.* It is a common human condition. Everyone experiences recovery at some point in their lives: when someone we love dies, when we experience other losses, traumas, illnesses, injuries.
- *Recovery is about taking back control.* Mental health problems are often presented and perceived as uncontrollable, or their control is seen as the province of experts. Recovery involves taking back control: over your problems, over the help and support you receive and your life.
- *Recovery is not a linear process.* Recovery is about trying and trying again. Relapse is not 'failure', but a part of the recovery process.
- *Everyone's recovery journey is different and deeply personal.* There are no rules of recovery, no formula for 'success'.

What might facilitate recovery?

The individual nature of recovery does not mean that recovery cannot be assisted or helped. Rather, it means that there is no one 'right' way. However, there are a number of things that service users often cite as important in the recovery process (Deegan 1988, 1993, 1996, Spaniol & Koehler 1994, Spaniol et al 1997, Vincent 1999, Young & Ensing 1999, May 2000). Underpinning the quest for renewed meaning, purpose, value and satisfaction, five key themes emerge: hope, relationships, understanding what has happened and grieving what has been lost, taking back control and opportunity.

Hope

Without hope – a vision of possibility – then recovery is impossible. If you cannot see any possibility of living a decent and valued life then there is no reason to do anything, no reason to get up in the morning, no reason to stay alive: the link between hopelessness and suicide has long been known (Beck et al 1990). There exists a considerable body of research into the importance of hope in health outcomes (Hickey 1986, Woodside et al 1994, Aguilar et al 1997, Kirkpatrick et al 2001). However, hope is generated in a social context: relationships are central to hope and recovery.

Relationships

Relationships with mental health workers can be important in fostering, or eroding, hope: if those people who are supposed to be helping you think that you will never amount to very much – what hope can there be? However, relationships with mental health professionals are not ones from which most people derive their sense of meaning and value: few people see their purpose in life as to be a mental patient. To be in a position where your only relationships are with a worker who is paid to be there is a demeaning position to be in and relationships with mental health professionals can never really be reciprocal. Always to be on the receiving end of help from others does little to inspire confidence and hope: people need relationships in which they can give as well as receive. Perhaps the effectiveness of relationships between professionals and service users might best be judged by the extent to which they enable a person to enter into those genuinely reciprocal relationships with family, friends, colleagues and other companions on which most people rely so heavily for their sense of value and self-worth.

Many people with mental health problems have found the support they receive from their peers invaluable in their recovery journey. People who have themselves faced the challenge of recovery are often in the best position to understand what the person is going through and provide inspiration and encouragement when the enormity of the challenge appears too great.

Understanding what has happened and grieving what has been lost

For many people, mental health problems represent a multi-faceted catastrophe. They represent a major bereavement and often involve multiple losses: loss of job, home, friends, family; loss of hopes and dreams; loss of all the 'privileges of sanity' like respect, being seen as a competent and valuable person, having what you say taken seriously, deciding what you want to do yourself.

As with any other bereavement – death, divorce, unemployment – people are likely to experience a range of emotions – shock, fear, denial, anger, despair, guilt. It is the sad reality that people with mental health problems too often find their experience of such emotions pathologised and dismissed as manifestations of their mental health problems.

> 'This has left many people with mental illness feeling devalued and ignored and has resulted in mistrust and alienation from the mental health system.'
>
> (Spaniol et al 1997)

Like anyone who has experienced a bereavement, someone grappling with life with mental health problems needs time, space and support to grieve what they have lost, find meaning in what has happened and answers to those 'why me?', 'what is the point?' type questions. Someone to share their pain and their search for an understanding that allows them a way forward – the possibility of continuing and rebuilding their life.

Taking back control

'We are learning that those of us with psychiatric disabilities can become experts in our own self-care, can regain control over our lives and can be responsible for our own journey of recovery.'

(Deegan 1992)

Recovery is not about passively sitting back and letting others do things for you . . . it is about taking back control. Mental health problems are often initially perceived as being uncontrollable and this sense of powerlessness is often exacerbated by disempowering mental health services that offer scant opportunity for choice and self-determination.

Different people derive meaning, value and purpose from different things, therefore the process of recovery centrally involves people deciding what they wish to do and what they wish to achieve rather than having these determined by others. However, two other domains are equally important: taking control of your problems and making your own decisions about the help and support you receive.

Self-management lies at the heart of the Department of Health 'Expert Patient Programme' (DH 2006d). This is a lay-led self-management programme designed to support people living with long-term health conditions such as heart disease, stroke, diabetes and mental illness to increase their confidence, improve their quality of life and better manage their condition. In the mental health arena self-management is often based on the Wellness Recovery Action Planning (WRAP; www.mentalhealthrecovery.com) developed by Mary Ellen Copeland (Copeland 1997):

'WRAP is a self-management and recovery system developed by a group of people who had mental health difficulties and who were struggling to incorporate wellness tools and strategies into their lives. WRAP is designed to:

- Decrease and prevent intrusive or troubling feelings and behaviours
- Increase personal empowerment
- Improve quality of life
- Assist people in achieving their own life goals and dreams.

WRAP is a structured system to monitor uncomfortable and distressing symptoms that can help you reduce, modify or eliminate those symptoms by using planned responses. This includes plans for how you want others to respond when symptoms have made it impossible for you to continue to make decisions, take care of yourself, or keep yourself safe.'

Increased choice and control over the support that you receive lie at the heart of the NHS reforms initiated with the NHS Plan (DH 2000 – see above). Increasingly people with mental health problems are being encouraged to access direct payments in order to enable them to make their own decisions about what support they need and who provides it (see DH 2006c) and the individualised budget pilot sites further elaborate and extend these possibilities for some disabled people, but all of this presupposes that people are able to access the opportunities that they seek.

Opportunity

Recovery is impossible without opportunity. If everywhere you turn you are excluded from those roles, relationships and activities that give your life value and purpose then it is not possible to sustain hope or rebuild a life that you find meaningful and satisfying. Social inclusion – the chance to participate in the social, economic and cultural life of the community of which you are a part – is critical.

Too often it is assumed that people with mental health problems have different needs from the rest of the population – needs for treatment, day centres, supported accommodation, assertive outreach in the community. However, it must be remembered that these are not needs in themselves but possible means of ensuring that needs – shared with everyone else – are met. Like anyone else, if people with mental health problems are to rebuild their lives they need somewhere decent to live, enough money to live on, things to do and people to do them with – friends, family, intimate relationships.

Equally, if not more importantly, people need the opportunity to contribute to the communities in which they live – either via paid employment or those myriad non-paid contributions on which our society depends like child-rearing, voluntary work, political activism. It remains the case that what we do affords us status and identity – a meaning and purpose in life.

It is the opportunity to access those opportunities that other citizens take for granted that lies at the heart of the social inclusion agenda. Indeed it is towards the participation and inclusion component of recovery that much recent government policy and guidance has been directed.

Social inclusion and recovery

There are two things that perpetuate the social exclusion of people with mental health problems:

- First there is prejudice and discrimination. People with mental health problems are distanced from other people – defined as 'other': one of 'them' rather than one of 'us'. In his book 'Shunned: Discrimination against people with mental illness' Thornicroft (2006) provides a comprehensive account of the extent of the prejudice and discrimination experienced by people with mental health problems.
- Second there is failure to provide the adjustments, help and support that a person needs to do the things they want to do.

Standard 1 of the National Service Framework for Mental Health (DH 1999) emphasises the importance of decreasing the discrimination and exclusion experienced by people with mental health problems. The major piece of work conducted by the Social Exclusion Unit (2004) both demonstrates the magnitude of the task and provides an action plan for approaching it. The report – 'Mental Health and Social Exclusion' – provides a comprehensive account of the evidence relating to the exclusion of people with mental health problems. It offers (p6) a vision of:

'a future where people with mental health problems have the same opportunities to work and participate in the community as any other citizen'

and offers a 27-point action plan that brings together different government departments and organisations in an effort to reduce the discrimination experienced by people, and provide the necessary support and adjustments to enable people to fulfil their aspirations and significantly improve their opportunities.

This was probably the first explicit recognition that mental health problems were not the exclusive preserve of the Department of Health and the health and social care services that it provides. As the lifetime prevalence of mental health problems is now estimated at some 50% of the adult population (Kessler et al 2005) there can be few citizens whose lives are not affected by such issues either via their own experience or that of people they know.

The 'social inclusion' of mental health can be seen in cross-sector initiatives both within government and outside. For example the 2006 Budget (for the first time) referred to the social exclusion experienced by people with mental health problems and the requirement for joint working between government agencies to reduce this (HM Treasury 2006). Similarly, since the publication of the 2004 Social Exclusion Unit Report, the need for action cutting across sectors can be seen in policy and guidance issued jointly by the Department of Health/Department of Work and Pensions, including 'Health Work and Well-being – Caring for our Future: A strategy for the health and well-being of working age people' (2005) and the 'Vocational Services for People with Serious Mental Health problems: commissioning guidance' (2006). Both of these documents identify the responsibilities not only of central government but also of employers, individuals, healthcare professionals, the employment service and other stakeholders in promoting opportunity and enhancing well-being. The 2006 action plan on social exclusion emphasises the need for a lifetime approach and prioritises the needs of a number of socially excluded groups. It includes the need to accelerate measures to encourage employment among those with severe mental health problems (Cabinet Office Strategy Unit 2006).

A recognition of the inclusion of mental health issues outside the traditional health and social care preserve has also been associated with a movement away from consideration of the rights of people with mental health problems solely in terms of compulsory detention and rights to treatment towards a consideration of the citizenship rights and the increasing inclusion of mental health service user/survivors in the broader Disability Rights agenda (see Chapter 5).

Recovery, rights and citizenship

The major changes in vision and purpose of health services heralded in the NHS Plan (DH 2000) and elaborated in subsequent policy and guidance require that health services are tailored around the wishes and concerns of those who use them. They move away from a sole focus on the treatment of illnesses towards a consideration of all facets of health and well-being, and increase the choice and control available to those who use them.

In mental health such changes are epitomised in the recovery agenda.

Sometimes recovery has been conceptualised purely in terms of an individual's journey of living with and growing beyond the limitations imposed by their mental health problems. This is a mistake. Fostering hope, developing ways of understanding and accommodating what has happened, and wresting control over problems and help received remain important, but alone they are not enough. Social exclusion – denial of access to those opportunities that most citizens take for granted – imposes insuperable barriers on the extent to which people are able to recover satisfying, meaningful and valued lives.

Attempts to reduce the barriers to recovery imposed by exclusion from the social, economic and cultural life of communities involve both the reduction of prejudice and discrimination and the provision of the adjustment and supports that people need to access the opportunities that they seek. They have taken the mental health agenda outside the realm of health and social care so that no longer is consideration of mental health issues the sole preserve of the Department of Health. Everyone – employers, housing authorities, schools, the providers of leisure and recreational services, the transport, physical health and criminal justice system, as well as the providers of health and social care services – are increasingly required to consider the support and adjustments they must make to accommodate people with mental health problems.

And at last, the opportunities available to people with mental health problems have moved beyond the moral or ethical imperative to the legal requirement. If people with mental health problems are to recover meaningful, valued and satisfying lives then this must be underpinned by rights: citizenship rights. The inclusion of mental health issues within a broader disability rights agenda can only enhance the possibilities of recovery. Indeed, if the vision of the Disability Rights Commission – a society in which all disabled people (both those with physical impairments and those with mental health problems) can participate as equal citizens (Disability Rights Commission 2001a,b) will there be anything to recover?

References

Aguilar E J, Haas G, Manzanera F J et al 1997 Hopelessness and first episode psychosis: a longitudinal study. Acta Psychiatrica Scandinavica 96:25–30

Anthony W A 1996 Recovery from mental illness: the guiding vision of the mental health system in the 1990s. Innovations and Research 2(3):17–24

Beck A T, Brown G, Berchick J, Stewart L B, Steer R A 1990 Relationship between hopelessness and suicide: a replication with psychiatric outpatients. American Journal of Psychiatry 147(2):11–23

Cabinet Office Strategy Unit 2005 Improving the life chances of disabled people. Cabinet Office Strategy Unit, London

Cabinet Office Strategy Unit 2006 Reaching out: an action plan on social exclusion. Cabinet Office Strategy Unit, London

Coleman R 1999 Recovery: An Alien Concept. Handsell Publishing, Gloucester

Copeland M E 1997 Wellness Recovery Action Plan (WRAP). Peach Press, Dummerston, VT

Deegan P 1988 Recovery: the lived experience of rehabilitation. Psychosocial Rehabilitation Journal 11(4):11–19

Deegan P 1989 A letter to my friend who is giving up. Paper presented at the Connecticut Conference on Supported Employment, Connecticut Association of Rehabilitation facilities, Cromwell, CT

Deegan P 1992 Recovery, rehabilitation and the conspiracy of hope: a keynote address. Center for Community Change Through Housing and Support, Burlington VT

Deegan P 1993 Recovering our sense of value after being labelled. Journal of Psychosocial Nursing 31(4):7–11

Deegan P 1996 Recovery as a journey of the heart. Psychosocial Rehabilitation Journal 19(3): 91–97

Department of Health 1999 National Service Framework for Mental Health. DH, London

Department of Health 2000 The NHS Plan: A plan for investment, a plan for reform. DH, London

Department of Health 2001a Safety First: Five-year report of the National Confidential Enquiry into Suicide and Homicide by People with Mental Illness. DH, London

Department of Health 2001b The Journey of Recovery: The government's vision for mental health care. DH, London

Department of Health 2004a NHS Improvement Plan 2004: Putting people at the heart of public services. DH, London

Department of Health 2004b National Standards, Local Action: Health and social care standards and planning framework 2005/06–2007/08. DH, London

Department of Health 2005a Creating a Patient-led NHS: Delivering the NHS Improvement Plan. DH, London

Department of Health 2005b Independence, Well-being and Choice: Our vision of the future of social care for adults in England. DH, London

Department of Health 2006a Our Health, Our Care, Our Say: A new direction for community services. DH, London

Department of Health 2006b Individual Budgets. DH, London

Department of Health 2006c Direct Payments for People with Mental Health Problems: A guide to action. DH, London

Department of Health 2006d The Expert Patient Programme. DH, London

Department of Health 2006e From Values to Action: The Chief Nursing Officer's review of mental health nursing. DH, London

Department of Health/Department of Work and Pensions 2005 Health, Work and Well-being – Caring for our Future: A strategy for the health and well-being of working age people. DH/DWP, London

Department of Health/Department of Work and Pensions 2006 Vocational Services for People with Severe Mental Health Problems: Commissioning guidance. DH/DWP, London

Disability Rights Commission 2001a Who We Are and What We Do. DRC, London

Disability Rights Commission 2001b Strategic Plan. DRC, London

Disability rights Commission 2006 Equal Treatment: Closing the Gap. DRC, London

Dunn S 1999 Creating Accepting Communities. Report of the Mind Inquiry into Social Exclusion and Mental Health Problems. Mind Publications, London

Hickey S S 1986 Enabling Hope. Journal of Cancer Nursing 9(3):133–137

Kessler R C, Demler O, Frank R G 2005 Prevalence and treatment of mental disorders, 1990 to 2003. New England Journal of Medicine 352(24):2515–2523

Kirkpatrick H, Landeen J, Woodside H, Byrne C 2001 How people with schizophrenia build their hope. Journal of Psychosocial Nursing 39(1):46–53

Leete E 1989 How I perceive and manage my illness. Schizophrenia Bulletin 15:197–200

May R 2000 My Recovery Journey. Paper presented at Strangefish Conference 'Recovery: An Alien Concept' at Chamberlin Hotel, Birmingham

Reeves A 1998 Recovery. A holistic approach. Handsell Publishing, Runcorn, Cheshire

Repper J, Perkins R 2003 Social inclusion and recovery. A model for mental health practice. Baillière Tindall, Edinburgh

Sayce L 2000 From psychiatric patient to citizen. Overcoming discrimination and social exclusion. MacMillan, London

Social Exclusion Unit 2004 Social Exclusion and Mental Health. Social Exclusion Unit, London

Spaniol L, Koehler M (eds) 1994 The experience of recovery. Center for Psychiatric Rehabilitation, Boston

Spaniol L, Gagne C, Koehler M 1997 Recovery from serious mental illness: what it is and how to assist people in their recovery. Continuum 4(4):3–15

Thornicroft G 2006 Shunned. Discrimination against people with mental illness. Oxford University Press, Oxford

Vincent S S 1999 Using findings from qualitative research to teach mental health professionals about the experience of recovery from psychiatric disability. Presentation at the Harvard University Graduate School of Education Fourth Annual Student Research Conference, Cambridge, MA

Woodside H, Landeen J, Kirkpatrick H 1994 Hope and schizophrenia: exploring attitudes of clinicians. Psychosocial Rehabilitation Journal 8:140–144

Young S L, Ensing D S 1999 Exploring recovery from the perspective of people with psychiatric disabilities. Psychiatric Rehabilitation Journal 22(3):219–231

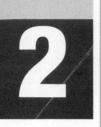

User involvement in 21st century mental health services:
'This is our century'

A. Faulkner

The term 'user involvement' often seems to give rise to anxiety and scepticism on behalf of both service users and professionals. The challenge is to make 'user involvement' vital and meaningful, introduce new ways of enabling people to appreciate it, and to understand the different agendas and pressures that fight over the idea of involvement. I hope to achieve some of this here. Under the following headings, this chapter traces the background policy framework to 'user involvement', covers the many different domains in which involvement takes place and takes us through some dilemmas through to the lessons learned for good practice:

- Background and policy framework
- Domains of involvement
- Dilemmas of involvement
- Learning the lessons.

First, however, here is a poem from Peter Campbell, whose contribution to user involvement and empowerment over the last few decades earned him a special award from the mental health charity Mind in 2006.

A Madman Teaching
A madman stands at the blackboard teaching.
He remembers the doctor had him there,
Pointing, questioning, silencing him
With his interpretations.
    Bowing ever so slightly
At his audience.
    A madman stands at the blackboard teaching.
He remembers the nurse putting the needle in,

Saying it was all for his own good, that he wasn't
Quite right.
Bowing ever so slightly
Towards the chargehand.
A madman stands at the blackboard teaching.
He remembers that the ward is closed,
The asylum shuttered.
A madman stands at the blackboard teaching.
This is our day.
This is our century.

(Campbell 2006a)

Background and policy framework

'It has been both a blessing and a curse that service user/survivor action
in the UK was engulfed so quickly in service-led enthusiasm for user
involvement.'

(Campbell 2006b)

The roots of user involvement can be traced back to evidence of dissatisfaction with mental health services voiced by individuals in the 19th century. Similar voices have been heard throughout the 20th century but it was not until the mid-1980s that voices of protest became more recognisably organised as a user or survivor movement. Initially the formation of hospital based Patients' Councils and a proliferation of user-led self-help and advocacy groups developed alongside the creation of more formally organised networks such as Survivors Speak Out, the Hearing Voices Network and the UK Advocacy Network. Other contemporaneous developments included campaigns for women-only services and advocacy, and against the use of ECT. The history of these initiatives is well documented by Peter Campbell in the Sainsbury Centre for Mental Health publication 'Beyond the Water Towers' (2005).

Much of the campaigning energy of the user/survivor movement in this country has been directed at existing psychiatric services and treatments, motivated by the desire to change and improve them, which is perhaps why 'user involvement' has become such a major development in the UK. Perhaps this is because Government policy has played a large role in legitimating user involvement. The NHS and Community Care Act 1990 and the Health of the Nation were amongst early documents that placed service users in a more central position within policy and planning of services. More recently there have been a number of policy initiatives that mention the role of service user (and carer) involvement in the planning and delivery of services: the NHS Plan, the National Service Framework for Mental Health England: 1999, the Healthcare Commission, Patient and Public Involvement (PPI) initiatives and the Research Governance Framework (DH 2001).

It is important to acknowledge that user involvement inevitably entails tensions: by its nature it assumes the power lies on one side of the involvement enterprise. Many service user groups are funded by statutory services in order that they provide 'involvement' in the form of service users attending numerous committees and planning meetings. This can produce an uncomfortable tension within a group that wants and needs to find ways of sustaining itself. At its worst, user involvement can become a battlefield where policy-makers, practitioners and service users fight over their competing agendas. At its best, it can become an integration of perspectives that leads to the achievement of shared goals.

Despite the increased recognition given over the years to the role of user involvement in the planning and delivery of services through Government policy, some of the core concerns of service users have seen little change or progress. Today, a visit to almost any user group throughout the UK will still find people talking with some distress about the lack of information about medication, the lack of choice or alternatives to medication, about bad experiences of coercive treatment, and the need for help in a crisis (see, for example, Rethink 2005, Faulkner 1997, Mental Health Foundation & Sainsbury Centre for Mental Health 2002). These issues still remain at the core of much user/survivor dissatisfaction, and are often motives for people wishing to become involved in attempts to change services. This lack of change is an important factor in understanding the sometimes frustrating situation that faces us all in making progress with 'user involvement'.

However, groups of mental health service users and survivors have taken some of these concerns – and others – and organised themselves independently to achieve them. These initiatives sometimes overlap with or inform developments in 'user involvement' and sometimes remain clearly separate from contemporary psychiatric services and policy. Fundamentally, this represents the familiar political debate about campaigning from the outside versus changing things from the inside. In general, it seems important to think of service user involvement as one part of the bigger picture of service user/survivor action, and to remember that there are many other activities and initiatives taking part on an independent basis. These can be about supporting each other, developing our own services or strategies for managing distress, or seeking creative outlets for expressing ourselves.

Domains of involvement

Given its many manifestations, it may be helpful to consider 'user involvement' within the following domains:

- Individual care
- Individual services
- Trust/organisation-wide
- Research and development
- National policy
- Training and education.

Individual care

'I am tired of being talked about,
treated as a statistic,
pushed to the margins of human conversation.
I want someone who will have time for me,
someone who will listen to me,
someone who has not already judged
who I am or what I have to offer.
I am waiting to be taken seriously.'

(excerpt from Nicholls et al 2002)

For many people, it is in individual care that we see the real test as to whether 'user involvement' is having an effect. Can an individual really contribute to decisions about their own care, feel seriously listened to and consulted by the relevant professionals involved? Or are we subject to the 'professional knows best' philosophy of care? The existence of the Mental Health Act clearly has its influence in this domain; unlike in any other area of health, we can be detained and treated against our will. This, though, is a domain where the service user/survivor movement has achieved some of its most notable successes: advocacy, crisis cards and advance statements were all first championed by service users and survivors.

The user/survivor movement has very much led the way in developing advocacy in mental health, recognising the unique position that people with mental illness diagnoses are in – primarily in relation to the Mental Health Act, but also in relation to the fundamental invalidation of our views through being deemed mentally ill. From early in the 1980s advocacy was a major issue for service users and survivors: finding ways to enable people to express their views within the individual care arena and in ward rounds about treatment issues, and then subsequently through Patients' Councils about more general service issues. The UK Advocacy Network (UKAN) originated at around that time, establishing a UK-wide system of representation and management (Wood 2004, Wood & Mullins 2004).

Crisis cards and advance statements were perhaps first developed by Survivors Speak Out, and are now becoming a more familiar and established concept (see www.mentalhealth.org.uk for information about the Mental Health Foundation project exploring advance statements). However, despite the fairly united opposition to any extension of compulsory powers by service users and survivors, little progress has been made in enabling these initiatives to overrule the Mental Health Act.

Research and much personal experience and anecdote demonstrate that there is still a long way to go in this domain. For example, many people are unaware of the Care Programme Approach, or indeed that they have a care plan – being involved in drawing up their care plan seems a distant goal (Rose 2001). Many people still report not being consulted about treatments and not being given information about services, medication and alternative treatments.

Fundamental to this and to all other areas of 'user involvement' is respect. Most of the Patients' Charters developed in the early 1990s started with establishing our right to respect as individuals, as citizens, as people with rights. This ostensibly simple value cannot be overstated. So many of us lose our self-respect when in hospital or in being treated against our will.

Individual services

Many mental health service users want to 'get involved' in order to change and improve services. Some very positive developments have occurred in this area in recent years. User involvement in individual services can manifest itself in a number of different ways, including basic feedback about services, evaluation and reviews, and involvement in service delivery.

One of the routes promoted and supported by the service user/survivor movement is Patients' Councils; these are normally based within hospitals to provide a forum for current and ex patients to voice their views about the service provided. They will normally have a route for these views to be fed back into the hospital management, whether via a joint meeting with staff or another method. Patients' Councils are as variable as their members and the services in which they are based, but they have received considerable support over the last two decades. Difficulties frequently concern the ability of a Patients' Council to ensure that the voices of marginalised groups of patients are heard, and there is tension around their ability to remain independent when based – and funded – within a large hospital service.

Another manifestation of user involvement in individual services is through involvement in the evaluation or monitoring of services. The Sainsbury Centre for Mental Health pioneered a methodology for 'user-focused monitoring', and distributed this widely through providing training and support to local service users to become involved in monitoring their own services. This gained some considerable credibility, and has spawned many service users skilled in interviewing others and groups dedicated to evaluating their local services (SCMH 2006). It has been shown that service users are likely to reveal more and to be more honest with interviewers who identify as service users themselves (Rose 2001).

Other examples of service users involved in individual services include:

- involvement in staff recruitment
- involvement in service delivery (e.g. code of practice for ward rounds)
- development of user-focused information packs (e.g. Camden Choices).

There still remain difficulties in understanding what 'user involvement' can or might be at this level. Staff 'on the ground' may well have been told to involve service users by managers, without very much assistance or groundwork undertaken to ensure that they understand why, what it might entail or how to go about it. There can often be resistance as a result of this.

Trust and organisation-wide initiatives

At the Trust or organisational level, service user involvement is beginning to become more systematic, largely due to the policy framework but also to a growing recognition that service user involvement can lead to an improvement in services. Service user representation can be seen on a plethora of committees and planning meetings, including, notably, on Local Implementation Teams (LITs) which exist to implement the National Service Framework.

To begin with, many Trusts and organisations believed that it was sufficient to have (often the same) one or two service users sitting on relevant planning forums or committees. This continues to some extent today, although there is widespread agreement that this approach does not work for many reasons. Not only will some managers express concern about individuals not being representative of the local service user population, but service users may become the subject of too many demands and become burnt out, ultimately voting with their feet to reject involvement. The attempt to implement user involvement then starts again from the beginning.

Successful initiatives include grassroots development work that ensures the growth and support of user groups to support individuals (usually at least two) to sit on the required committees and planning forums, support and training to enable them to take part with equal membership, and the production of accessible and jargon-free information. Examples suggested to me include: the Service User Reference Group in Camden; Brent User Group linking with local LIT structures; Westminster Consultation Project; West Dorset Mental Health Forum (see 'Best Practice in Mental Health in the South West', a document currently accessed on the Sainsbury Centre for Mental Health website).

Research carried out at the Sainsbury Centre for Mental Health (Wallcraft 2005) found the following activities being carried out by 300 service user groups across England:

- 79% self-help and mutual support
- 72% service user involvement
- 69% education and training
- 41% creative activities
- 38% advocacy
- 28% service user-run services.

Here, service user involvement was defined as 'taking part in some form of consultation with mental health professionals and decision-makers'. To what extent this kind of involvement is making a difference is harder to identify. Crawford et al (2001) found a relatively small number of reports that attributed changes in services to the involvement of service users. Simpson & House (2002) carried out a systematic review to determine the effect of involving service users in the delivery and evaluation of mental health services. For the most part their conclusions are positive, although they identified few studies to fit their criteria. They found that the influence of trainers who had been users on the attitudes of trainees was positive; also that service user interviewers may have brought out more negative opinions of services than non-user interviewers. Several studies from the US indicated that where service users were employed as case managers, outcomes for their clients were positive.

User involvement in research

Department of Health guidance in the form of the Research Governance Framework for Health and Social Care was published in April 2001. The framework comprises two areas of relevance to service users: a call for the active involvement of service users and carers at every stage of the research cycle; and a move towards greater openness about research undertaken by organisations. The organisation INVOLVE was established in 1995 as an advisory group to the Department of Health, with the aim of promoting public involvement in health, social care and public health research. The impact of these developments has been to introduce into a range of public funding streams requirements on researchers to demonstrate in funding applications how consumers will be involved in their research projects, as well as to put user involvement on the agenda of NHS R&D frameworks.

The involvement of service users as active participants in the research process is not a new idea. In the disability field and in feminist research ideology, emancipatory research – research that has the aim of empowerment at its core – has been around for some time. In these fields it has become commonplace for research to be undertaken by people with the relevant disability under investigation, by women with women, and by people from black and minority ethnic communities where the research involves their community. This has meant the introduction of new challenges to the subjects being researched, but also to the methodologies being used and the aims of the research process (see, for example, Barnes & Mercer 1997).

Service user involvement in research has increased incrementally in the last decade – many service users have chosen research as their core endeavour for involvement and change (see Lindow 2001, 2002, Beresford & Wallcraft 1997, Rose 2003, Faulkner 2002, 2005).

Several units or departments dedicated to user involvement in research have become established in the last few years: for example, SURESearch at the University of Birmingham, and SURE (Service User Research Enterprise) at the Institute of Psychiatry in London. Some voluntary organisations, such as the Mental Health Foundation and the Sainsbury Centre for Mental Health, established programmes of work dedicated to 'user-led' research which recognised and supported the potential of service users to undertake their own research. At a national level, the Mental Health Research Network has a 'hub' dedicated to service user involvement in research adopted by the network: the Service User Research Group, England or SURGE. SURGE has published guidance for researchers about how to involve service users in research and is monitoring progress (SURGE 2005).

User involvement in national policy

This is perhaps the area that has attracted greatest controversy amongst service user and survivor groups. The difficulty of whom and how to involve service users at this level has often been the subject of debate and disagreement. Despite Government policy on user involvement in service planning, research and delivery, national policy initiatives have frequently adopted inappropriate methods for user involvement; for example, recruiting known and trusted individuals in preference to approaching networks recognised by the wider service user/survivor movement. This gives rise to familiar complaints about tokenism, and the failure to be inclusive or to have a feedback route to other service user and survivor groups about what is going on. An example of this was the formulation of the National Service Framework (England), where a number of service users rejected the process and/or spoke out about its failures (Read 2001, Trivedi 2001).

When it was first established as CHI, the Healthcare Commission adopted a user-focussed approach to monitoring mental health trusts, making a real attempt to ensure that the voices of service users are heard through the nation-wide reviews of clinical governance. They involved two service users in each local review to carry out interviews with service users, building on the knowl-edge gained through user involvement in research and monitoring. Their meth-ods have changed but elements of the approach remain, and the Commission is working in partnership with Mind to continue this work.

Service user involvement in NIMHE was evaluated by HASCAS and as a result has been taken forward in the Making a Real Difference work undertaken across a number of different regional development centres (RDCs). Service users are involved in most of the RDCs to a variable extent and with variable success.

User involvement in training and education

According to Peter Campbell (2006b), 'involvement in the training and educa-tion of mental health workers is a good example of the willingness to attempt change through collaboration'. User involvement in training and education is a key feature of the service user/survivor movement in the UK, as opposed to other countries where user-controlled services have been a more obvious focus. National training bodies, such as CCETSW (Central Council for the Education and Training of Social Workers) require service users to be involved in their training programmes, and training materials have been developed with the sig-nificant input of service users (e.g. Certificate in Community Mental Health Care; Mental Health Foundation/Pavilion).

A significant advantage of involvement in the training and education domain lies in its potential for empowerment for service users and survivors; developing the skills with which to train others can be an important achievement for many people, and enables us to value our own experience in a new and powerful way. Furthermore, the value of seeing service users in a powerful role may well alter the perceptions of the trainees; certainly it is often recorded as an appreciated part of a course (Repper & Breeze 2006).

Dilemmas of user involvement

Service user involvement presents us with a number of dilemmas, some of which are outlined below.

Different agendas

A fundamental difficulty with 'user involvement' is that the people who will be coming together to put it into effect are likely to have different aims or goals in mind. As suggested above, the different stakeholders may have different ideas of what constitutes 'user involvement' and of how to go about it. For some people, the process is all and the outcomes are not given sufficient emphasis; for others, the frustration of not being able to bring about change through involvement is ever-present. Agreeing goals and acknowledging different underlying agendas in an atmosphere of co-operation at the outset is essential.

One of my most informative experiences involved supporting the re-establishment of a local user group. The failure of local commissioners and providers to acknowledge their own needs for 'user involvement' and hence offer to support the needs of the user group meant that the process was painful and ultimately not successful. It is not enough to simply require service users to sit on committees and forums and attend meetings; these individuals have to come from somewhere and to return there to feed back what is going on in these meetings. Hence the need to first support the development of the user group and then to come to a joint understanding of what 'user involvement' might mean to all of the relevant stakeholders.

Diversity

One of the keys to success of 'user involvement' is whether we have achieved the full and comprehensive inclusion of diverse groups of service users. Service user groups have traditionally been white and also often male-dominated, so service users as well as professionals face this particular dilemma. Black and minority ethnic service users have tended not to organise in this way or to feel excluded by the groups that do.

'It is not our duty to be involved but our right. Through enabling, empowering and encouraging our self-expression, user involvement can be rewarding, stimulating and relevant to us.'

(Veronica Dewan in 'Diverse Minds')

Where groups or organisations have been successful in reaching a diverse mix of service users, it is usually by adopting a flexible approach to involvement – not requiring everyone to turn up for meetings, but going to meet people where they are and in the ways that make sense to them.

Representation and tokenism

Concerns that have been raised amongst 'involved' service users include marginalisation, tokenism and burn-out. All too often, the few able and articulate service users who are chosen or recruited to user involvement projects then receive criticism – from professionals – for being atypical and non-representative. Some of these issues were explored in some depth at the Survivor Workers Conference held in 2001 co-ordinated by Rose Snow. This touches on a more complex issue. With the proportion of people who are known to experience mental health problems at one time or another, it is clear that many will be workers within the health and social care professions. For someone to assume an identity of 'service user' or 'survivor' (or, indeed, another related term), it is likely that they have taken on something of that role and status and have some connection with the wider community of service users and survivors.

Incorporation

Related to the concept of 'different agendas' is the notion that to be involved assumes some measure of acceptance of the existing mental health service structures or models. People employed as User Involvement workers may feel compromised, because they are seen to be incorporated into the system by one side and perhaps as an interloper by the other. This is particularly true in research, where acceptance of the medical model may be almost a pre-requisite for becoming involved in much research. Thus, service user researchers need to be able to select where and with whom they will and will not become involved; alternatively, clinical academic researchers may need to revise their own theoretical perspectives and ideas about the research process. This is not to say that it cannot work, however – far from it. But these issues do need to be honestly stated and shared.

Empowerment

For 'user involvement' to be meaningful and effective, mental health service users need to be offered opportunities for empowerment. This may mean substantial grassroots capacity-building to enable local service users to first find and support each other, before deciding if they wish to become involved in local services and go on to develop the skills required. It can be empowering just to have an opportunity to tell your story and be heard, whether within the context of a user group, a planning forum, or a training exercise. However, without the opportunity for analysis, this can equally end up being a disempowering experience.

Empowerment is a difficult word to grasp in many ways. It is often said that no-one can empower another person, but they can offer opportunities for empowerment. In research, empowerment may be found through the opportunity to gain skills and to feel a valued member of a team, but it can also be found through adopting the 'research gaze'. In other words, through looking at the wider experience of service users and services through the prism of research, an individual can gain a valuable opportunity to see their own personal experiences within a wider context.

Grassroots capacity-building

This has been touched on elsewhere, but it is a continuing dilemma: how can small local user groups – which remain at the heart of the service user/survivor movement and of 'user involvement' – best develop and support their members, managing through periods of distress and with limited or inadequate funding? Capacity-building needs to be funded if service user involvement is to be sustained.

Learning the lessons

What, then, have we learnt to take forward user involvement into the 21st century? The question is no longer 'why user involvement?' but 'how to do it'. I think we have learnt that service user involvement needs:

- adequate resources
- payment for involvement
- transparent and clear goals and objectives
- benefits for everyone involved
- adequate practical and emotional support
- training in relevant skills for service users and staff/professionals
- equal access and accessibility
- involvement of diverse communities and marginalised groups
- respect for everyone
- good communications and feedback about progress and results.

There are a number of resources which address effective user (and carer) involvement from different perspectives. Box 2.1 shows the key chapter headings from a guide to involving service users and carers in voluntary organisations. Some of these headings will appear again and again in documentation and guidelines about user involvement, particularly adequate resourcing and payment for involvement, support and training, offering choices, and the need to be clear about why you want to involve service users/carers and who you want to involve. Some of the underlying principles are drawn out in more detail in the guidance produced by SURGE (Service User Research Group England) (Box 2.2).

We have also learnt that involvement can have a significant effect on people. In the field of research, where most of my experience comes from, I have seen many people gain skills which have enabled them to lead workshops, give presentations, interview others and gain confidence. The lesson I have learnt is

---

Box 2.1

User and Carer Involvement: a good practice guide (Hanley & Staley 2005)

- Preparing your organisation for involvement
    - Being clear about why you want to involve service users and carers
    - Being clear about who you want to involve
    - Ensuring you have the appropriate policies and procedures in place
    - Resourcing involvement
    - Challenging people's attitudes and beliefs
- Involving service users and carers in practice
    - Giving people a choice about how they get involved
    - Involving people who may be marginalised
    - Providing training and support for staff, service users and carers
    - Ensuring user and carer involvement has an impact
    - Communication and feedback
    - Involving service users in measuring the success of involvement

---

Box 2.2
....
Guidance for Good Practice: service user involvement in the UK Mental
Health Research Network (SURGE 2005)

- Literature review
  - Benefits of involvement
  - Power and negotiation
  - Clarity/transparency
  - Early involvement
  - Accessible language
  - Flexibility
  - Support
- Training
  - Payments
  - Resources
- Guidance for good practice
  - Underlying principles
  - Capacity building
  - Identifying priorities
  - Commissioning research
  - Ethical Approval and Research Ethics Committees
  - Undertaking research
  - Dissemination and Implementation
  - User controlled research

---

never to underestimate anyone. Everyone has something to say and something to contribute to the endeavour.

References

Barnes C, Mercer G (eds) 1997 Doing disability research. The Disability Press, Leeds

Beresford P, Wallcraft J 1997 Psychiatric system survivors and emancipatory research: issues, overlaps and differences. In: Barnes C, Mercer G (eds) 1997 Doing disability research. The Disability Press, Leeds

Campbell P 2006a Brown linoleum green lawns. Hearing Eye, London

Campbell P 2006b Some things you should know about user/survivor action. A Mind resource pack. Mind Publications, London

Crawford M J, Rutter D, Manley C et al 2001 User involvement in the planning and delivery of mental health services. Report to London Region NHSE

Department of Health 2001 Research governance framework for health and social care. DH, London

Faulkner A 1997 Knowing our own minds. Mental Health Foundation, London

Faulkner A 2002 Things have really changed. Openmind 116 (July/August)

Faulkner A 2005 Institutional conflict: the state of play in adult acute psychiatric wards. Journal of Adult Protection 7(4):6–12

Hanley B, Staley K 2005 LMCA user and carer involvement: a good practice guide. Long-term Medical Conditions Alliance, London

Lindow V 2001 Survival research. In: Newnes C, Holmes G, Dunn C (eds) This is madness too. PCCS Books, London

Lindow V 2002 Being ethical, having influence. Openmind 116:18–19

Mental Health Foundation and Sainsbury Centre for Mental Health 2002 Being there in a crisis. MHF and SCMH, London

Nicholls V & the Somerset Spirituality project research team 2002 Taken seriously: the somerset spirituality project. Mental Health Foundation, London

Read J 2001 Dazed and annoyed. Openmind 115 (July/August)

Repper J, Breeze J 2006 User and carer involvement in the training and education of health professionals: A review of the literature. International Journal of Nursing Studies, Volume 44, Issue 3. Pages 511–519

Rethink 2005 Future perfect: mental health service users set out a vision for the 21st century. Rethink, London

Rose D 2001 Users' voices: the perspectives of mental health service users on community and hospital care. The Sainsbury Centre for Mental Health, London

Rose D 2003 Collaborative research between users and professionals: peaks and pitfalls. Psychiatric Bulletin 27(11):404–406

SCMH 2006 Guide to user-focused monitoring: setting up and running a project. Sainsbury Centre for Mental Health, London

Simpson E, House A O 2002 Involving users in the delivery and evaluation of mental health services: systematic review. British Medical Journal 325:1265

SURGE 2005 Guidance for good practice: service user involvement in the UK Mental Health Research Network. UKMHRN/SURGE, London

Trivedi P 2001 Never again. Openmind Issue 10 (July/August)

Wallcraft J 2005 On our own terms. Sainsbury Centre for Mental Health, London

Wood P 2004 Advocacy standards: standards for advocacy in mental health. UK Advocacy Network, London

Wood P, Mullins G 2004 Advocacy today and tomorrow: the UK Advocacy Network training tool. UK Advocacy Network, London

Useful resources

Campbell P 2006 Some things you should know about user/survivor action. A Mind resource pack. Mind Publications, London.

Faulkner A 2004 The ethics of survivor research: guidelines for the ethical conduct of research carried out by mental health service users and survivors. Policy Press on behalf of the Joseph Rowntree Foundation, Bristol.

UFM Network 2003 Doing it for real: a guide to setting up and undertaking a User Focused Monitoring project. Sainsbury Centre for Mental Health, London (www.scmh.org.uk)

Resources on payment

A guide to paying members of the public who are actively involved in research. Involve, October 2003 (www.invo.org.uk)

Hanley B et al 2003 Involving the public in NHS, public health and social care research: briefing notes for researchers (second edition). Involve (www.invo.org.uk)

A fair day's pay: a guide to benefits, service user involvement and payments. Mental Health Foundation, July 2003 (www.mentalhealth.org.uk)

Turner M 2007 Contributing on equal terms; getting involved and the benefits system. Report to Dr Stephen Ladyman, Minister for Community. Shaping Our Lives/Social Care Institute for Excellence, London

Carers of people with mental health problems

J. Repper

Background

There are almost three million people in the UK who provide support for a family member or friend who has mental health problems (Office for National Statistics 2003). Up to 175,000 of these carers are under the age of 16, often unsupported by formal services (Aldridge & Becker 2003). As mental health services have moved into the community, so much of the responsibility for providing care – emotional and practical support, subtle monitoring of the health of the person they care for, and co-ordination of input from formal services – has shifted onto informal carers, usually family members. This contribution goes largely unrecognised and, at least from carers' points of view, largely under-valued by statutory services.

Research into the lives and experiences of family carers of people with mental health problems has repeatedly described their feeling that they have to 'battle' with the system (Veltman et al 2002), that there is little acknowledgement of their point of view (Jeon & Madjar 1998) and that professionals adopt a 'blaming' perspective (Pejlert 2001). It has even been suggested that professionals rarely, or never: help carers identify resources that might help them; assist them to plan for the future; help them reflect on what they do well; give them respect for what they do (Doornbos 2001).

This chapter reviews policy and legislation relating to carers of people with mental health problems and refers to the literature on carers' needs. It considers the progress and impact of the implementation of carer policy.

The policy and legislative context

The last 20 years has seen an increasing range of legislative initiatives designed to improve the situation of carers. Successive governments have introduced a series of legislative changes (Box 3.1) including formal assessment of carers as a means of ensuring their needs are adequately addressed and that partnerships between family and formal care giving systems are created

Box 3.1

Summary of Carer Legislation (adapted from Simpson et al 2007)

- 1995 The Carers (Recognition and Services) Act
  People providing 'substantial care on a regular basis' have the right to request an assessment of their needs.
- 2000 The Carers and Disabled Children Act
  Ensures access to services for carers in their own right – even if the person they care for is not receiving support.
- 2001 The Health and Social Care Act (Section 1)
  Requires commissioners and service providers to consult patients and public about carers' issues.
- 2002 The NHS Service Reform and Health Care Professionals Act
  The Commission for Patient and Public Involvement in Health required to set up forum and independent complaints and advocacy service for patients and carers.
- 2003 The Community Care (Delayed Discharge etc) Act
  Gives carers right to own assessment and to request home visit to assess their needs before a patient can be discharged from hospital.
- 2004 The Carers (Equal Opportunities) Act
  Assessments to include work, training, leisure needs. Requires local health services to work with local authorities and collaborate with education, housing, social care, etc, in providing support to carers.

(DH 1999a). These began in 1995 with the passing of the Carers (Recognition and Services) Act (DH 1995) which, according to Clements (2006), contains 'the core statutory responsibilities' towards carers and introduced the concept of a 'carer's assessment'. This entitled carers who provided, or were intending to provide, 'a substantial amount of care on a regular basis' to a separate assessment of their needs providing that the person they were supporting was also having an assessment. In order to further enhance the status of carers the UK Government introduced the 'Carers National Strategy' (DH 1999a) intended to provide specific services for carers, notably in the form of 'short breaks'. To facilitate this strategy an annual 'carers grant' was given to local authorities in order to promote the more widespread and innovative provision of such breaks.

The rights of carers were further enhanced by the Carers' and Disabled Children's' Act (DH 2000a) which afforded carers the right to an assessment, even if the person they were caring for was not receiving one. Furthermore, in 2004, the Carers (Equal Opportunities) Act mandated that local authorities inform carers of their right to an assessment and extended the focus of the assessment to specifically include issues to do with work, education and leisure.

Carers supporting people with mental health problems have the same rights as other carers but their situation received particular recognition in the National Service Framework for Mental Health (DH 1999b). Standard 6 focussed specifically on the needs of carers and stated that:

All individuals who provide regular and substantial care for a person on CPA (Care Programme Approach) should have an assessment of their caring, physical and mental health needs, repeated at least on an annual basis, and they should have their own written care plan, which is given to them and implemented in discussion with them.

This care plan should include 10 key action points:

- Identify carers of people with mental health problems
- Provide carers with the information they need in order to help them to provide care
- Listen to what carers have to say
- Consider whether carers are providing regular and substantial care
- Assess carer's needs
- Co-ordinate with carer, service user and other agencies to meet Standard 6
- Formulate carer's care plan
- Review annually or if circumstances change significantly
- Consult with carers about the services they receive
- Involve carers in the planning and development of services.

The legislative focus on carers *assessment* provides a means of ensuring that services engage with carers in a manner that is measurable and audited through social services performance indicators. However, this focus on carer assessment (potentially a one-off or annual event carried out quite separately from mental health service provision) can obscure the fundamental role that carers play in the lives of many people with mental health problems and the crucial contribution they make to communities:

'Carers play a vital role in helping support users of mental health services and those with mental health problems not in touch with services. Providing help, support and advice to carers can be one of the best ways of helping people with mental health problems. Support for carers must be mainstreamed into the activities of all health and social care mental health services.'

(DH 2002, p23)

In order to be effective and meaningful, carer assessments need to be seen as just one part of the partnership between formal and informal systems of care. Rather than a one-off event conducted quite separately from the person with mental health problems, they must be collaborative and ongoing. Repper et al (2007) have suggested a number of principles for good practice in carer assessment arising from the Partnerships in Carer Assessment Project (PICAP), a 3-year DH funded study of assessing carers of people with mental health problems. These include:

- Assessment must be part of an ongoing partnership between carers and services, where there is regular contact with a known person.
- Contact with carers should be initiated as early as possible and the carer engaged as an equal partner from the outset.

- The carer's role and expertise must be fully explored, recognised and respected (equally, areas where carers may lack knowledge and expertise should be acknowledged and addressed).
- Carers should be involved in planning and agreeing the care plan for the person for whom they care.
- Carers must receive the information and support they need in order to help them to care most effectively.
- A carer's willingness or ability to care must not be taken for granted.
- Assessment should start by exploring carers' understanding of what the assessment involves.
- Assessment must be proactive and planned rather than crisis driven.
- Assessment should focus on the outcomes or goals that are important to carers.
- Assessment should take an holistic approach and recognise the needs and preferences of both the carer and the person they care for.
- Assessment should result in a care plan developed in collaboration with the carer that makes clear the type and level of support to be provided, when and by whom.
- Assessment must take account of differing cultural, ethnic or other beliefs and value systems in families.
- First language preferences of carers should be respected.
- Good carer assessment requires assessors to have specialised and broad ranging knowledge and highly developed interpersonal skills.

There also exist numerous national guidelines on 'good practice' with carers that go far beyond the annual assessment required in policy and legislative terms. These include the National Institute for Clinical Excellence (NICE) guidelines on schizophrenia, dementia, eating disorders and depression; the Mental Health Policy Implementation Guidance (PIG) on community mental health teams, acute in-patient units, low secure units and intensive care units; the best practice guidance for GPs and primary care services produced by the Princess Royal Trust for Carers in partnership with the Royal College of General Practitioners; and 'Good Psychiatric Practice' guidance on confidentiality and information sharing produced by the Royal College of Psychiatrists (RCP 2006).

As a backdrop to these carer specific requirements, all recent health policy, particularly mental health policy (Box 3.2), has emphasised the need for service user *and carer* involvement in decision-making at all levels of service commissioning, delivery and evaluation. As the NHS Plan (DH 2000b) clearly states, 'services will be shaped around the needs and preferences of individual patients, their families and carers'. The implications of this consumer orientated approach are discussed more fully in Chapter 1.

Implementation of policy relating to carers of people with mental health problems

There is some evidence that carers are beginning to be involved in service planning, commissioning, delivery and evaluation: several NHS Trusts have

---

Box 3.2

Summary of Mental Health Policy related to Carers (adapted from Simpson et al 2007)

- 1999 National Service Framework (MH)
  Standard 6 – Caring about Carers
- 1999 National Strategy for Carers: Caring about Carers
  Considers needs of carers in three areas: information, support and care
- 2000 The NHS Plan: a plan for investment, a plan for reform
  Based on principle of user focussed services; pledged 700 carer support workers, increased carer breaks, better carer support networks.
- 2001 The Capable Practitioner: a framework and list of practitioner capabilities required to implement the NSF
  Identifies values, attitudes, knowledge, and specific capabilities for communicating with service users and families; plus capabilities for partnership working and for collaborating across agencies.
- 2001 NSF (Older People)
  Builds on principles in NHS Plan and includes specific standard for older people with mental health problems including importance of good information for carers and support to be partner in care.
- 2002 Developing Services for carers and families of people with mental illness
  Provides guidance for implementation of Standard 6 of NSF (MH) and for developing mental health carer support services.
- 2005 NSF (Children, Young People and Maternity Services)
  All children and parents or carers require access to information and support to ensure mental health is promoted; recognises that untreated mental health problems can cause distress for them, their family and in long term.
- 2005 Every Child Matters: Change for Children
  Recognises role played by parents and carers. Makes support for parents and carers routine, particularly at transition points in child's life.
- 2005 Ten Essential Shared Capabilities: A framework for the whole mental health workforce
  Carers and families acknowledged throughout all 10 capabilities; stresses need for partnerships and to work positively with conflict and tensions between service users and carers.
- 2005 Health, Our Care, Our Say
  Pledges help for carers including: better information, emergency respite care, expert carers programme and direct payments.
- 2005 From Values to Action: CNO's review of Mental Health Nursing
  Emphasises the importance of mental health nurses working positively with service users and carers

---

carer representatives at Board level, carers are involved in most Patient Advice and Liaison Services, and carers are beginning to find a voice in the evaluation of services. However, it is difficult to quantify the level or impact of this involvement – certainly, there is a long way to go before the involvement and support of families and carers becomes a core component of high quality, effective mental health care (Hervey & Ramsey 2004).

Even though carer assessments form the mainstay of carer legislation and policy, there is little evidence available about their implementation and impact.

Appleby's review of the implementation of the National Service Framework (NSF) over its first five years (Appleby 2004, p74) concluded that, with respect to Standard 6: 'we have too little to report on improving the support we provide to carers ...'

The data cited in the report were minimal, indicating an increase in support services for carers, and modest success in ensuring that carers of people on enhanced CPA had a care plan, but giving no information at all on the provision or uptake of carer assessments.

It is important to set such scant progress in the overall context of developments for carers in general, and for carer assessments in particular. Despite the numerous policy initiatives designed to ensure that services engage with informal carers, recent evidence indicates that the uptake of carer assessments has been very limited. The policy guide on implementing the Carers (Equal Opportunities) Act 2004 notes that 'progress in carrying out carer assessments is slow, and few separate assessments are carried out' (SCIE 2005, Section 2, p2). Similarly, in reviewing the success of several initiatives designed to promote stakeholder participation in England, Wales and Northern Ireland Roulstone et al (2006, p69) concluded that carer assessment represents 'one of the least consistent and least satisfactory elements'. Their report highlights the continued uncertainty and lack of clarity surrounding carer assessments, stressing the low awareness and uptake of assessments and the fact that even carers who have had an assessment are often unaware of this and/or receive little or no feedback and subsequent support. The recent review of the Modernising Adult Social Care (MASC) (Newman & Hughes 2007) research programme reaches a remarkably similar conclusion.

Clearly, therefore, the challenge of providing a comprehensive assessment of carers' needs is not unique to mental health, nor is it confined to the UK, with several studies and reports noting similar issues in a number of countries, including the USA (National Carers Alliance 2006), Canada (Guberman 2005) and Australia (Guberman et al 2003). Whilst this would suggest the existence of shared and enduring issues, it has long been recognised that difficulties relating to carers generally are exacerbated:

- for those supporting people with mental health problems (Hogman & Pearson 1995) because of the isolation experienced by carers (Karp 2002) and the stigma associated with mental illness (Reifer & Cox 2001)
- by the unpredictable nature of many mental illnesses (Jeon & Madjar 1998, Newbronner & Hare 2002) fuelling fears of relapse and of services not responding 'until something dreadful has happened' (Howe 1995)
- by the guilt and blame carers may feel for the mental illness of their family member – a feeling that, arguably, has been reinforced by services (Hatfield 1994)
- by potential conflict between carers and service users about appropriate care, particularly at times of crisis (Pinfold et al 2004).

In the PICAP study of carer assessments in mental health services, one of the main findings was just how few carer assessments were completed: even in sites with reputedly good practice in carer assessments, very small numbers of carers were identified by services and even fewer were offered carer assessments (Repper et al 2007). The reasons cited for this included:

- Carers are not identified through the service users' assessment. Although the care programme assessment documents used with service users do include questions about informal carers, this relies on service users informing their assessor about the people who provide emotional and practical support for them. Service users may consider themselves to be fairly independent; they may not mention the support they receive from others. They may, understandably, not be aware of the stress they can create for family members and genuinely feel that that they do not have 'carers' – the term itself is problematic as it implies a dependent role for the 'cared for'. There may be some disruption within the family so that they are reluctant to involve family members in their care, or they may actively request that family members are not consulted or contacted with regard to their needs.
- Where carers are identified they are often not considered eligible for assessment as they have a limited caring role. Eligibility criteria varies with different formal interpretations of the legal term 'regular and substantial caring role' as well as variation between the different worker's interpretations of the term.
- Carers themselves may be reluctant to accept the offer of an assessment of their needs. Carers referred for an assessment after long contact with services may have lost faith in services' ability to make a difference, many feel 'traumatised' by their contact with services and reluctant to get involved with services further. Carers may also have concerns about the responsibilities that they perceive to run alongside formal identification as a carer. They may not understand, or even object to, the term 'carer' – seeing themselves as a mother, father, sibling or friend rather than a 'carer'. They may also misunderstand the meaning of the term 'assessment' perceiving it to be an assessment of their ability to care. For some carers, the assessment form can be a barrier, seeming like yet more bureaucracy.

This situation is not confined to carers' assessment: even when the person with a mental health problem is on enhanced CPA and carers want to be involved and have regular contact with the service user (Krupnik et al 2005, Wynodin & Orb 2005), very few are engaged as active participants in sharing their knowledge and expertise, leaving them frustrated and resentful (Wynodin & Orb 2005).

The roots of carers' exclusion may lie in early – but lingering – theories about the role of the family in either the aetiology of mental illness (particularly schizophrenia), or as a major cause of relapse (Lefley 1990, Jungbauer et al 2004, Shooter 2004, Krupnik et al 2005, Sjoblom et al 2005). There are, moreover, several additional barriers to greater partnership working between professionals and carers, including:

- The continued adherence to a model of care based on symptoms and medical treatment (Godfrey & Wistow 1997) in which the professional is seen to be the expert (Hatfield 1990), holding specialist knowledge

(McCann & Clark 2003). Treatments therefore tend to be given **to** people rather than developed **with** them (Anderson 2000). Accepting carers as 'co-experts' (Nolan et al 2003) poses a threat to professional status (Walker & Dewer 2001, Lloyd & Carson 2005).

- The focus of professional interventions is primarily on the user/client (Karp 2002, McCann & Clark 2003), and this can result in a conflict of loyalty (Sjoblom et al 2005) and fosters the belief that involving carers may threaten or compromise the care that the user receives (Kaas et al 2003).

- The above situation is exacerbated by the thorny issue of patient/client confidentiality. This is widely recognised as a significant impediment to the greater involvement of family carers (Godfrey & Wistow 1997, Rethink 2003, Wynoden & Orb 2005, Pack 2005, Sjoblom et al 2005, Cormac & Tihanyi 2006) that requires urgent attention (Hervey & Ramsay 2004, Pinfold et al 2004, DH 2006). Whilst guidance is available this is often interpreted in a 'conservative' fashion (Marshall & Solomon 2005). Recent extensive research has argued for the need to find ways of reducing the limitations imposed by a strict adherence to confidentiality in order to promote open and honest communication between carers and professionals (see Pinfold et al 2004), but it is still recognised that individually tailored solutions requiring a 'carefully weighted judgement' are needed (DH 2006).

- Professionals lack the training and skills to work collaboratively with families (Kaas et al 2003, Sin et al 2003, Pack 2005). Improved training is seen as a prerequisite (Thomas et al 1999) if professionals are better to understand carers' perspectives and to this end the greater involvement of families in professional education is now widely promoted.

Although formal family psychosocial interventions are not the focus of this chapter, there are important lessons to learn from them. Despite their effectiveness in reducing relapse (Fadden 1998), the fact that the National Institute for Clinical Effectiveness concludes that they should be a routine intervention in the treatment of schizophrenia, and the significant investment in training staff in the use of these skills (Brooker & Brabban, 2004) they remain largely unavailable to families and informal carers. Very few PSI trainees work with families (Fadden 1998) due to lack of confidence, lack of time/resources, lack of managerial support – and apparent difficulty identifying 'appropriate' families. Thus the majority of families and informal carers of people with mental health problems are receiving neither assessment of their needs nor the support and interventions that might meet their needs.

How can services improve support for carers?

Notwithstanding the 'uniqueness' of each caregiving situation, literature on the experiences of carers of people with mental health problems suggests the emergence of common themes which can help to inform the accessible, appropriate and acceptable support of carers. These include:

The importance of understanding the 'meanings' that carers of people with mental health problems ascribe to their situation (Jeon & Madjar 1998, Rhoades &

McFarland 1999), and the impact such meanings have on their sense of identity (Tuck et al 1997, Karp & Tanarugsachock 2000). This suggests that the support offered should take a carers' perspective and explore carers' understandings of what has happened if acceptable support is to be provided. At the same time carers, and particularly new carers, value help in understanding and interpreting both the mental illness and their responses to it (Rose 1998).

The temporal nature of caring and the changing demands, understandings and feelings of control that carers develop over time (Jeon & Madjar 1998, Rose 1998, Karp & Tanarugsachock 2000). A number of authors have adopted a temporal perspective in an effort to better understand the changing nature of the caring experience in mental illness so that support can be tailored to their changing needs and relationships (Godfrey & Wistow 1997, DH 2002, Pagnini 2005, Walton-Moss et al 2005). As Dawson et al (2004) suggest, support should be '*choreographed*' to match carers' unfolding needs. However, this rarely seems to be the case, especially in the early stages of caring when contact with professionals is often limited (DH 2002, Rethink 2003, Sin et al 2003) with the result that carers are rarely able to choose to care or not (Rethink 2003), and are frequently poorly prepared for their role (Chien et al 2004).

One of the most comprehensive descriptions of the 'caring career' is provided in a study to identify '*turning points*' in the joint experiences of both carer and the cared-for person (Karp & Tanarugsachock 2000, Karp 2002). Karp & Tanarugsachock (2000) describe four '*interpretive junctures*' with associated emotional reactions:

- Before diagnosis – when carers experience a sense of '*emotional anomie*' characterised by uncertainty and confusion as they are confronted by unexplained behaviours that make no sense within existing frames of reference.
- Diagnosis – is seen as a '*pivotal*' moment when a potential explanation, albeit in medical terms, is available. At this point carers crave information and actively work to 'learn' about the 'illness'. This is a period in which carers usually embrace their role enthusiastically in the belief that they can 'save' or 'cure' their loved one. At the same time carers may find it difficult to fully empathise with their relative, and can feel frustration when there is little apparent reciprocity in their relationship.
- Realisation of permanency – as time passes there is increasing recognition that carers' initial hopes for a 'cure' will not be realised and this is often a period of deeply conflicting emotions when the 'permanency' of the illness is acknowledged. Carers can feel anger, resentment, loss and grief as their own hopes/aspirations are put on hold and there is little apparent focus on their needs.
- Acceptance that they cannot control the illness – eventually most carers come to accept that much of the illness is outside of their control and they may begin to decrease their involvement without feeling guilty. Their ability to do so depends on achieving what Karp & Tanarugsachock (2000) call the 4 'c's:

  - I did not **cause** this
  - I cannot **control** this

– I cannot **cure** this

– I can only **cope** with this.

For Karp (2002, p200) tensions between carers and professionals are most profound at key transition points, especially during crises, because:

'... *what family members experience as traumatic and chaotic turmoil, they [professionals] experience as routine, even boring ... this ritualisation of their crisis feels callous to them [carers].*'

To compound matters, carers' need for information, especially in the early stages, are often ignored and they feel marginalised and disregarded. In such circumstances carers soon become 'cynical' about the whole system, and lose trust, which subsequently can be very hard, if not impossible, to re-establish. Such dynamics are typified in carers' contact with psychiatrists who, according to Karp (2002), tend to base their therapeutic model on a 'two-person social system only – doctor and patient'. Consequently carers often see psychiatrists as:

- being unwilling to listen to them
- decontextualising treatment by disregarding their expert knowledge
- making 'snap' judgements without sufficient knowledge
- behaving in a callous way and making carers' pain worse
- being quick to blame carers.

Recognition that caring, while often difficult and stressful, is not a universally negative experience (Veltman et al 2002) and that assessment should promote a strengths-based approach (Rose 1998) that acknowledges experienced carers as co-experts (Newbronner & Hare 2002). Several commentators have called for a focus on potential satisfactions of caring (Rose 1998, Arksey et al 2002) and, in particular, an appreciation of the strengths, resources, competence and resilience that carers may possess or be helped to develop (Cleary et al 2003, Saunders 2003, Schulze & Rössler 2005, Addington et al 2003, 2005).

'*In psychiatric research we are unaccustomed to examining positive aspects of functioning, we would do well to recall that caregivers of relatives with serious mental illness cope effectively with taxing and enduring problems. In attempting to measure the experience we should resist the tendency to pathologise; identifying and understanding coping is as pertinent as detecting psychopathology.*'

(Szmukler et al 1996)

The combination of a focus on the 'burden' of caring – with implied blame of the individual service user – with the considerable focus on expressed emotion (EE) – with the implied blame of the family (Rose et al 2002, Jeon 2003, Mubarak & Barber, 2003) has laid the foundations for the strained and often negative interactions that occur between carers and mental health professionals. A more balanced relationship is unlikely to emerge until there is a significant shift away from the preoccupation with burden:

'towards more positive formulations of the caring experience, recognising that it can be a fulfilling aspect of a relationship and therefore both good and bad effects need to be taken into account.'

(Wooff et al 2003, p30)

Taking account of carers' unique situations and experiences as determined, for example, by their age, gender, general health, relationship with the care recipient, cultural background, employment situation, housing, financial resources and other responsibilities. It is such factors that shape and define carers' identities and perceived obligations, suggesting the potentially conflicting demands they may face.

Much of the existing literature in caring in mental health focuses primarily on the experience of schizophrenia with limited attention given to depression, eating disorders, anxiety and substance abuse (see, for example, Winn et al 2004). Other notable gaps are apparent in respect of carers from black and minority ethnic (BME) groups (Ho et al 2002, Rungreangkulkij et al 2002, DH 2002, Schulze & Rössler 2005); rural carers (DH 2002); young carers (DH 2002, Pagnini 2005); carers of people with obsessive compulsive disorders (Laidlaw et al 1999); sibling carers (Hatfield & Lefley 2005); carers of adults with attention deficit disorder (Hare et al 2004); carers of people with HIV/AIDS (Flaskerud & Lee 2001); carers of people with Huntington's disease (Lowit & Teijlgen 2005); carers of people with mental health problems in older age (Horton-Deutsch et al 2002, Ferguson & Keady 2001, Jeon 2003, Bartels 2005); young carers (for exceptions see Dearden & Becker 1999, Aldridge & Becker 2003, Gladstone et al 2006); and carers from different ethnic groups. The limited work on ethnic diversity suggests that black carers receive less assistance and are less involved with treatment plans (Leavey et al 1997), that they perceive less burden and stigma but are more likely to disagree with professionals about the most appropriate forms of help (Reifer & Cox 2001).

In a widespread consultation with carers about what they want from mental health services, Newbronner & Hare (2002) identified four key characteristics that were prioritised and stressed that quality is as much about the 'process' of service receipt, as the service itself. Carers wanted services that are:

- Positive and inclusive – so that carers are seen as an integral part of the system, rather then being marginalised or blamed. A willingness to share information is essential, as is acceptance of carers as partners/co-experts.
- Flexible and individualised – services that are person-centred, delivered on time and are consistent with existing routines, cause minimum disruption and provide as normal a life as possible for their relative.
- Accessible and responsive – services that are reliable, available outside 'office' hours, provide rapid access in a crisis, and have a low trigger threshold so that they can be genuinely preventative.
- Integrated and coordinated – services that cut across agency boundaries, and provide 'seamless' access and delivery.

In addition, carers value time and continuity in their contact with services (Rose 1998), a non-judgemental and non-blaming attitude (Doornbos 2001,

Reifer & Cox 2001), acknowledgement of their expertise (Newbronner & Hare 2002) and service responses that are consistent with their routines and ways of working (Rose 1998, Newbronner & Hare 2002).

Conclusion

'A cultural shift within mental health is required: professionals must change their attitudes towards working with families. Carers ask for professionals to respect their expertise and knowledge.'

(DH 2006, p5)

Progress in the implementation of mental health policy relating to carers has been slow, and this reflects the wider situation of carers generally, who remain fairly marginal figures. In the field of mental health Simpson & House (2005) contend that it is time to move beyond the rhetoric of partnerships, but paradoxically the NSF has 'too little to say' about good practice for working with carers (Hervey & Ramsay 2004). Indeed, whilst the NSF is putatively based on the best available evidence, that supporting Standard 6 is scant, with there only being eight references cited, four of these from official DH or SSI sources.

The importance of family and professional carers working together in a reciprocal relationship in which the strengths, resources and expertise of both family and professional carers are valued (Biegel et al 1995), is now recognised. Indeed, such is the importance of a change in professional culture that it has been argued that modifying attitudes towards carers may well be preferable to the development of carer-specific services (Newbronner & Hare 2002). Indeed, even where effective family interventions skills have been developed and staff are trained in using these skills, they are not being implemented. It appears that a shift in attitudes is required before carers are routinely identified, engaged, involved, informed and worked with, as partners in care. The main difficulty for services and providers seems to lie not in *how* to work with carers, but in working with them at all.

References

Addington J, Coldham E L, Jones B, Ko T, Addington D 2003 The first episode of psychosis: the experience of relatives. Acta Psychiatrica Scandinavica 108:285–289

Addington J, McCleary A, Addington, D. 2005 Three year outcome of family work in an early psychosis programme. Schizophrenia Research 79:107–116

Aldridge J, Becker S 2003 Children caring for parents with mental illness: perspectives of young carers, parents and professionals. The Policy Press, Bristol

Anderson M 2000 A strain towards consensus? The individual, the family, and New Zealand's Mental Health (Compulsory Assessment and Treatment) Amendment Bill 1999. Psychiatry, Psychology and Law 7(1):111–118

Appleby L 2004 The NSF for Mental Health – 5 years on. Department of Health, London

Arksey H, O'Malley L, Baldwin S, Harris J, Mason S 2002 Services to support carers of people with mental health problems: literature review. NCCSDO, London

Bartels S J 2005 Improving the system of care for older adults with mental illness in the US. American Journal of Geriatric Psychiatry 11(5):486–497

Biegel D E, Song L-Y, Milligan S E 1995 A comparative analysis of family caregivers' perceived relationships with mental health professionals. Psychiatric Services 46(5)

Brooker C, Brabban A 2004 Measured success: a scoping review of evaluated psychosocial interventions training for work with people with serious mental health problems. NIMHE/ Trent WDC, Nottingham

Chien W-T, Norman I, Thompson D R 2004 A randomized controlled trail of a mutual support group for family caregivers of patients with schizophrenia. International Journal of Nursing Studies 41(6):637–649

Cleary M. Freeman A, Hunt G, Walter G 2003 What patients and carers want to learn: an exploration of information and resource needs in adult mental health services. Australian and New Zealand Journal of Psychiatry 39:507–513

Clements, L 2006 Carers and their rights – the law relating to carers. Carers UK, London

Cormac I, Tihanyi P 2006 Meeting the mental and physical health care needs of carers. Advances in Psychiatric Treatment 12:162–172

Dawson S, Kristjanson L J, Toge C M, Platt P 2004 Living with Huntington's disease: need for supportive care. Nursing and Health Science 6:123–130

Dearden C, Becker S 1999 The experiences of young carers in the UK: the mental health issues. Mental Health Care 2(8):273–276

Department of Health 1995 Carers (Recognition and Services) Act. HMSO, London

Department of Health 1999a The Carers National Strategy. HMSO, London

Department of Health 1999b National Service Framework for Mental Health. DH, London

Department of Health 2000a Caring About Carers, Carers and Disabled Children Act. HMSO, London

Department of Health 2000b NHS Plan. HMSO, London

Department of Health 2002 Developing services for carers and families of people with mental illness. HMSO, London

Department of Health 2006 Sharing mental health information with carers: points to good practice for service providers. NCCSDO, London

Doornbos M M 2001 Professional support for family caregivers of people with serious and persistent mental illnesses. Journal of Psychosocial Nursing 39(12):39–45

Fadden G 1998 Family intervention. In: Brooker C, Repper J (eds) Serious mental health problems in the community: policy practice and research. Baillière Tindall, Edinburgh

Ferguson C, Keady J 2001 The mental health needs of older people and their carers: exploring tensions and new directions. In: Nolan M R, Davies S, Grant G (eds) Working with older people and their families: key issues in policy and practice. Open University Press, Buckingham, p120–138

Flaskerud J H, Lee P 2001 Vulnerability to health problems in female informal caregivers of persons with HIV/AIDS and age-related dementias. Journal of Advanced Nursing 33(1):60–68

Gladstone B M, Boydell K M, McKeever P 2006 Recasting research into children's experiences of parental mental illness: beyond risk and resilience. Social Science and Medicine 62:2540–2550

Godfrey M, Wistow G 1997 The user perspective on managing for health outcomes: the case of mental health. Health and Social Care in the Community 5(5):325–332

Guberman N, Nicholas E, Nolan M R, Rembecki D, Lundh U, Keefe J 2003 Impacts on practitioners of using research-based carer assessment tools: experiences from the UK, Canada, Sweden, with insights from Australia. Health and Social Care in the Community 11(4):345–355

Guberman N (Convenor) 2005 Who's supposed to care? Changing norms and values with regard to family responsibility for the frail elderly. Symposium at 18th Congress of the International Association of Gerontology, Rio de Janeiro, Brazil, 26–30 June 2005

Hare D J, Pratt C, Burton M, Bramley J, Emerson E 2004 The health and social care needs of family carers supporting adults with autistic spectrum disorders. Autism 8(4):225–444

Hatfield A B 1990 The social context of helping families. In: Lefley H P, Johsson D L (eds) Families as allies in the treatment of mental illness: new directions for mental health professionals. American Psychiatric Press, Washington, p77–89

Hatfield A B 1994 Family education: theory and practice. New Directions for Mental Health Services 62:3–12

Hatfield A B, Lefley H P 2005 Future involvement of siblings in the lives of persons with mental illness. Community Mental Health Journal 41(3):327–338

Hervey N, Ramsay R 2004 Carers as partners in care. Advances in Psychiatric Treatment 10:81–84

Ho G J, Weitzmann P F, Lui X, Leukoff S E 2002 Stress and service use among minority caregivers to elders with dementia. Journal of Gerontological Social Work 33(1):67–88

Hogman P, Pearson G 1995 The silent partners: the needs and experience of people who provide informal care to people with severe mental illness. National Schizophrenia Fellowship, London

Horton-Deutsch S L, Farran C J, Choi E E, Fogg L 2002 The PLUS Intervention: a pilot test with caregivers of depressed older adults. Archives in Psychiatric Nursing XVI(2):61–71

Howe G 1995 Working with schizophrenia: a needs based approach. Jessica Kingsley, London

Jeon Y-H 2003 Mental health nurses work with family caregivers of older people with depression: review of the literature. Issues in Mental Health Nursing 24: 813–828

Jeon Y-H, Madjar I 1998 Caring for a family member with chronic mental illness. Qualitative Health Research 8(5):694–706

Jungbauer J, Stelling K, Dietrich S, Angermeyer M. 2004 Schizophrenia: problems of separation in families. Journal of Advanced Nursing 47(6):605–613

Kaas M J, Lee S, Peitzman C 2003 Barriers to collaboration between mental health professionals and family in the care of persons with serious mental illness. Issues in Mental Health Nursing 24:741–756

Karp D A 2002 The burden of sympathy. How families cope with mental illness. Oxford University Press, Oxford

Karp D A, Tanarugsachock V 2000 Mental illness, caregiving, and emotion management. Qualitative Health Research 10(1):6–25

Krupnick Y, Pilling S, Killaspy H, Dallan J 2005 A study of family contact with clients and staff of community mental health teams. Psychiatric Bulletin 29:174–176

Laidlaw T M, Falloon I R H, Barnfather D, Coverdale J H 1999 The stress of caring for people with obsessive complusive disorders. Community Mental Health Journal 35(5):443–450

Leavey G, King M, Cole E, Hoar A, Johnson-Sabine E 1997 First-onset psychosis psychiatric illness: patients' and relatives' satisfaction with services. British Journal of Psychiatry 170(1):53–57

Lefley H P 1990 Research directions for a new conceptualisation of families. In: Lefley H P, Johsson D L (eds) Families as allies in the treatment of mental illness: new directions for mental health professionals. American Psychiatric Press, Washington, p127–163

Lowit A, Teijligen E R van 2005 Avoidance as a strategy of (not) coping: qualitative interviews with carers of Huntington's disease patients. BMC Family Practice 6:38

Lloyd M, Carson A 2005 Culture shift: carer empowerment and co-operative inquiry. Journal of Psychiatric and Mental Health Nursing 12:187–191

McCann T V, Clark E 2003 A grounded theory study of the role that nursing plays in increasing clients willingness to access community mental health services. Journal of Mental Health Nursing 12:279–287

Marshall T, Solomon P 2005 Professionals' responsibilities in releasing information to families of adults with mental illness. Psychiatric Services 54(12):1622–1628

Mubarak A R, Barber J G 2003 Emotional expressiveness and the quality of life of patients with schizophrenia. Social Psychiatry and Psychiatric Epidemiology 38:380–384

National Carers Alliance 2006 Caregivers Count Too! A toolkit to help practitioners assess the needs of family caregivers. National Carers Alliance, London

Newbronner E, Hare P 2002 Services to support carers of people with mental health problems. Consultation Report for the National Coordinating Centre for NHS Service Delivery and Organisation R & D. NCCSDO, London

Newman J, Hughes M 2007 Modernising adult social care: what's working? Department of Health, London

Nolan M R, Lundh U, Grant G, Keady J (eds) 2003 Partnerships in family care. Open University Press, Buckingham

Office for National Statistics 2003 www.dh.gov.uk/en/Publicationsandstatistics (accessed 8 October 2007)

Pack S 2005 Empowering families to care for people with schizophrenia. Nursing Times 101(30):32–34

Pagnini D 2005 Carer life course framework: an evidence-based approach to effective carer education and support. Carers NSCI, Sydney

Pejlert A 2001 Being a parent of a son or daughter with severe mental illness receiving professional care: parents' narratives. Health and Social Care in the Community 9(4):194–204

Pinfold V, Farmer P, Rapaport J et al 2004 Positive and Inclusive: Effective ways for professionals to involve carers in information sharing. Research Report for NCCSDO. NCCSDO, London

Reifer B V, Cox N 2001 Caring and mental illness. In: Cluff L E, Binstock R H (eds) The lost art of caring: a challenge to health professionals, communities and society. John Hopkins University Press, Baltimore, p55–74

Repper J, Nolan M, Grant G, Curran M, Enderby P 2007 Family carers on the margins. Draft Report submitted to Service Delivery and Organisation Research and Development Programme. LSHTM, London

Rethink 2003 Who cares? The experiences of mental health carers accessing services and information. Rethink, London

Rhoades D R, McFarland K F 1999 Caregiver meaning: a study of caregivers of individuals with mental illness. Health and Social Work 24(2):291–298

Rose L E 1998 Benefits and limitations of professional–family interactions: the family perspective. Archives of Psychiatric Nursing XII(3):140–147

Rose L E, Mallinson R K, Walter-Moss B 2002 A grounded theory of families responding to mental illness. Western Journal of Nursing Research 24(5):516–526

Roulstone A, Hudson V, Keaney J, Allison M, Warren J 2006 Working together: carer participation in England, Wales and Northern Ireland. SCIE, London

Rungreangkulkij S, Chafetz L, Chesla C, Gilliss C 2002 Psychological morbidity of Thai families of a person with schizophrenia. International Journal of Nursing Studies 39(1):35–50

Royal College of Psychiatrists 2006 Good psychiatric practice guidance on confidentiality and information sharing. RCP, London

Saunders J C 2003 Families living with severe mental illness: a literature review. Issues in Mental Health Nursing 24:175–198

Schulze B, Rössler W 2005 Caregiver burden in mental illness: review of assessment, findings and interventions in 2004–2005. Current Opinion in Psychiatry 18:684–691

Shooter M 2004 Partners in care: who cares for carers? Psychiatric Bulletin 28:313–314

SCIE 2005 The health and well-being of young carers. Research Briefing 11. www.scie.org.uk/
publications/briefings/briefing11/index.asp (accessed 23 October 2006)

Simpson A, Benn L 2007 Scoping exercise to inform the development of a National Mental
Health Carer Support. City University, London

Simpson E L, House A O 2005 User and carer involvement in mental health services: from
rhetoric to science. British Journal of Psychiatry 183:89–91

Sin J, Moore N, Wellman N 2003 Developing services for the carers of young adults with early
onset psychosis: listening to their experiences and needs. Journal of Psychiatric and Mental
Health Nursing 12:589–597

Sjöblom L-M, Pejlert A, Apslund K 2005 Student nurses view of the family in psychiatric care.
Journal of Clinical Nursing 14:562–569

Szmukler G I, Herrman H, Colusa S, Benson A, Bloch S. 1996 A controlled trial of a
counselling intervention for caregivers of relatives with schizophrenia. Social Psychiatry and
Psychiatric Epidemiology 31:149–155

Thomas C W, Guy S M, Ogilvie L P 1999 An evaluation of a practitioner training program
designed to assist families of people with severe psychiatric disorders. Psychiatric
Rehabilitation Journal 23(1):34–41

Tuck I, du Mont P, Evans G, Shupe J 1997 The experiences of caring for an adult child with
schizophrenia. Archives of Psychiatric Nursing 9(3):118–125

Veltman A, Cameron J I, Stewart D E 2002 The experience of providing care to relatives with
serious mentalillness. The Journal of Neuroses and Mental Disease 190(2):108–114

Walker E, Dewar B 2001 How do we facilitate carers' involvement in decision making? Journal
of Advanced Nursing 34(3):329–337

Walton-Moss B, Gerson L, Rose C 2005 Effects of mental illness on family quality of life.
Issues in Mental Health Nursing 26:627–642

Winn S, Perkins S, Murray J, Murphy R, Schmidt U 2004 A qualitative study of the
experience of caring for a person with Bulimia Nervosa, Part 2: carers' needs and
experiences of services and other support. International Journal of Eating Disorders
36:269–279

Wooff D, Schneider J, Carpenter J, Brandon T 2003 Correlates of stress in carers. Journal of
Mental Health 12(1):29–40

Wynoden D, Orb A 2005 Impact of patient confidentiality on carers of people who have a
mental disorder. International Journal of Mental Health Nursing 14:166–171

Supporting equal citizenship and inclusion

E. Sayce

Introduction

For over 100 years, and more intensively for the last 30, the discrimination faced by people with a diagnosis of mental illness has been repeatedly documented in gory detail. It has been voiced by mental health service users (see Campaign against Psychiatric Oppression bulletins from the 1970s), described by voluntary organisations (Camden Consortium 1989, Beeforth et al 1990), explored by academics and senior clinicians (Link et al 1997, Link & Phelan 2001, Sartorius & Schulze 2005, Thornicroft 2006) and acknowledged by Government (ODPM 2004).

We no longer need to describe an injustice that is recognised. We need to understand how to be effective in overcoming it. To that end it is useful for mental health practitioners, service users and policy makers to consider how a rapidly changing citizenship and equality policy agenda can be used to promote equality on mental health grounds. Practitioners can provide information and active support to service users in securing rights and opportunities in employment, education, travel and services. They can also provide expert advice on how to change whole organisational systems to achieve greater equality.

A brief history

In 1978 Mind argued for legal protection against discrimination on mental health grounds in employment and sent a dossier of discrimination cases to the (Labour) Employment Minister. He replied saying he doubted there was sufficient discrimination of this kind to merit new law (Bynoe et al 1991). Less than 30 years later beliefs had shifted. Mainstream leaders in Government and psychiatry argued strongly that discrimination was the – or at least a – major priority.

Professor Graham Thornicroft from the Institute of Psychiatry found discrimination to be both common and severe and argued that there was a need 'to demolish both direct and structural discrimination against people with mental illness' (Thornicroft 2006). Professor Norman Sartorius of the World Psychiatric Association stated 'there is no greater problem in the field of mental health internationally than stigma' (Sartorius 2001).

In 2004 the British Government's Social Exclusion Unit (SEU) found that over 80% of mental health service users thought stigma was a major problem, higher than any other single issue. The SEU created a major national action plan to reduce social exclusion, building on the National Service Framework commitment to reduce stigma and discrimination.

The policy response

In Britain, the USA and most European countries discrimination against mental health service users is debarred through disability discrimination law. This is a recent development: in Britain discrimination was entirely legal until 1996. It only became illegal because mental health organisations involved themselves in coalitions for lobbying, against considerable policy resistance. The following US Senate debate on the Americans with Disabilities Bill gives a flavour:

> Mr Helms: Does the list of disabilities include paedophiles?
> Mr Harkin: What?
> Mr Helms: P-a-e-d-o-p-h-i-l-e-s
> Mr Harkin: I can assure the Senator, no
> Mr Helms: How about schizophrenics?
> Mr Harkin: Schizophrenics, yes...
> Mr Helms: Homosexuals?
> Mr Harkin: No; absolutely not...
> Mr Helms: A schizophrenic is covered, the senator said. I want to know if an
>   adoption agency is forbidden to take that into account if the prospective
>   adopter is a schizophrenic or manic depressive ... If this were a bill
>   involving people in a wheelchair or those having been injured in the war,
>   that is one thing ... But how did you get into the business of classifying
>   people who are HIV positive, most of whom are drug addicts or homosexuals
>   or bisexuals, as disabled?
>
> (Americans With Disabilities Act Senate Floor Debate, 7 September 1989)

Against an attack that aimed to separate 'deserving' impairments (wheelchair use, war wounds) from 'undeserving' (psychiatric impairment, AIDS), it was the solidarity amongst disability and mental health organisations that kept people with mental health problems covered by the Bill.

Similar strategies were used by different disability and health condition groups in relation to Britain's Disability Discrimination Act 1995 (DDA), which again resulted in coverage of both psychiatric impairments and AIDS, despite opposition; although in Britain, unlike the USA, those with drug and alcohol problems were never included, as their organisations did not get involved in the lobbying coalitions.

The role of mental health voluntary and professional organisations to achieve rights has been critical. People with personality disorders would not have been included in the DDA without the 1990s lobbying and coalition building of Mind and service user groups like Survivors Speak Out. In 2005 organisations including the Royal College of Psychiatrists, Disability Rights Commission and voluntary organisations representing HIV/AIDS, cancer, MS and mental health jointly secured improvements to the DDA – coverage of HIV/AIDS, cancer and MS from the point of diagnosis; and removal of the discriminatory requirement that someone must prove their mental illness 'clinically well recognised' to get protection under the DDA, when this did not apply to people with physical impairments.

Why bother with rights?

Legal rights to equality are a profound statement of a society's values. They often result from campaigns that take new ideas from minority concerns to a big shift of mind-set: witness the movements for votes for women, the end of Apartheid in South Africa or gay civil partnership in Britain. Once new laws are passed and publicly debated, they further reinforce and spread the change of view. The mid-point of public opinion changes – as more and more people accept that women should have the vote, or gay partnerships be recognised. It took less than 20 years, and a fair policy wind, for Stonewall to be set up and achieve civil partnerships, an equal age of consent and a shift in public opinion.

Mental health service users and disabled people more broadly have sought to benefit from a similarly profound shift. Despite recognition of discrimination, a substantial public opinion shift has not yet occurred; indeed discriminatory attitudes have got worse since the 1990s (Thornicroft 2006). But a quiet revolution may be beginning, with more people deciding to 'come out' as mental health service users, from the famous (Stephen Fry, Dame Kelly Holmes, Frank Bruno) to people in ordinary jobs or none. And although the employment rate of people with schizophrenia is lower in Britain than elsewhere in Europe (Thornicroft, 2006) the rate for people with long-term mental health problems generally has grown modestly, from 14.5% in 1998 to 20.2% in 2005 (DRC 2007a).

Legal rights matter not only as a potent cultural symbol, but as a source of power to challenge discrimination. Link & Phelan's reassessment of the concept and evidence on stigma argue that 'stigma is entirely dependent on social, economic and political power' (Link & Phelan 2001). The only ways to challenge it effectively are to limit the exercise of power – for instance by passing and enforcing anti-discrimination laws – and/or to transform the beliefs of those who hold power. Educational initiatives alone are unlikely to change discriminatory attitudes and behaviour. What is needed is an 'iron fist' of power within the educational velvet glove. It was not enough in 1960s America to agree that black people were equal; laws had to be passed to sweep away white-only universities, lunch counters and the like.

How have legal rights worked in practice?

The terms 'disability access' and 'disability equality' conjure up visions of ramps, lifts and re-designs of the physical environment. This is a misunderstanding of current legislation. Access and equality for 'disabled people' go far beyond the physical environment. Adjustments required include changes in service systems, schools, colleges and workplaces of direct benefit to people with long-term physical or mental health conditions, autistic spectrum disorders, learning disabilities and more. For example:

> Ms Beartt worked for the prison service. She was sacked whilst on sick leave with depression. She argued that the prison service had failed to make a reasonable adjustment – namely to relocate her, in line with medical advice. Her claim of disability discrimination was successful. She was awarded around half a million pounds in compensation for lost earnings.

In Britain the Disability Discrimination Act 1995 (DDA) protects the following people from discrimination: anyone with a physical or mental impairment, which has a substantial and long-term adverse effect on a person's ability to carry out normal day-to-day activities. Where treatment mitigates the adverse effect the person is still covered. Case law to date shows that people found to be disabled under this definition include those with schizophrenia, clinical depression, clinical anxiety, bipolar affective disorder, agoraphobia, post-traumatic stress disorder and bulimia nervosa. 'Long-term' is defined as having lasted, or expected to last, for at least 12 months.[1] This includes people who had a long-term mental health problem in the past – and are still facing discrimination because of it.

The DDA also requires employers, service providers and educational bodies to make 'reasonable adjustments': for instance, an employer would be expected to offer gradual return to work to someone coming back to work following depression, or flexible hours so they could see a psychiatrist or counsellor.

The law has been used by a number of people with mental health problems to get redress; and gradually the law itself has been somewhat strengthened, both through Parliament and through precedents set in the courts and tribunals.

In education, cases have demonstrated the requirement for schools and colleges to make adjustments: for instance, requiring a university to provide accommodation on campus for someone with mental health-related difficulties in travelling. In goods and services there have been some limited successful legal challenges in housing – stopping evictions – and insurance – stopping blanket exclusion of people with mental health problems (though insurers will still generally only pay out for situations unrelated to pre-existing conditions; or will load premiums).

The law against employment discrimination, implemented from 1996, is several years more developed than on goods and services (1999) or education

---

[1] An episodic condition in which each episode lasts less than 12 months is covered, as long as the overall condition has lasted or is expected to last for more than 12 months.

(2002). It therefore merits more detailed scrutiny. Soon after the employment provisions came into force in 1996, it became clear that the law could be useful in challenging overt discrimination against people with mental health problems by employers. Yet, even by the late 1990s it was still assumed in many quarters that the law was 'really' for people with physical impairments. By the turn of the century it was clear that 23% of DDA employment cases were brought by people with mental health problems (DWP/DRC 2004). There were further landmark cases, including Ms Melanophy's successful 2001 case against a publishing company for sacking her when her normally high performance was temporarily affected by a 'high' period.[2]

Other cases were more problematic. For instance:

Ms Marshall, with a good Cambridge degree and relevant employment experience, applied for a job as a police finger-printing officer and was offered the job – only to have the offer withdrawn when occupational health screening revealed her diagnosis of manic depression. In 2001 she won her DDA case and received nearly £20,000 in compensation. She went on to work successfully elsewhere. However, the police force later appealed and won, in a decision that sent shock waves through mental health circles.

This decision was possible because tribunals had (since an important non-mental health case, Jones v Post Office 2001) started taking narrow decisions on employers' responsibilities. Basically, as long as they obtained occupational health advice (even poor advice) from a suitably qualified person, and as long as this produced an answer 'which was not irrational' the tribunals could not disagree with the risk assessment the employer reached. This was widely viewed as a discriminators' charter.

However, in 2004 the DDA was amended in line with European requirements: direct employment discrimination became illegal; it could no longer be justified. The new Code of Practice stated that if an employer rejected someone without proper consideration of the impact of the particular person's disability on whether s/he could do the particular job, that would be unlawful. This is likely to mean the Marshall decision would have been different, post 2004.

A 1995 Mori poll found that the public was most likely to accept people with mental illness as road-sweepers, actors, comedians or farm workers; and least likely to accept them as doctors, child-minders, police officers or nurses. It seems madness co-exists in the public mind with the most menial and the most creative jobs – but not with jobs requiring responsibility.[3] Hence perhaps a decision that someone with depression can be an odd job man but not a supervisor (as happened in the case of Paul Vs probation service – subsequently more progressively overturned on appeal). In reality, decision-makers from Winston Churchill to Alistair Campbell have had mental health problems; and the law is beginning to catch up with that reality.

---

[2] Details of all legal cases cited here can be found at www.drc-gb.org.
[3] MORI (1995) Public Attitudes Survey commissioned by Mind. Reported on 20 March 1995.

A man was offered a job as a care worker by a local authority. He had a history of mental health problems, but did not disclose that fact in response to a medical questionnaire. Between accepting the job and starting work, he experienced a severe episode of depression. When the local authority got to hear of that, the offer of employment was withdrawn, notwithstanding the view of the occupational health officer that the client was fit for work. The client brought a disability discrimination claim and lost – because the tribunal found his depression did not have a substantial and long-term adverse effect on his ability to carry out normal day-to-day activities.

This and other similar cases reveal a continuing weakness in the DDA. If someone is not quite 'disabled enough' to qualify for protection under the DDA, they can still be viewed as too 'disabled' by an employer to do a job and therefore refused work. This leaves people in a catch-22 situation and means employers are free to discriminate, paradoxically, against people who do *not* have major impairments.

Different lobbying approaches have been used to try to overcome this barrier to justice. One approach is to change the time limit, so people with (for instance) depression would be covered if the depression had lasted or was likely to last for 6 months: lobbying for this was unsuccessful in 2004–5. Another is to make any discrimination on disability/mental health grounds illegal, irrespective of how 'disabled' the person is, thereby removing the first challenge in taking a case – proving you are 'disabled' in the meaning of the Act. This was discussed by the Disability Rights Task Force in 1997–9 but rejected by Ministers and some disability organisations and has now been promoted by the DRC (2007a); but has not been implemented.

Other cases have extended the interpretation of the law. Hewett versus Motorola established that the ordinary 'day to day activities' used to define whether someone is disabled do include understanding of social interaction. The particular case concerned experiences of Asperger's and autism but the conclusion is highly relevant for mental health service users.

Another case, involving someone with epilepsy, established that requiring a driving licence for a job where driving is not integral, can be discriminatory; this too could be very helpful to mental health service users.

A House of Lords case involving a mental health service user and others, established that discrimination is illegal even after a person has left the job (for instance, in the provision of references).

Other cases have concluded that the causes of an impairment are not relevant – for instance, if alcohol consumption (not covered by the DDA) leads to depression the person is covered as long as the depression meets the DDA definition.

This short history of how the DDA has been used shows there has been some progress in legal terms – albeit often through 'two steps forward, one step back'. Some of the significant weaknesses have been remedied, others not. But there are also wider concerns, beyond legal precedent.

Firstly, there are formidable barriers for individuals in securing redress. DWP and DRC found the Disability Discrimination Act difficult to use: from

realising a 'disability' law might apply to you (since 52% of DDA-disabled people do not consider themselves disabled), to getting advice, proving you are
'disabled' (without undermining your claim to be able to do a job) and accessing
the tribunal process itself (DWP/DRC 2004) – and those facing greatest barriers are people with mental health problems. Secondly, even where people
bring successful legal challenges, this does not necessarily change the organisation let alone the sector.

For these reasons individual legal redress has been supplemented by a range
of more strategic and systemic approaches to securing equality:

- 'Strategic' legal interventions, like formal investigations into an organisation
  or sector, resulting in robust recommendations for change. The DRC
  undertook such investigations into website accessibility; and health
  inequalities experienced by people with mental health problems and/
  or learning disabilities (see below).
- A positive duty on public sector organisations, in force from 2006, to
  promote equality – not redressing discrimination after the event, but taking
  active steps to promote equal outcomes, through the core methods of
  evidence gathering, involving disabled people, impact assessments and
  action plans. This covers an organisation's whole business, from policy to
  procurement and commissioning decisions, employment, service provision
  (and more).
- Communications and good practice that demonstrate to people with rights
  and/or duties under the DDA the full range of people covered (i.e. not just
  those who see themselves as 'disabled'). And then give them the
  information and tools they need to take proactive action to secure their
  rights or to meet good practice. This is about using the law as backdrop,
  without ever having to go near a court or tribunal.
- Putting 'disability and long-term health conditions', including mental health
  conditions, at the heart of public policy. Demonstrating how inclusive
  policies and delivery benefit Britain as well as people directly affected by
  disability or long-term health conditions.

Strategic legal enforcement

From 2004–6 the DRC ran a general Formal Investigation into physical health
inequalities experienced by people with mental health problems/and or learning
disabilities. Methods used included the most comprehensive study of primary
care records and mental health issues in the world (8 million primary care
records), coupled with Area Studies in four areas, extensive consultation with
service users and providers, evidence reviews and written and oral evidence
taken by a high level Inquiry Panel who made recommendations designed to
work in the newly configured NHS. The investigation findings included
(DRC 2006):

- People with schizophrenia, bipolar disorder or depression have significantly
  higher rates of obesity, smoking, heart disease, hypertension, respiratory
  disease, diabetes, stroke and breast cancer than other citizens.

- The investigation also made an internationally completely new finding, that people with schizophrenia are almost twice as likely to have bowel cancer.
- They are more likely than others to get illnesses like strokes and coronary heart disease (CHD) before 55. Once they have them they are less likely to survive for 5 years.
- All these facts mean they die younger than others. Social deprivation is one important factor but the differences cannot be explained by social deprivation alone.

'Five year survival rates show lower survival rates for patients with mental health problems for almost all key conditions.'

(Hippisley-Cox et al 2006)

- Despite these risk factors these groups are actually less likely to get some of the expected evidence based checks and treatments. As the authors of the investigation's clinical data analyses put it:

'CHD patients with schizophrenia have higher risks (as reflected in the higher prevalence of smoking), but are less likely to be screened for raised cholesterol and less likely to be in treatment so there is a need to raise awareness among general practitioners and consider ways in which this shortfall can be addressed.'

(Hippisley-Cox et al, cited in DRC 2006)

- Mental health service users experience 'diagnostic overshadowing', with physical health problems being viewed as part of the mental health problems and not fully explored or treated.
- Whereas mental health service users – and mental health practitioners – saw access difficulties as the responsibility of the service, primary care practitioners tended to see the problems as inherent to the individual (not attending because of a chaotic lifestyle).

'In almost all interviews with primary care staff we heard about patients from these groups who don't follow advice as given, don't attend for appointments and who can't cope with the implications of the advice they have been given. There did not seem to be any strategies in place to support these groups to follow any advice or guidance they might have been given.'

(Semele et al Area Studies cited in DRC 2006)

- The investigation also identified low expectations – the attitude that people with mental health problems 'just do' die younger or 'just won't participate in health services designed to improve physical health'. And it found non-compliance with DDA duties to make reasonable adjustments; and a lack of policy impetus and leadership to create change right through the health system.

The investigation made recommendations designed to challenge low expectations, give service users more power through information on rights and give service providers and commissioners tools to support work to reduce these particular health inequalities. The recommendations range from the practical – enabling people to record their access needs on the patient record and then meeting them – to the strategic. For instance, assessing the physical health needs of people with mental health problems as part of local strategic needs assessments, commissioning new service models that meet the whole community's needs and tracking over time whether important health outcomes like early death from coronary heart disease are becoming more equal.

The Formal Investigation report was given formally to the Secretary of State for Work and Pensions and the Secretary of State for Health and Welsh Minister of Health. Progress in implementing the outcomes will be assessed by a reconvened Inquiry Panel and thereafter it is hoped that health inspection bodies and the new Commission for Equality and Human Rights Commission (EHRC) will track progress.

In 2006 the DRC launched another Formal Investigation, into whether Fitness Standards required for people to work in nursing, social work or teaching discriminate against disabled people and/or those with long-term health conditions. This investigation will be significant to mental health service users. For instance, Peter van der Gught, a social worker of 17 years' experience, challenged a decision that because he had a diagnosis of bipolar disorder he should be subject to extra scrutiny and checks on his fitness to practise, when no problems had occurred. The General Social Care Council withdrew the requirement on him in 2006.

The EHRC, which replaces the existing equalities commissions (including DRC), will be able to undertake formal investigations. They could be an important lever for systemic change. It will also, like the DRC, have other strategic powers at its disposal – for instance, entering into enforceable action plans with organisations where there is evidence of patterns of discrimination.

The Disability Equality Duty

The Disability Equality Duty, in force since December 2006, is a vital tool to ensure proactive, systemic action to promote equality between disabled and non-disabled people. Similar to the Race Relations Amendment Act in purpose, it requires public organisations to gather evidence, involve disabled people, undertake disability equality impact assessments and take action.

Guidance on the DED (available at www.drc-gb.org) advises that organisations should consider monitoring by broad impairment group: for instance, mental health problems, sensory impairments, learning disabilities. This means the disparities between impairment groups – as well as between 'disabled' people overall and non-disabled – will be revealed, offering more scope to take and monitor action over time. This is an important step forward from the more generic approach to 'disability rights' in vogue previously which suggested people were 'disabled' by the society around them, and that their specific 'impairment' was insignificant.

The Statutory Code of Practice on the new Disability Equality Duty suggests that public sector organisations may prioritise remedial action in relation to groups facing particular exclusion. For instance a mental health NHS Trust could take active steps to recruit people with mental health problems, as part of their core business of remedying social exclusion and promoting employment opportunities for people with mental health problems.

Lessons from the (somewhat similar) Race Relations Amendment Act suggest that whilst some public agencies had effective leadership and experienced benefits from taking action (CRE and Schneider Ross 2002), in others – and in the media – there was little more than lip service, with authorities meeting only minimum paper-based requirements (Cohen 2006, personal communication). For the DED to be embedded and to be fully inclusive of equality on mental health grounds will require active engagement by mental health experts (service users, professionals, commissioners, policy makers).

Communicating and embedding equality on mental health grounds

Communications initiatives to improve attitudes and behaviour towards people with mental health problems have a mixed history. Some programmes have not been based on evidence – and assumed, for instance, that giving the public information (on its own) or explaining how common mental health problems are, or saying they are an 'illness', will change attitudes. None of these particular strategies is based on positive evidence – and all strategies can backfire spectacularly, potentially actually entrenching discriminatory attitudes (Sayce 2000). More effective are contact between service users and others on at least equal terms that moderately disconfirm stereotypes (Hewstone 2003) and emotionally impactful communications.

Some of the approaches that can be effective include: people with mental health problems providing training, working, going to school or college, being involved in community activities alongside other citizens, on at least equal terms. An emotionally impactful mental health campaign in New Zealand used TV slots featuring a famous rugby player (amongst others), posters highlighting the achievements of people with mental health problems and linked local activities. Public attitudes measurably improved (although more towards people with depression than schizophrenia); evaluation showed that discussion of the campaign in families was common, thereby potentially powerfully breaking down taboos. Campaigns that include positive imagery/messages of active contribution and participation – rather than highlighting that people are victims (whether of the 'illness' or of discrimination) – seem most promising (Sayce 2000, 2007, Thornicroft 2006).

Given the international wheelchair symbol to denote disability, and the ubiquitous use of wheelchairs and white sticks as ready visual markers, it is no surprise that the public – and key audiences like 'disabled people' themselves – do not understand 'disability' to include diabetes, depression or heart disease (DWP 2004). It is critical that mental health service users be informed of their status as disabled and their subsequent rights – however they choose to define themselves. It is also important that employers and service providers understand that the DDA requires them to eliminate discrimination and promote equality for mental health service users alongside other 'people with disabilities or long-term health conditions' (those considered 'disabled' by the DDA).

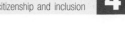
Employers and service providers (including the NHS, according to DRC evaluation in 2005) tend to think 'disability access' means lifts and ramps. One simple step to broaden their horizons, implemented by the DRC, is always to list the unexpected adjustment first – for the person with schizophrenia or dyslexia – and only mention at the end the expected physical adjustments.

Putting mental health and disability at the heart of public policy

Arguably the interests of mental health service users, and disabled people more broadly, will be embedded into practice across sectors most effectively once they are seen not only as a niche special rights issue – but as developments that matter to Britain and to mainstream delivery targets (DRC 2007a, 2007b).

Take child poverty. One-third of children living in poverty have at least one disabled parent. In 2006 Secretary of State for Work and Pensions John Hutton stated that child poverty 'is a disability issue'. If Governments (and both Labour and Conservative parties support this objective) are to meet their goals to halve and then abolish child poverty they cannot ignore 'disabled' parents, often someone with a mental health problem.

Imaginative approaches to reducing poverty in families with parents with mental health problems is vital to meeting child poverty targets: through relaxing benefit regimes so people can work when well and for hours that suit them; and meeting needs for childcare and parenting support as a core part of Pathways to Work and mental health care planning.

The same arguments can be made in relation to employment policy. In 2007 40% of people on incapacity benefit had a mental health problem as their primary 'disability'. Britain cannot meet its 80% overall employment rate target unless people with mental health problems are effectively supported to get and keep jobs. This in turn can only happen through evidence based individual placement and support; opportunities for careers, not just jobs; and serious action by employers to root out discrimination and share best practice in recruitment, retention, promotion, development, occupational health and more. That way we might move away from the shocking 2001 figure that only 37% of employers would employ someone with a mental illness (DWP 2001).

Similarly, if the recommendations of the DRC's formal investigation on health inequalities were implemented, it would help meet existing Government targets: to reduce health inequalities and premature death from conditions like cancer and heart disease, to increase cost effective early interventions, to improve flexibility and the patient experience overall.

Conclusions: implications for mental health practitioners, policy makers and service users

Since 2007 the EHRC has been championing equality and tackling discrimination – replacing the separate Commissions for disability, race and gender. It is vital that people with mental health expertise (as service users, practitioners, managers, commissioners, advocates) engage with the new Commission if it is to prioritise mental health. Mental health could – should – be viewed as a core dimension of the EHRC's work. Since discrimination (from racism to homophobia) damages mental health, and people with mental health problems are amongst the most excluded in Britain, mental health threads through every strand of its operation.

In the DRC, it was leadership that gave equality for people with mental health problems priority, for instance:

> *'As someone with personal experience of depression I've been delighted to work with users and survivors of mental health services from around Britain to help the DRC address the particular types of discrimination we face. We are breaking down fear and prejudice.'*
>
> (Richard Exell, DRC Commissioner, cited in DRC Annual Report 2001)

Mental health service users and professionals can stimulate and demonstrate leadership and take forward the citizenship inclusion agenda at different levels:

In policy: for instance, influencing the EHRC leadership or giving expert evidence on putting mental health at the heart of policies from child poverty to skills. This might involve making links between mental health and other policy and delivery areas (education, employment, housing); and improving our collective evidence on what works to embed equality, transform cultures, give service users greater power and tackle discrimination effectively. It might involve influencing Government (for instance, the Office for Disability Issues that works across Government Departments to improve disabled people's life chances) and working with disability and mental health professional and voluntary sector organisations through networks on social inclusion.

In service development: in public sector organisations, and those contracted by the public sector, practitioners can contribute expertise to the Disability Equality Duty – making sure that the whole organisation's thinking includes the equality of people with mental health problems alongside other disabled people; and advising on what this means in practice, from being exemplary in employing people with mental health problems, to working for equal outcomes through service provision.

In practice:

- Building into care planning questions about people's aspirations, ensuring the team is equipped to support people to meet their aspirations (for instance, having vocational workers in the team to support people to get and keep education or jobs), ensuring people can get basic rights met and measuring team performance by how far those aspirations and rights are met.

- Supporting people individually to achieve citizenship, recognising when they have a DDA case and recommending that they seek legal advice. There is no need to know the legal detail – but to advise people where to seek help could embolden them to challenge unfairness, not to give up.

- Familiarising themselves with the types of 'reasonable adjustment' that people with mental health problems have found helpful – from being able to travel outside the rush hour to avoid panic, to gradual return to work – and provide this information to service users. This can make a huge difference to what people can then negotiate for, with their employer, or college.

- Providing expert opinion on who can or cannot work or take on a particular professional training. By knowing what others with mental health problems have achieved, and what can be achieved with adjustments, practitioners can guard against the assumption that someone will not be able to hold down a responsible job, or enter a career.

- Raising expectations. It is not inevitable that people with mental health problems are poor, out of work and living with poor physical health; it is imperative to demonstrate the changes that are possible and to lead service developments to make them happen. Everyone involved in mental health has a core role in supporting that cultural shift.

References

Beeforth M, Conlon E, Field V, Hoser B, Sayce L (eds) 1990 Whose service is it anyway? Research and Development for Psychiatry, London

Bynoe I, Oliver M, Barnes C 1991 Equal rights for disabled people: the case for a new law. Institute for Public Policy Research, London

Camden Consortium 1989 Treat me well. Camden Consortium, London

Commission for Racial Equality and Schneider Ross 2002 Towards equality. An evaluation of the public duty to promote race equality and good race relations in England and Wales. CRE, London

Department of Work and Pensions 2001 Recruiting benefit claimants: qualitative research with employers in ONE pilot areas. Research Series Paper No 150, prepared by Bunt K, Shury J and Vivian D. DWP, London

Department of Work and Pensions and Disability Rights Commission 2004 Monitoring the Disability Discrimination Act 1995 Phase 3. DWP, London

Disability Rights Commission 2006 Equal treatment: closing the gap. A formal investigation into physical health inequalities experienced by people with learning disabilities and/or mental health problems. DRC, London 2006 (all research carried out for the investigation is available on the DRC website at www.drc-gb.org/health)

DRC 2007a Coming together: mental health service users, equality and human rights. Disability Rights Commission Mental Health Action Group, London

DRC 2007b The disability agenda. Disability Rights Commission, London

Exell R 2001 DRC Commissioner. Cited in DRC Annual Report 2001. Disability Rights Commission, London

Hewstone M 2003 Intergroup contact: panacea for prejudice? The Psychologist 16(7):352–355

Hippisley-Cox 2006 Cited in: DRC 2006 Equal treatment: closing the gap. A formal investigation into physical health inequalities experienced by people with learning disabilities and/or mental health problems. DRC, London

Link B G, Struening E L, Rahav M, Phelan J C, Nuttbrock L 1997 On stigma and its consequences: evidence from a longitudinal study of men with dual diagnoses of mental illness and substance abuse. Journal of Health and Social Behavior 38:177–190

Link B G, Phelan J C 2001 On the nature and consequences of stigma. Annual Review of Sociology 27:363–385

MORI 1995 Public Attitudes Survey commissioned by Mind. Reported on 20 March 1995. MORI, London

Office of the Deputy Prime Minister 2004 Mental health and social exclusion. Social Exclusion Unit Report. ODPM, London

Sartorius N 2001 Global programme against stigma and discrimination because of schizophrenia. Paper to World Psychiatric Association Conference, Leipzig, 2001

Sartorius N, Schulze H 2005 Reducing the stigma of mental illness: a report from a global programme of the World Psychiatric Association. Cambridge University Press, Cambridge

Sayce L 2000 From psychiatric patient to citizen: overcoming discrimination and social exclusion. Macmillan, London

Sayce L 2007 Tackling social exclusion across Europe. In: Knapp M, McDaid D, Mossialos E, Thornicroft G (eds) Mental health policy and practice across Europe. Open University Press, Buckingham

Semele et al 2006 Area studies. Cited in: DRC 2006 Equal treatment: closing the gap. A formal investigation into physical health inequalities experienced by people with learning disabilities and/or mental health problems. DRC, London

Thornicroft G 2006 Shunned: discrimination against people with mental illness. Oxford University Press, Oxford

Black and minority ethnic issues

J. Bennett

Introduction

Evidence of inequalities in mental health services for people from Black and minority ethnic (BME) communities was first highlighted in the early 1960s. Initial research pointed to the over-representation of people of African-Caribbean and Irish descent and the under-representation of Asian people within institutional settings. For three decades evidence continued to demonstrate that BME groups had a differential and negative experience of mental health services. The most consistent evidence was, and still is, associated with the negative experience of the African-Caribbean community. The first one-day census (MHAC 2005, 2006) revealed that African-Caribbean people are three times more likely to be admitted to hospital, up to 44% more likely to be sectioned under mental health legislation, and that Black and mixed heritage service users report a far worse experience of hospital care than other ethnic groups.

The initial response to suggestion of inequalities focused primarily on producing research evidence of ethnic differences in diagnosis and utilisation of mental health services. The cause for these differences was seen to be primarily due to the misinterpretations of the cultures of Black and minority ethnic groups. Cultural awareness or multicultural training was introduced to enable mental health practitioners to provide more appropriate services (Luthra & Oakley 1991).

The 1980s saw ethnic minority groups developing alternative services to those provided in the statutory sector and many Black and Asian mental health professionals and service users began to campaign for change in statutory services. By the 1990s there was evidence of even higher rates of diagnosed schizophrenia amongst second generation African-Caribbeans, aversive pathways to care and poorer outcomes (Sashidharan 2001). At the same time there was growing dissatisfaction, fear and mistrust of mental health services among BME service users and their communities (SCMH 2002), fuelled by the deaths of African-Caribbean men in mental health services. The inquiry report

'Big, Black and Dangerous' (Prins 1993) investigated the deaths of three Black men in Broadmoor hospital. Although it raised a number of concerns including the disproportionate use of restraint, drug treatment and racism, the recommendations were largely ignored by the Government and mental services. In 1998, one year before the National Service Framework (NSF) was published, the death of David Bennett, whilst being restrained by mental health nurses, once again raised significant concerns about the treatment of BME groups.

The National Service Framework published in 1999 set out a 10-year vision and a comprehensive framework to improve mental health care in England (DH 1999). Whilst it acknowledged that BME groups were disadvantaged and dissatisfied with mental health services, the NSF did not include any specific interventions to address these issues.

The review of the NSF five years on (DH 2004) makes little mention of BME groups. Although much emphasis has been placed on the achievement of targets to set up specialised community mental health teams including home treatment teams, no outcome data were reported for minority groups. This is despite the suggestion made in the NSF that home treatment teams were more acceptable and accessible to these groups. Indeed, a recent study of the impact of functionalised community services including home treatment teams (Commander & Disanyake 2006) found an overall decrease in hospital admissions, yet the proportion of Black (as opposed to Asian) people admitted increased. Further, a significantly higher percentage of Black people received a diagnosis of schizophrenia and were detained compulsorily both before and after the introduction of specialist teams. Thus these new service models appear unlikely to improve Black people's experience of in-patient services.

The NSF progress review acknowledged the need for urgent improvements in the experience of people from ethnic minority groups. It proposed to address this in the next five years through the Delivering Race Equality programme launched in 2005 – essentially the 'NSF for BME groups'.

This chapter outlines the background to Delivering Race Equality and the central elements of the action plan. The appropriateness of the action plan to address race inequality and the progress in implementation are discussed.

Background to the Delivering Race Equality action plan

The Macpherson inquiry, into the police investigation of the racist killing of Stephen Lawrence, published its report in the same year (1999) as the NSF for mental health set out its recommendations. The central conclusion was that institutional racism was the main cause of unequal treatment for people from BME groups by the police service and that this was a problem within all public bodies. According to Sashidharan (2001), the assertion of institutional racism made it easier to talk about race and racism and 'set down a defining marker in the discourse about race'. It also shifted the discourse on race relations from 'individual prejudice and ethnic need to systemic, institutional racial inequality and injustice'.

In response to the recommendations of the Macpherson report, the Race Relations (Amendment) Act (RRAA) (2000) extended the Race Relations Act 1976 to cover the functions of all public bodies, including the NHS. The Act set out a general duty for all public bodies to eliminate unlawful discrimination and promote equality of opportunities and good relations between differing ethnic groups. This includes publication of a Race Equality Scheme (RES); producing employment data by racial groups and using this data to identify differences between ethnic groups, investigate causes and address discrimination.

The government and public bodies, including the NHS, for the first time acknowledged that there was an urgent need to address racism. However, policy developments within the NHS focused on equality and diversity in the workforce and little action was taken to address institutional racism in service delivery. This inertia was reflected in the NSF, which, although acknowledging the poor experience of BME groups, did not set out any actions to address racism in mental health services.

The inquest into the death of David Bennett (Allison 2001) was to become the watershed for change. The coroner passed a verdict of accidental death aggravated by neglect and stated that he felt the NHS was not taking the issue of racism seriously enough despite the extensive evidence from similar deaths. He made public a number of recommendations, which he felt the NHS needed to take seriously, including the need to address racial abuse in service delivery. This outcome resulted in public and political pressure for an inquiry into the case and the wider issues of BME communities' experience of mental health services.

Around the same time, a paper entitled 'Institutional Racism in British Psychiatry' was published in the British Medical Journal (Sashidharan 2001). Professor Sashidharan argued that, until racism is addressed in psychiatry, there is unlikely to be significant progress in improving services for minority groups. He called for a national strategy for mental health and ethnic minority groups. This view was supported in a commentary on the paper by the President of the Royal College of Psychiatry (Cox 2001).

The demand for change was further reinforced by the damning findings of a review of the relationship between mental health services and African and Caribbean communities (SCMH 2002) and the Government's approval of a part-public inquiry into the death of David Bennett. The National Mental Health Taskforce set up an Ethnicity and Mental Health reference group, to draw up proposals to improve mental health services to Black and minority ethnic communities in England. The resulting report, 'Inside Outside' (NIMHE 2003a), emphasised the need to accept that institutional racism existed in mental health care and the recommendations and objectives set out were a direct and practical response to the problems experienced by BME groups within psychiatry.

The report of the Independent inquiry into the death of David Bennett was published in 2004 (Norfolk, Suffolk and Cambridgeshire Strategic Health Authority 2004). A core recommendation was the need for acknowledgement of the presence of institutional racism in mental health services and a commitment to eliminate it. Whilst the Government rejected the finding of institutional racism, it acknowledged that direct and indirect racial discrimination existed in the NHS and specifically in mental health services. A commitment was made to root out racism, tackle inequalities and improve the experience of BME groups. The Government's formal response to the inquiry recommendations was published together with an action plan to deliver race equality in mental health services (DH 2005).

Delivering Race Equality: the action plan

The Delivering Race Equality (DRE) action plan was a development on the initial publication, Delivering Race Equality: A framework for action (NIMH 2003a). DRE is a five-year action plan which proposes that should this and other reforms in health and social care be successful, mental health services will significantly improve for BME groups. Improvement is to be judged on 12 characteristics (Box 5.1).

The action plan outlines three building blocks for change:

- Appropriate and responsive services to be achieved through improvement in direct clinical care, developing a more culturally capable workforce, and developing organisations to deliver non-discriminatory recovery-orientated care.
- Engaged communities to enable an influence on policy and provision – achieved through engaging communities in building capacity to facilitate change at the local level, supported by 500 new community development workers and 80 community engagement projects.

Box 5.1

Delivering Race Equality: characteristics for change in mental health service by 2010

- Less fear of mental health services among BME communities and service users
- Increased satisfaction with services
- A reduction in the rate of admission of people from BME communities to psychiatric in-patient units
- A reduction in the disproportionate rates of compulsory detention of BME service users in in-patient units
- Fewer violent incidents that are secondary to inadequate treatment of mental illness
- A reduction in the use of seclusion in BME groups
- The prevention of deaths in mental health services following physical intervention
- More BME service users reaching self-reported states of recovery
- A reduction in the ethnic disparities found in prison populations
- A more balanced range of effective therapies, such as peer support services and psychotherapeutic and counselling treatments, as well as pharmacological interventions that are culturally appropriate and effective
- A more active role for BME communities and BME service users in the training of professionals, in the development of mental health policy, and in the planning and provision of services
- A workforce and organisation capable of delivering appropriate and responsive mental health services to BME communities

- Better information on service use and needs – achieved through improved monitoring of ethnicity, better analysis and dissemination of information, and an improvement in available knowledge about effective services. This will include the evaluation of the action plan.

The Department of Health BME Mental Health Programme Board is responsible for the delivery of both the action plan and the response to the death of David Bennett. The Board is accountable to the BME national steering group co-Chaired by the Minister of State for Health. The National Institute for Mental Health England (NIMHE) has appointed a National Director and eight Race Equality Leads (RELs) to take national and regional leadership on implementation of the action plan. Focused implementation sites (FISs) across the country were identified to demonstrate how change can be achieved. Each site will implement action in different ways, depending on local needs.

Appropriateness of the Delivering Race Equality action plan

Conceptual framework

The DRE action plan is based on three reports: Inside Outside (NIMH 2003a), Delivering Race Equality: A framework for action (NIMH 2003b) and the report of the Independent inquiry into the death of David Bennett (Norfolk, Suffolk and Cambridgeshire Strategic Health Authority 2004). However, Bhui and colleagues (2004) have suggested that there is some contradiction between these foundational documents. Whilst the aim of Inside Outside was on tackling institutional discrimination and motivating and educating the workforce to improve clinical practice with diverse cultural groups, Delivering Race Equality, intended to be the implementation guide, has 'changed the emphasis from clinical effectiveness and equity to strategic and organisational change' (p364). The DRE action plan is not based on a conception of racism as the cause of inequalities in mental health. Having rejected the Bennett inquiry's finding of institutional racism, the Secretary of State for Health in collaboration with the Chair of the Commission for Racial Equality (CRE) set out the initial thinking that was further developed to form the conceptual framework for DRE (Reid & Phillips 2004). The problem of racial inequality is seen as a result of ineffective management of the diversity and difference presented by BME groups' diverse cultures and backgrounds. Whilst not totally rejecting individual racism, it is argued that this is not a problem as individual racist acts are rarely recognised as such by the victim or perpetrator. It is suggested that systemic bias accounts for 99% of racial inequality. This systemic bias is seen as the result of insufficient leadership focused on effecting change. Managing diversity is thus seen as the key to success. This requires organisational leadership to effect change including the development of more BME leaders.

Additionally, mainstreaming race equality is seen as a fundamental principle. That is, building race equality into all that is done including local delivery plans, commissioning and inspection of services and local performance management systems. Although the DRE proposes a comprehensive plan of action the refusal to accept institutional racism raises questions about the Government's commitment and the adequacy of the proposed plan to eliminate racial discrimination. Sashidharan believes that having diversity management and policy changes does not make health care organisations like the NHS really challenge discrimination. He believes change will only be achieved if specific targets are set for improvements in clinical services (MacAttram 2005). This is reinforced by Bhui et al (2004) who suggest that the lack of explicit guidance in DRE on the improvement of clinical services could lead to the action plan being seen as another strategic plan with little clinical impact. Moreover, the Macpherson Report (1999) states that, 'there must be an unequivocal acceptance of the problem of institutional racism and its nature before it can be addressed'.

Bhui et al (2004) suggest that DRE expects that compliance with Race Relations legislation (RRAA 2000) will persuade NHS Trusts to implement the DRE programme. This does not appear to be happening. The RRAA requires all public bodies to publish a Race Equality Scheme (RES), outcomes of race equality impact assessments and employment monitoring statistics. However a quantitative audit by the Healthcare Commission (March 2006) found that only 1% (7/570) of Trusts have fully met the Act's requirement in this area. Further, the DH carried out a Strategic Health Authorities (SHAs) review of NHS Race Equality Schemes (DH 2006a). Surprisingly no question was asked about the number of Trusts that had met the RRAA requirement of publishing a RES. However, the data indicated that 68% of the 28 SHAs 'do not ensure that regular reporting on race equality targets forms part of the Local Delivery Plan (LDP) between them and their Trusts or PCTs' (DH 2006a).

Despite the above scenario no Trust or PCT had been served a compliance notice by the CRE.

Whilst the RRAA sets a framework for compliance addressing organisational systems and processes, the content of the RES embodies the action needed to improve care delivery, particularly the role that healthcare professionals' perception and clinical judgement play in racial disparities. This element will be dependent on the DRE action plan, which is proposed to be inadequate.

Oakley (2003) suggests that whilst racial equality may need to be enforced by legal measures and the outcomes of cases, it:

'must be achieved by leaders with vision, and supported by managers with the ability to implement organisational change, who themselves must be supported by effective programmes in fields such as staff training and development.' (http://www.errc.org/cikk.php?cikk=1191).

He believes that 'without this type of back-up, there is a danger that legal action alone can result in increased resistance to change, because organisations and their staffs become pushed into defensive positions in which they cannot see any alternative way forward'.

It is clear that use of the law to address racial disparity in mental health care can be effective – but only if appropriate targets are set to improve clinical services and there is proper monitoring and enforcement. This does not appear to be happening currently.

Appropriate and responsive services

Training is the main approach proposed by DRE to develop appropriate and responsive services. Bhui and colleagues (2004) suggest that the cultural capability framework outlined in Inside Outside has not been adopted by the DRE action plan. They believe that this is the most appropriate approach to motivate and equip mental health professionals with relevant skills and is vital in order to eradicate inequalities.

Bhui and colleagues' criticism is unclear, as DRE has adopted the two approaches advocated in Inside Outside to achieve cultural competence and capability. The first being the need for staff to receive mandatory training in cultural awareness and the second that there should be an emphasis on ensuring the workforce is diverse reflecting the population it serves. DRE proposes that all mental health practitioners will receive training in cultural competence. The problem here is that both publications appear to have adopted a very narrow definition of cultural competence as a single programme of training. The most commonly used definition and conceptual framework of cultural competence is based on the work of Cross et al (1989) who define cultural competence as:

> 'a set of congruent behaviours, attitudes and policies that come together in a system, agency or among professionals and enable that system, agency or those professionals to work effectively in cross cultural situations'.

In this definition cultural competence refers to the development and provision of systems of care, which demonstrate an awareness and integration of the health-related beliefs and cultural values of diverse populations. Training is only one element of the cultural competence framework. The real question is whether cultural competence training proposed by DRE has been shown to be effective in reducing racial disparities in healthcare.

Cultural competence training describes a vast array of educational activities that are aimed at enhancing the capacity of service delivery systems to meet the needs of different racial and ethnic populations. In the US significant resources have been invested in developing and delivering cultural competence training. A review of training programmes and curricula in cultural competence (US DHSS/OMH 2001) found that in academic settings, cultural competence training ranged from semester-long courses to discrete components that are part of a broader course outline. Outside academic settings, continuing education courses and courses designed for organisations and staff range from a few hours to a few days.

Training is delivered by a range of consultants and trainers. Each trainer developing the content and teaching approach, and both content and approach varies widely. Generally the content includes an overview of the role of culture in health service delivery, and on the health beliefs and behaviours of specific ethnic groups. Evaluation of this training concluded that cultural competence training can have an effect of increasing general knowledge about an ethnic population, but can lead to facile stereotyping if improperly conducted or understood (Fortier et al 1999). However given the absence of any standardised curriculum elements or evaluative measures for content or quality, it is impossible to discern the relative quality of one training program over another.

In addition a systematic review (Beach et al 2005) sought to synthesise the findings of studies evaluating interventions to improve the cultural competence of health professionals. The conclusions of the review were that cultural competence training might improve the knowledge, attitudes and skills of health professionals. However, evidence that it improves health outcomes and equity of services across racial and ethnic groups is lacking. Despite extensive application of cultural competency frameworks in the US, cultural competence in general suffers from a lack of agreed upon definition and there is an array of differing approaches to training.

A second issue of concern with the focus on cultural competence is the emphasis on culture. Gregg (2004) suggest that whilst it is encouraging that there is an increasing recognition of the importance that culture may play in health related behaviours, there is concern that the cultural competency literature tends to present this framework as a panacea against racism and health care inequality. Gregg argues that research concluding that minority patients' reports of feeling disrespected and of receiving poorer care represents a lack of cultural competence in the health care system is problematic. He suggests that questions about disrespect and lack of care based on how a person looks and sounds are questions of racial bias. He further states that 'race is not culture and racism is not simply a lack of cultural competence'. Thus taking this approach dilutes the importance of racism in perpetuating disparities and suggests the problem of inequalities is one of cultural dissonance. Thus the locus of the problem is considered to be a result of the person's cultural difference and not in the racial bias of the institution. He believes that lumping racism under cultural competence makes it more palatable and much easier to ignore.

In addition, Manthorpe & Iliffe (2004) claim that cultural competence and cultural capability run the risk of presenting culture in a simplistic way. They suggest this approach often focuses on the superficial manifestation and older definitions of culture including health beliefs, values, and communal rituals and shared traditions.

Over the last two decades the concept of culture has been radically transformed through work in anthropology and sociology. Cortis (2004) cites work by Hall (1993), which suggests that culture cannot be viewed as a finite set of customs, traditions and beliefs. Culture is viewed as more than an expression of group identity but is dynamic, changeable and affected by a range of factors including social conflicts and power relations. The simplistic use of culture in public policy suggests that ethnic groups categorised as African-Caribbean, Asian or White are made up of people who are all the same, in a static culture. Manthorpe & Iliffe (2004) suggest that whilst culture may have some relevance in health disparities, it is also important to consider intra-cultural differences. They believe that what professionals need is competence to see when and how ethnicity and culture is relevant in their practice.

Bennett (2006) suggests that training to address race inequality cannot be seen as a single event delivered within a given model or framework that is appropriate for all personnel within an organisation.

Whilst it may be useful for training to include elements on race and culture, essentially the evidence available indicates that 'training for race equality' in mental health services should focus on the problems of inequality in mental health such as diagnosis and compulsory detention, reducing fear etc. It should also be based on the needs of the particular organisation and grounded within a wider framework of race equality.

Better information

A central element of the DRE action plan is an improvement in the collection, analysis and dissemination of ethnicity data to inform the process of developing a more equitable mental health service. Aspinall (2006) has assessed how successfully DRE is likely to deliver the information base and analytical resources necessary for the implementation of the action plan. He outlines an array of recommendations for improving the collection of ethnicity data from published policy documents. This includes the Department of Health's data set on hospital in-patients, primary care data and data from specialist mental health and social care services. Additionally, recommendations on the specific data to be collected are extensive, including referral rates, hospital admission, pathways to care diagnosis, restraint and seclusion, deaths racial incidents etc.

Aspinall (2006) examines how much of this data is available through current and planned data collections. In terms of primary care, he argues that whilst DRE recommends that mental health services should record data of users' ethnicity, language and religion, no specific targets are set for primary care. This is seen as a serious omission given that services are primary care led and commissioned, and it is a lost opportunity for linking ethnicity data to morbidity and prescribing practices. In relation to treatments Aspinall highlights the wide concern regarding the overuse of medication and poorer access to psychological treatments for BME groups. He argues that although there is a lack of data on these therapies within key routine data sets and that patient surveys by the Healthcare Commission resulted in a very low response rate from minority groups, DRE does not endorse ethnic monitoring with respect to these treatments. The decision is left to commissioners and service providers according to their perception of whether this will be useful in developing local services. This, Aspinall suggests, is not in keeping with DRE's recommendation that organisations should have information by ethnicity on medication.

Aspinall concludes that DRE is often not clear on the specifics of monitoring ethnicity and service use or on how routine data can be used. In terms of the annual census, he argues that this is 'stock data', which offers a snapshot at a single point in time while what is needed is 'flow data' that are collected routinely and continuously.

Engaging communities

One of the few areas that received specific funding within the DRE action plan is 'engaging communities'. This involves funding for 80 community engagement projects and the recruitment of 500 community development workers. Thomas et al (2006) evaluated the effectiveness of a community development project in

Bradford to overcome inequalities in mental health for BME groups. The findings indicated that participants in the project valued the support they received. They wanted their needs to be met in ways that are generally not available within mainstream services, including 'shared spiritual, creative, fitness, social and learning activities, help to get work and a wish to help and be helped by their peers'.

The project was found to be useful in facilitating a dialogue between local communities and statutory services. However Thomas et al (2006) suggest that there is a need to distinguish community development from community engagement. Community engagement is seen as being at the lower end of approaches enabling community participation as the agenda is set by statutory organisations and there is little exchange of power or influence. With community development, the community identifies the problems and helps to shape the solutions. This approach requires statutory organisations to acknowledge and prioritise local concerns. Not surprisingly, the project concluded that whilst community development is possible and effective, most primary care trusts (PCTs) will find it a challenge to fit this approach into their tight framework of accountability and performance.

Progress on the Delivering Race Equality action plan

The DRE action plan is only in the second year of implementation. Therefore there is a limited amount of information available to the public on progress to date. According to the Department of Health's progress report (June 2006; DH 2006b) the following key components of the five-year action plan are already operating:

- Seventeen focused implementation sites (FISs) are up and running at Strategic Health Authorities across the country.
- The first annual Count Me In Census was taken in March 2005, covering all in-patients in mental health facilities. The purpose is to better monitor the mental health service experience of BME service users. The findings underline the urgent need to implement DRE.
- Eighty community engagement projects in PCTs are helping to build capacity in non-statutory sector and partnerships between the non-statutory and statutory sectors.
- 500 community development workers (CDWs) are being recruited.

There has been some criticism of progress with implementing the DRE action plan. Of significance is a letter from the Minister of Health Rosie Winterton to Strategic Health Authorities outlining her concerns about the implementation of the BME programme. She pointed out that services are discriminating against BME groups in a way that is unethical and unlawful. She raises concern about the delay in recruiting of community development workers despite £16million a year being made available in PCTs baseline budgets (DH 2006b). The target was to recruit 500 community development workers by 2006 but to date only 170 are in post. The deadline has been shifted to 2007. It appears that the financial problems of the NHS have resulted in monies being diverted to other areas of service provision.

Sashidharan (2004) has commented on the resources allocated through DRE suggesting that this has been taken up by further layers of bureaucracy and more committees and working groups, rather than devoted to comprehensive reform of mental health service. Fernando (2006) has also criticised progress with the implementation of DRE. He highlights the poor progress made by Race Equality Leads (RELs) in delivering change in service delivery, ineffective use of resources and poor leadership of the programme.

Significantly, the Department of Health's lead and architect of the DRE action plan resigned his position. He criticised the delays in implementation of the action plan, claiming this is due to inadequate resources and a lack of central leadership (Brody 2006).

Conclusions

For over three decades evidence has shown racial inequalities in the experience and outcomes for people from Black and minority ethnic communities, particularly those of African and Caribbean descent. Despite this evidence the NSF 10-year plan to improve mental health services failed to set any specific targets to address inequalities and discrimination for BME groups.

Delivering race equality (arguably the 'NSF for BME groups') was developed as a direct result of consistent pressure from minority communities, BME service users and carers, and mental health professionals. This pressure culminated around the death of David Bennett and the subsequent public inquiry. The added political pressure generated by the Bennett inquiry led to the policy on delivering race equality.

The DRE action plan is in the early stages of implementation and proposed evaluation data will not be available for some time. However a number of weaknesses have been highlighted both in the conceptual framework and the key 'building blocks' of the action plan. Progress with implementation of the action plan has been widely criticised, particularly in terms of adequacy of resources and the lack of central leadership and commitment to the programme.

The evidence from the first BME census shows that Black and minority service users continue to experience racial discrimination in their use of mental services. People of African and Caribbean descent still seem to get the worst deal. In addition, recent evidence questions the value of intensive community services in reducing the over-representation of Black people in in-patient settings.

There is extensive evidence of the problems faced and numerous recommendations on how these problems can be addressed. The DRE action plan does not appear to be the solution and the fear is that it will be another 'token' programme with little impact on racial inequalities in mental health services.

References

Allison R 2001 System failed patient who died under restraint. Guardian, May 18, p6

Aspinall P J 2006 Informing progress towards race equality in mental healthcare: is routine data collection adequate? Advances in Psychiatric Treatment 12:141–151

Beach M C, Price E G, Gary T L et al 2005 Cultural competence: a systematic review of health care provider educational interventions. Medical Care 43:356–373

Bennett J 2006 Achieving race equality through training: a review of approaches in the UK. Journal of Mental Health Workforce Development 1(1):5–11

Bhui K, McKenzie K, Gill P 2004 Delivering mental health services for a diverse society. British Medical Journal 329–364

Brody S 2006 Kamlesh Patel quits Department of Health role to pursue call for inquiry. www.communitycare.co.uk/ (accessed 30 November 2006)

Commander M, Disanyake L 2006 Impact of functionalised community mental health teams on in-patient care. Psychiatric Bulletin 30:213–215

Cortis J 2004 Managing society's difference and diversity. Multicultural Nursing (sample issue) 13–18

Cox J L 2001 Commentary: Institutional racism in British psychiatry. Psychiatric Bulletin 25:248–249

Cross T, Brazen B, Dennis K, Isaacs M 1989 Towards a culturally competent system of care, volume 1. Georgetown University Child Development Center, Washington DC

Department of Health 1999 The National Service Framework for Mental Health; modern standards and service models. DH, London

Department of Health 2004 The National Service Framework for Mental Health – five years on. DH, London

Department of Health 2005 Delivering race equality in mental health care, an action plan for reform inside and outside services and the Government's response to the Independent inquiry into the death of David Bennett. DH, London

Department of Health 2006a SHA's review of NHS Race Equality Schemes – DH analysis of returns. DH, London

Department of Health 2006b BME mental health progress report. DH, London http://www.dh.gov.uk/PolicyAndGuidance/HealthAndSocialCareTopics/MentalHealth/BMEMentalHealth/BMEMentalHealthArticle/fs/en?CONTENT_ID=4114939&chk=NCk1ii

Department of Health 2006c Black and minority mental health. Minister of State for Health Services. DH, London

Fernando S 2006 Delivering Race Equality plan: Is it falling apart? http://healthweb.blink.org.uk/index.php?option=content&task=view&id=108

Fortier J P, Convissor R, Pancheco G 1999 Assuring cultural competence in health care: recommendations for national standards and an outcomes-focused research agenda. US Department of Health and Human Services Office of Minority Health, Washington DC

Gregg J 2004 Letter to the editor. Journal of General Internal Medicine 19:900

Healthcare Commission 2006 Race Equality audit. Healthcare Commission, London

Hall S 1993 Culture community nations. Cultural Studies 7(3):349–363

Luthra M, Oakley R 1991 Combating racism through training: a review of approaches to race training in organisations. Policy paper in Ethnic Relations, No. 22. Centre for Research in Ethnic Relations, Coventry

MacAttram M 2005 Census reveals unprecedented levels of racism within the NHS, National BME Mental Health Network http://www.bmementalhealth.org.uk/index.php?option=com_content&task=view&id=46&Itemid=1

Macpherson W R Rt. Hon the Lord 1999 The Stephen Lawrence Inquiry. HMSO, London

Manthorpe J, Iliffe S 2004 Capacity and competence. Rapid response, British Medical Journal 329–364

Mental Health Act Commission 2005 Count me in: results of a national census of in-patients in mental health hospitals and facilities in England and Wales. Healthcare Commission, Mental Health Act Commission, Care Services Improvement Partnership and National Institute for Mental Health England, London

- Mental Health Act Commission 2006 Count me in: the national mental health and ethnicity, 2005 service user survey. Mental Health Act Commission, London

National Institute for Mental Health England 2003a Delivering Race Equality, A Framework for action. NIMHE, London

- National Institute for Mental Health England 2003b Inside Outside, Improving mental health services for Black and minority ethnic communities in England. NIMHE, London

Norfolk, Suffolk and Cambridgeshire Strategic Health Authority 2004 Independent Inquiry into the death of David Bennett

- Oakley R 2003 Institutional racism: lessons from the UK. European workshop on Roma-police relations, March 1999. http://www.errc.org/cikk.php?cikk=1191

Prins H (Chairman) 1993 Big Black and Dangerous. Report of the Committee of Inquiry into the Death in Broadmoor Hospital of Orville Blackwood and a Review of the Deaths of Two Other Afro-Caribbean Patients. SHSA, London

Race Relations (Amendment) Act (2000) HMSO, London

Reid J, Phillips T 2004 The best intentions: race, equity and delivering today's NHS. Fabian Society, London

Sashidharan S 2001 Institutional racism in British psychiatry. Psychiatric Bulletin 25:244–247

Sashidharan S 2004 NHS lacks the commitment and leadership to root out racism in mental health services. Rapid response, British Medical Journal 329–364

SCMH 2002 Breaking the circles of fear, a review of the relationship between mental health services and African and African Caribbean communities. SCMH, London

Thomas P, Seebohm P, Henderson P, Munn-Giddings C, Yasmeen S 2006 Tackling race inequalities: community development, mental health and diversity. Journal of Public Mental Health 5:13–19

US Department of Health and Human Services, Office of Minority Health 2001 National Standards for Culturally and Linguistically Appropriate Services in Health Care: Final Report. US Department of Health and Human Services, Washington DC

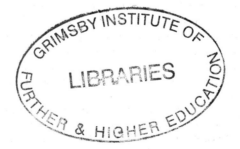

6

Women and mental health

J. Carlisle

The nature and course of mental ill health, pathways into care, and treatment differ between women and men. This chapter will briefly review the context of services for women, and ways in which the National Service Framework for Mental Health (NSFMH) addressed the specific needs of women. In reviewing the policy recommendations, the chapter will also look at case studies of organisations attempting to implement appropriate services.

Mental ill health in women and men

Published rates on mental illness have shown significant differences between women and men. The 2001 Office for National Statistics (ONS) household survey of psychiatric morbidity reported rates of all neurotic disorders to be more common in women than men (with the exception of panic disorders, which had equal prevalence). Women also exhibit higher rates of eating disorders and are at twice the risk of developing post traumatic stress disorder (PTSD) than men after a traumatic event. Higher rates of personality disorder, substance misuse and alcohol dependence are observed in men (ONS 2001). In addition to these differences, there is a range of mental disorders that can only be experienced by women such as perinatal disorders or syndromes associated with reproductive/hormonal changes.

Differences also exist between women and men in the way they access services. Due to high rates of drug and alcohol problems in men, more men than women use specialist services for these problems (along with accident and emergency services). For women, their socioeconomic realities (such as being a primary carer, issues of poverty) lead them to use primary care or community services.

Historical context

The wider National Service Framework was published in 1999 (DH 1999a), yet the strategy for women was not formalised until 2002 with the publication of 'Women's Mental Health: Into the Mainstream' (DH 2002a). This was the result of many years campaigning by health organisations and charities such as Mind and WISH that highlighted the neglect and paucity of services for women with mental illness. In 1992, Mind ran a 'Stress on Women' campaign that raised the profile of inequality and abuse suffered by women whilst seeking help from mental health professionals. This was further supported by proposals aimed at developing services that were more responsive to women's needs.

Lart et al (1999) conducted a systematic review (commissioned by the NHS Executive High Secure Psychiatric Services Commissioning Board – HSPSCB) that examined the literature on secure psychiatric service for women. The findings revealed that treatment regimes for women were the same as for men (i.e. not specific to women or tailored to their needs). Further, that provision of secure psychiatric services tended to either have women as an afterthought or be gender blind. The former detailed services that provided wards for men differentiated by legal category, diagnosis or function. Wards for women did exist, but were not differentiated in the same way – all health and legal categories of women were held together on the same ward regardless of treatment needs. Services which were gender blind just had mixed-sex wards. Neither of these options addressed the specific needs of women in an appropriate manner.

Lart et al (1999) also found that no studies looked at how the service models they defined impacted on women, or examined issues such as diversity, discrimination or oppression. Often studies did not report findings by gender, or they did report that data was collected from women, but the numbers were too small to be scientifically viable and therefore were excluded from analysis. Thus neglect of women regarding service provision transcended into research. The systematic review did however highlight gaps in knowledge including the examination of gender and social inequalities, the experiences of women, and the need to involve women in the planning of new service provision.

Whilst Lart et al (1999) focussed on women in secure psychiatric care, Mind and WISH continued to campaign to open up the debate and identify service needs for women at a wider level; for women inappropriately placed in secure care, and those that could receive better care in the community than was available at that time; considering social and economic realities of women; and diversity issues, including specific groups of particularly vulnerable women (i.e. vulnerable to mental health problems as well as vulnerable to exclusion from services), and the impact of mixed-sex wards.

'Secure Futures for Women' (see DH 1999b) conducted a listening exercise, expanding on the areas identified above to assess what women and other stakeholders thought of women's services, and how they could be made more effective for women. This landmark document highlighted the fact that women bear the brunt of poverty and social isolation and that the need to provide women-only services is imperative to the physical and mental safety of female service users.

Why 'women-only' services?

Women-only services are not merely required because of the differing treatment needs of women and men, but also because the multiple roles women have, and adverse life experiences, can lead to a negative impact on mental health and well-being: factors that need to be addressed in a forum that is specific to women.

It has been highlighted through the aforementioned reports and campaigns that key socioeconomic, physiological and psychological risk factors can impact on poor mental well-being. These include: poverty, employment, women's work in the family, physical ill health, blighted childhood, life events, social isolation, and experiences of violence and abuse. These factors and circumstances not only impact on mental health, but impact also on the ability of the individual to access services. In addition to this, there are certain groups of women whose experiences make them more vulnerable to illness, or more likely to be excluded from obtaining appropriate care. Specifically the identified groups are women who are mothers and/or carers, older women, women from Black and minority ethnic (BME) groups, lesbian, bisexual, and transsexual women, women involved in prostitution, women offenders, women with learning disabilities and women who misuse alcohol and/or drugs. Thus service provision must consider the treatment needs of women in the context of their lives and experiences.

Current service provision

Services provided exclusively for women do exist. However, many exist within the voluntary sector or are quite specific (such as secure care). Voluntary sector provision is not always recognised as a typical 'mental health' service, but it is acknowledged that they do provide the vast majority of 'women-only' day services, and are able to adequately address many of the needs of its service users. Current statutory service provision specifically for women is scant on a national level. The DH's service mapping exercise in 2001 revealed that only 20% of day hospitals and 25% of day centres provided women-only sessions. Acute services and some secure services are still mixed sex, but have single sexed sleeping accommodation and bathing facilities. In part, as a consequence of the paucity of gender specific services, there is little research evidence of 'what works' to model future service development on. It has rather been left to a 'what doesn't work' framework on which to begin attaching needs led services. For example, concerns raised about mixed sex wards posing a threat to the safety of women for reasons such as coercion, violence and abuse, have led to the recognition that a single sex service is likely to be more beneficial to the mental health and physical security of the individual. Without substantial needs led research in this area, the bottom-up approach to service development could miss out on more appropriate or potentially effective ways of providing care for women with mental health problems.

Service user involvement

'Into the Mainstream' has used evidence from small scale research on what women want from mental health care. In general this is provided by services users, survivors and carers, and there are common themes. Women want services that:

- promote empowerment, choice and self determination
- give equal credence to the context and underlying causes of mental ill health as to the symptoms
- provide responsive support to the roles that women have through safer housing, education, training and work opportunities
- focus on positive aspects of their lives to assist with abilities and potential for recovery.

Recommendations of mental health policy: implementing 'Into the Mainstream'

The implementation guidance for mainstreaming women's mental health sets few explicit targets in terms of volume of services or provision of explicit staffing levels. The following summary of the recommendations of the policy objectives demonstrates that the key to implementation lies (as the title suggests) in 'mainstreaming' mental health services for women, i.e. moving away from services for women being 'special' or 'bolt-on' towards gender specific services as the norm. A gendered (and ethnically sound) 'whole person' approach to care is implicit to service planning and delivery, no longer merely considered as an objective in a care plan.

The guidance is underpinned by essential organisational principles which form a theoretical framework for all agencies involved to use in the development of services. Briefly, these principles are:

- Mainstreaming gender and the specific needs of women. Ensuring that all organisations are sensitive to gender (and ethnicity) as an integral part of the service development process, not as an afterthought. Gender sensitive mental health care will acknowledge the experiential and perspective differences between women and men in relation to:
  – childhood and adult life experiences
  – social, family and economic realities
  – expression and experience of mental ill health
  – pathways into service
  – treatment needs and responses.
- Involving women through a 'whole person' approach. Listening to and validating the experience of women and developing services that foster safety, promote empowerment and provide choice and self-determination. Women require services that acknowledge their economic realities and can support their role within the family or society. Putting the service user at the forefront of planning is essential to tailoring services to needs. There is a requirement for consultation with 'hard to reach' women who are vulnerable to mental ill health, but also vulnerable to exclusion from services due to the context of their lives.

- Whole system approach. Robust planning and commissioning of services which includes genuine service user and carer involvement will impact positively on effectiveness and continuity of services. All inter-agency working should offer the same quality of seamless, general support, thus the whole system becomes focused on appropriately gendering each aspect of service delivery.
- Partnerships and multi-agency working. This links in with the previous point that a holistic approach to care planning will transcend traditional healthcare providers and include social care, voluntary and private sectors. In planning community services, social and economic factors that impact on health and mental well-being must be addressed to the advantage of women with mental health problems.
- The voluntary sector. It is acknowledged that some of the 'best practice' evidence of service provision has come from the voluntary sector. This valuable source of expertise must be maintained as an integral part and lead provider of women-only services where PCTs can establish service level agreements on standards of care.

Planning services for women at a local level

Given existing core priorities and pressures on health care services, the development of services for women is proposed in solid incremental steps rather than all at once. The recommendation in the guidance is that every PCT will have a three-year plan on implementation that is informed by relevant stakeholders. The planning must establish a conducive context (consisting of a senior lead, a steering group, multi-agency forum, and women's service user group). The planning must also: incorporate resource mapping, identify gaps in service provision, link in with an appropriate voluntary or private service, review the safety and appropriate sensitivity of existing mixed-sex services, and establish service evaluation/audit/governance to ensure that gender is implicit in all service models.

Essential to the effective delivery of appropriate mental health services are cross-cutting issues such as:

- Workforce development to include gender awareness training, staff support, and identifying leaders with a clear commitment to addressing gender.
- Governance to ensure quality and equality in service provision, which formally includes gender (and ethnicity) in all reporting procedures, reviews and actions.
- Research to focus explicitly on women, and where data sets have low statistical power, other analysis techniques should be considered (such as combining study results and conducting meta-analysis). The principle for research should be one of inclusion, with a greater emphasis on user led/ focused research.
- Service evaluation and monitoring must include a gender (and ethnicity) dimension.

- Service standards must be created so that the continuing development and effectiveness of services for women can be monitored.
- Mental health promotion within society in general as well as in secondary mental health services (including early intervention and appropriate discharge planning) are likely to impact positively on future mental health. Thus public health measures including staff training in health promotion in relation to the context of women's social environment is of importance in planning services for women.

In terms of service delivery, the key issues are those of individual assessment and care planning, and the provision of medical and psychological therapies.

- Assessment and carer planning. The Care Programme Approach (CPA) holds services users needs central, and assessment must consider gender, ethnicity, and the broader context of women's lives (i.e. family, social and economic realities, strengths, aspirations and competencies).
- Care and treatment. A range of therapies should be made available to women so that medication is not the only treatment option. Women services users have expressed a desire for more 'talking therapies' and to reduce reliance on medication. Whatever the treatment option, there must be scope for the woman to exercise choice, embracing principles of empowerment, providing the most appropriate environment, pace and progress of the therapeutic process.
- Primary care issues. Early detection and intervention of illness relies on primary care practitioners being alert to the specific needs of women in relation to the context of their lives (family, social and economic realities).

Non-specialist mental health services: extending women-only community day services

In acknowledging that the needs of women will change over time, the provision of women-only community services must be developed in a range of settings (DH 2003). Whilst PCTs have a role in service commissioning and redesign, utilising the expertise and experience of established voluntary sector services is key to the success of providing women-only facilities.

Service specification from the initial guidance does not recommend services by volume or staffing levels, but suggests ways in which models can be developed based on who the service is for, what it should do, service principles, planning and commissioning, staffing, hours of operation, referral criteria, assessment of risk and policy on violence, providing information to women who may be interested in using the service, and continual service improvement.

In addition to women-only community day services, there is a need to provide safe and supported housing to provide assistance during times of greater illness or pressure, and to promote recovery from mental illness. This requires commissioning from local housing authorities, social services and other linked public and voluntary organisations.

Specialist mental health services: extending women-only provision

The guidance for implementing acute and secure care (DH 2003) is similar in format to that of non-specialist community women-only services – recommending actions rather than volume of services or targets.

For acute services, the aim is to provide a self-contained women-only unit (or ward) by re-configuring in-patient services, and also to provide women-only crises houses in the community as an alternative to in-patient stays. Community based residential acute care should have the potential to accommodate women's children if that is deemed appropriate.

For women's secure services, specific guidance is provided to assist with the development of services which have a safe, validating and self-affirming environment; are conducive to a therapeutic milieu; provide no greater physical security than the individual requires; and are flexible and responsive for full integration into the wider mental healthcare system.

It is acknowledged that there are gaps in services providing low level secure provision; high support community residential settings, and for those with learning and associated disabilities. Importantly, there is an emphasis on enabling women to be detained as close to their originating authority as possible. This should assist in creating a sustained pathway through to community care and eventual discharge. Where women are provided for in mixed-sex environments, women must be kept safe from intimidation, coercion, violence and abuse by other patients, visitors, intruders or members of staff.

The service specification for dedicated secure care provision has an overarching framework that can be applied to the development of all mainstream women-only services. Again, the implementation objective, whilst being specific, does not dictate volume. The exception to this is that 95% compliance with 'Guidance on Safety, Privacy and Dignity in Mental Health Units' (DH 2000) requiring trusts to eliminate mixed-sex accommodation, bathing and toilet facilities by 2002.

Meeting the needs of specific groups of women

'Women's mental health: Into the mainstream' (DH 2002a) acknowledges that there are women who are vulnerable to mental ill health, and who may have particular difficulty accessing appropriate, gender (and ethnically) sensitive services. These groups are:

- Women who have experienced violence and abuse. Traditionally, services for women who have experienced violence and abuse have been provided by the voluntary sector. In mainstreaming women's mental health, the impact of violence and abuse has to become a core mental health issue. The service development recommendation is that a lead person at a senior level within every mental health trust is appointed to co-ordinate appropriate staff training and support, facilitate inter-agency working, develop specific interventions, and provide assessment and care planning with respect to violence and abuse on a routine and consistent basis.

- **Women from Black and minority ethnic communities.** For these women, it is a requirement under the Race Relations (Amendment) Act (2000) for public authorities to promote race equality and positive community relations. This includes: consulting with different racial groups on policy/ services, assessing the potential impact of new proposals on different racial groups; taking remedial action where adverse impact is identified, making information on services accessible to the public (including minority ethnic groups), and monitoring workforce by ethnicity. The appointment of 500 community development workers will foster relationships with women of the same ethnicity in the community in which they live, assisting with access to appropriate mental health services.

- **Women who are mothers.** In addressing service needs for women who are mothers, there is an emphasis on partnerships with Children and Family Services enabling and supporting women in maintaining their parenting role wherever possible. This includes: access to community support services such as Sure Start; ensuring children are safely looked after if the mother is admitted to in-patient care (and that contact is maintained where possible); that discharge plans consider the parenting role and welfare of the children; having designated family areas (for in-patient care) and crèche facilities/ family friendly appointments (for out-patient care); acknowledging the potential for respite or 'time out' away from children or residential support where children can also stay; and support also for children who may become young carers.

- **Women offenders.** The individual and social cost to women and their families due to imprisonment has led the DH and Home Office to recommend that custody should only be used as a last resort (for serious offences and public protection). For those women vulnerable to mental illness, an early intervention approach should be adopted which allows (i) care to be managed in the community, and (ii) the option of appropriate community disposal. Key to this recommendation is the development of joined-up services allowing for care packages to be delivered in the community that are tailored to the needs of the individual. Of those women needing mental health care who remain in prison, seamless care should be established on resettlement to their original trust area. Care for women in prison should be equivalent to that expected in the community. The NSF recommendation is that local PCTs along with mental health trusts develop in-reach services, provide prison healthcare staff with training, support and supervision, appropriately transfer women with severe mental illness out to secure mental health services, and make sure that healthcare trusts are identified and can locate women (given the movement of prisoners) to enable continuity of care. However, the high rates of psychiatric morbidity among prisoners requires policy change in mental health care provision for women, including service redesign, not just a philosophical adjunct to the mainstreaming document (DH 2002a). Seamless through-care is almost impossible to achieve, especially if women are sentenced to lengthy prison terms then held out of their originating health trust area. The frequent movement of prisoners across the prison estate (either because of change in security category, point in sentence, changing role/function of the prison) makes lead responsibility for healthcare obscure, robust service provision difficult, and healthcare record keeping fragmented. Ultimately the women pay a heavy price with the negative impact of poor continuity of care both in prison, and on release from prison.

- Women who self harm. Staff should be trained in routinely assessing the possibility of self harm. Protocols should be developed for staff training and support in helping women who self harm. These policies should be informed by women service-users and for the care model to take a 'harm minimisation' approach rather than the 'prevention' of self harm behaviours.

- Women who receive a diagnosis of Borderline Personality Disorder. Recommendations for implementing care for women is more extensively cited in 'Personality Disorder: No longer a diagnosis of exclusion' (NIMHE 2003).

- Women with dual diagnosis, with substance misuse. Recommendations for implementing care for women can be found in 'Dual diagnosis: good practice guide' (DH 2002b).

For the latter two groups of women above, the complex nature of illness of severity of need require specialist sensitive, tailored services.

- Women with perinatal ill health. The recommendations for implementation are based on whether a woman has a previous history of mental ill health or not. For those with a history (including family history) advice should be made available on the potential effects on mental health that exist during pregnancy and following birth. Specialist mental health services should be involved with antenatal care and be continuous post delivery. For women with no previous history of mental ill health, the early detection during antenatal or at postnatal stages is important. It is recommended that all staff in primary care, midwifery and health services should be alert to the detection of depression. Staff training should be explicit in this area. Women should also have access to information though public health initiatives on mental health and pregnancy and how to access help.

- Women with eating disorders. Recommendations are aimed at PCTs to commission collaborative work with general mental health trusts and specialist services in: early detection, increased awareness of eating disorders in schools and communities through public health initiatives, and to improve the service user experience by considering community day programmes as an alternative to in-patient care.

Challenges to mainstreaming women's mental health

Whilst 'Women's Mental Health: Into the Mainstream' (DH 2002a) is a landmark document displaying a concerted effort by the current Government to address issues for women and developing gendered services, it is not without criticism. Newbigging (2006) has concerns that whilst the principles behind the policy are to be taken in good faith, the differing perspectives of various stakeholders might lead to some not having the complete understanding of the changes that are needed, still less of how to go about effecting them. Moving on from philosophy to action the principles in the real world is a demanding task. Undoubtedly, it will be difficult to persuade some services to embrace the recommendations, and at worst, some sectors might be actively resistant to implementing policy. Indeed, some of the recommendations within the implementation guidance are vague, yet this non-prescriptive method could allow for creativity in service development.

Newbigging (2006) identifies factors that influence successful implementation of the policy. Importantly, implementing such strategy is not a linear process. Previous attempts at developing services for women have explored 'in-house' alterations (such as segregating the bathing and sleeping areas of women and men), or developing 'bolt-on' options – where new services are attached to existing services/models/frameworks. However, mainstreaming women's mental health requires a cultural shift in thinking, explicitly forcing women's mental health onto the commissioners' agenda on par with factors such as staffing and treatments. Far from implementing policy on women's mental health at one time point (as legislation), it is more likely to occur in stages. The development at each stage however will be made by local authorities in relation to other service priorities and pressures. Further to this, funding/resource availability to implement the changes needed has not been made clear by Government.

Somewhat echoing concerns raised by Newbigging (2006), Rachel Perkins (2005) is cynical about the translation of policy into practice. Her experiences both as a service-user and commissioner revealed conflicting perspectives on meeting the needs of women in providing women-only day services. Perkins (2005) makes two main points: (i) that developing services has become target driven; and (ii) that meeting the targets may compromise the ethos of the policy itself. For example, policy dictates that separate washing and sleeping facilities must be made available for women. However the reality of this might be that access to the facilities for women are via areas used by men. An audit of procedure would deem the policy requirement to be fulfilled, yet it negates the principles on privacy, safety and dignity (i.e. the sentiments behind the principle of the policy are lost).

In her capacity as commissioner of services, Perkins (2005) argues that the delivery of women-only services is not straightforward, and is compromised by the conflicting wants and needs of various stakeholders. Included in this are:

- Some women do not want to be on a women-only unit.
- Lack of flexibility with bed numbers means that once a women-only service has reached capacity, available beds in other areas will make wards 'mixed-sex' again. The use of 'swing-beds' (which are multi-use) may destabilise care.
- There is a general lack of nursing staff support for women-only wards.
- The low numbers of ICU beds needed for women make the service resource intensive.

The decisions that have to be made by those both commissioning and pur-chasing services must be needs led, but it can be seen that the needs of women service users are varied, both in what they desire for themselves and what is required at each stage of their care. This makes structuring service provision difficult, and even if money and resources were no obstacle, the range of ser-vices required to provide choice and meet the needs of the service users would be extensive. However, both money and available resources *are* real obstacles, which further compound the elusiveness of achieving appropriate care for women.

Implementing mental health policy

From April 2007 there has been a *Public Sector Duty* to promote gender equal-ity, in policy, workforce and service delivery. In addition to this new legislation, active social inclusion of people vulnerable to mental ill health has been promoted by the 'Day services commissioning guidance: From segregation to inclusion'. Leading on from this, Newbigging & Abel (DH, 2006) developed 'Supporting Women Into the Mainstream: Commissioning women-only day services', with the aim that the two implementation documents work in tan-dem. The latter provides excellent 'practical pointers' to assist those commis-sioning and developing services. The emphasis on listening to women and involving women in each step of the service development process in maintained throughout the guidance.

Women-only community day services provide the best opportunities to sup-port women whilst they maintain their usual roles in the family or employment (or both). The success of such services has been borne out by women who have utilised day support in the voluntary sector (DH 2006). Maintaining support and links with such services whilst extending them throughout the wider NHS is an important part of mainstreaming women's mental health services. Day service options will be able to reach out to groups of women who previously would have either been reluctant to, or had difficulty in accessing care. An impor-tant part of day service provision is the emphasis on 'key people' rather than overt services or buildings (DH 2006). The individual needs of women service users should dictate the use of resources, which might be local befriending or shopping assistance or outreach, rather than attendance at a 'day centre'.

Achievement

In 2003/4 the National Institute for Mental Health in England (NIMHE) began a programme in which to support the implementation of the National Service Framework to mainstream women's mental health. Key to this support is the identification of six priority areas which aim to enhance the progression of development of services for women:

- improving the experience of mental healthcare
- improving choices into psychological therapies
- improving support in relation to perinatal mental health

- equality for Black and Asian women
- improving care and support for service users surviving sexual and other abuse
- improving mental health support for women in the criminal justice system.

NIMHE facilitates the Mental Health Trusts Collaboration Project in which nine Trusts are involved in piloting implementation of policy on violence and abuse (Section 8.1 of the implementation guidance; DH 2003), the results of which will inform DH practice guidelines for service providers to encourage a gold standard delivery in England and Wales.

Allied to NIMHE, CSIP (Care Services Improvement Partnership), hosted by local NHS organisations and consisting of eight regional development centres have the core remit of providing support to local trusts in implementing policy. Each of the CSIP regional centres have begun developing strategies to enable the practical implementation of policy now that guidance has been given. It is too early to judge whether the Government's 10-year target will be adequately met, or if the challenge of addressing the cultural shift of listening to and pro-actively responding to the mental healthcare needs of women could be done in the time projected. It does appear however that there is a concerted effort by Trusts and partner agencies to (i) acknowledge and (ii) plan to work out how and when the much needed changes will be made.

An example of some progress made can be seen on the website of West Midlands CSIP (http://www.westmidlands.csip.org.uk/). A key aim of 'Into the Mainstream' (DH 2002a) has always been to involve service users and carers in the design and implementation of policy. West Midland's CSIP hosts a 'Users in Partnership Women's Mental Health Group' (UiP) which has worked closely with each Trust's Women's Lead. The involvement of UiP cor-ner-stoned their expertise, provided peer support for current service users and survivors and aimed to promote women's mental health issues both locally and nationally. Their strategy has been to provide training for user group members in mainstreaming gender equality, support the development of women-only acute in-patient services in Dudley, and provide training on gender equality and diversity to nursing students in the area. There has been a positive impact in implementing policy as a direct result of the collaboration between UiP and the PCT leads.

The objective of delivering single sex accommodation has been largely suc-cessful (DH 2005). There are three key objectives to meeting this target:

- to ensure that appropriate organisational arrangements are in place to secure good standards of privacy and dignity for hospital patients
- to achieve the Patient's Charter standard for segregated washing and toilet facilities across the NHS
- to provide safe facilities for patients in hospitals who are mentally ill which safeguard their privacy and dignity.

Nationwide, the DH report those trusts that have complied with the above objectives (DH 2005). However their report is not specific to mental health services or services for women. Gathering such information is left to discrimi-nate reporting by individual Trusts.

An example of this is that of Ealing PCT who in 2005 were able to report:

- The savings accruing from the ward closure will in 2006/07 produce an Early Intervention Service (EIS) and the three major 'secondary care' service developments demanded by the NSF and other policy initiatives will have been delivered.
- The resources freed up by the ward closure will additionally allow the development of a high dependency women's service that will reduce, if not remove, female PICU outliers; a child friendly visiting area and a women-only day area and women-only dining facilities.
- A proportion of the savings made in PCT contract negotiations will be re-invested in new primary care mental health workers. Four Gateway Workers (wholly meeting the target) will be employed to facilitate the interface working between primary and secondary care. Each worker will be based in primary care as was the first such worker, employed since late 2004. Each will relate to one of the four WLMHT CMHRC sectors. Seven Graduate Primary Care Mental Health Workers (against a target of nine) will be employed offering CBT to mild and moderately depressed primary care patients in each EPCT neighbourhood.
- A proportion of the savings made in PCT contract negotiations will be re-invested in Carers' Workers (wholly meeting the target) and in BME Community Development workers (wholly meeting the target).

Thus, there are examples of good practice with respect to services for women. Some information can generally be found within the initial documents such as 'Into the Mainstream' (DH 2002a) and 'Secure Futures' (DH 1999). However, due to the magnitude of change needed, it is difficult to assess whether services for women have been amended or developed across the breadth of mental health services as not enough is reported about meeting targets in line with 'Mainstreaming Gender and Women's Mental Health' (DH 2003), leading to the assumption that in effect, little progress is actually being made. To ensure that the implementation of policy is being complied with in an effective manner, a comprehensive review of service development in line with strategy conducted by an agency such as the Healthcare Commission would be very welcome.

References

Department of Health 1999a National Service Framework for Mental Health. HMSO, London

Department of Health 1999b Expert Project Group Secure Futures for women: Making a difference. Available electronically only via http://www.dh.gov.uk/en/Publicationsandstatistics/Publications/PublicationsPolicyAndGuidance/DH_4077724

Department of Health 2000 Guidance on Safety, Privacy and Dignity in Mental Health Units: guidance on mixed sex accommodation for mental health services. HMSO, London

Department of Health 2002a Women's Mental Health: Into the Mainstream. Strategic Development of Mental Health Care for Women. HMSO, London

Department of Health 2002b Dual diagnosis: good practice guide. HMSO, London

Department of Health 2003 Mainstreaming Gender and Women's Mental Health: Implementation Guidance. HMSO, London

Department of Health 2005 Elimination of Mixed Sex Hospital Accommodation. Available electronically only via http://www.dh.gov.uk/en/Publicationsandstatistics/Publications/PublicationsStatistics/DH_4112140

Department of Health 2006 Supporting Women into the Mainstream: Commissioning women-only day services. HMSO, London

Ealing PCT 2005 (http://www.ealingpct.nhs.uk/content/downloads/board_papers/June2005/Mental%20Health%20Services%20Report.doc)

Lart R, Payne S, Macdonald G, Beaumont B, Mistry T 1999 Women and secure psychiatric services: a literature review. York NHS Centre for Review and Dissemination, University of York, York

NIMHE 2003 Personality disorder: no longer a diagnosis of exclusion. National Institute for Mental Health in England, London

Newbigging K 2006 Unpicking 'Into the mainstream': presentation given to North West Forensic Academic Network Conference (available via http://www.medicine.manchester.ac.uk/NWFAN/conferences/)

Office for National Statistics 2001 Psychiatric morbidity among adults living in private households, 2000. HMSO, London

Perkins R 2005 A clinical and social perspective. Social Perspectives Network. SPN Paper 7 (www.spn.org.uk)

7

Implementing National Service Frameworks for mental health:
dual diagnosis

H. Wells • R. Gray

Introduction

One of the major areas of concern in mental health services is the impact psychoactive substance use has on a person's mental health (Gournay et al 1997). The relationship between substance use and mental health problems is now well recognised (Farrell et al 2001). Studies have shown that substance misuse by patients with mental health problems is negatively correlated with medication compliance (Olfson et al 2000). It has been found that people with co-occurring mental health and substance misuse disorders have approximately twice the readmission rates compared to singularly diagnosed patients (Hunt et al 2002), make greater use of emergency services (Cantwell 2003), have increased incidents of violence and suicidal behaviour (Cantwell 2003), and poor prognosis of both mental health and substance use disorders (Hunt et al 2002).

Various researchers have studied the prevalence rates of dual diagnosis, problematic substance use and mental health. In the USA, the Epidemiological Catchment Area (ECA) survey (Regier et al 1990) found that 47% of those with a schizophrenic disorder also had a substance use problem, and that 53% of drug dependents and 37% of alcohol dependents had a lifetime prevalence for at least one mental health problem. These findings, however, cannot easily be generalised to the UK due to the differences between cultures and services (Weaver et al 2003). Research in the UK reported prevalence rates of dual diagnosis as high as 52% (Menezes et al 1996, Kamaili et al 2000, Wright et al 2000, Duke et al 2001, Graham et al 2001). A UK study of comorbidity of substance use and mental illness (COSMIC – Weaver et al 2003) found that approximately 75% of service users in drug services and 85% of service users in alcohol services experienced mental health issues. Of these, 39% reported that they were receiving no treatment for their mental health issues. In mental health services, 44% of service users reported problematic substance use in the previous 12 months. The study found that people with dual diagnosis had poor overall functioning, more unmet needs than those with a single diagnosis, and that services were not identifying and treating comorbidity effectively (Weaver et al 2003).

One of the reasons that dual diagnosis is not correctly identified or treated is due to the lack of training and specialist knowledge in dual diagnosis. Walsh & Frankland (2005) surveyed mental health service staff, asking whether they felt competent to complete a substance misuse assessment, to which the majority of staff replied 'no'. When asked to complete a mental health assessment, an equal number of substance misuse service staff replied 'no'. This suggests that staff in both mental health and substance misuse services do not have sufficient knowledge and training to be able to identify issues of comorbidity.

When dual diagnosis is correctly identified and treated, improvement in mental heath functioning in patients with dual diagnosis, as compared to patients with a mental health diagnosis alone, appears to occur more rapidly. One study found that for patients with schizophrenia and comorbid substance use the length of stay in hospital was 30% shorter and they demonstrated more pronounced improvements in their symptoms compared with patients with a single diagnosis of schizophrenia (Ries et al 2000). The researchers concluded that the substance use may have temporarily exacerbated their mental health condition and then stabilised more rapidly with a respite from substance misuse.

The existing framework for dual diagnosis

There is currently no National Service Framework (NSF) specifically for dual diagnosis. Elements of the NSF for mental health have therefore been identified as being pertinent to the area of co-occurring mental health and substance misuse. The NSF for mental health (DH 1999) made a number of recommendations for the provision of mental health treatment. Some of these recommendations are directly relevant to service users with dual diagnosis.

What has been achieved since the National Service Framework for mental health (1999)?

A number of documents have been published in order to summarise the needs of clients with dual diagnosis and the staff that work with them. These documents provide guidance to practitioners and services based upon the best available evidence. The two main publications, to date, are the 'Dual Diagnosis Good Practice Guide' (DH 2002) and 'The Capable Practitioner' (SCMH 2001).

The Department of Health's 'Dual Diagnosis Good Practice Guide' (DH 2002) was developed in support of the NSF for mental health. It has been the most significant document in dual diagnosis in the UK. It highlighted that people with dual diagnosis 'deserve high quality, patient focused, integrated care'. The guide stated that services for this client group should be 'mainstreamed' – delivered through existing mental health services. The guide recognised that, unless both mental health and substance misuse services work effectively, people with dual diagnosis will drop out of care.

The guide identified one area for improvement in the delivery of dual diagnosis services: multi-agency collaboration and training for all staff who are working with people with dual diagnosis. Mental health services and substance misuse services have developed separately, with few services specifically designed to help people with dual diagnosis. These fields have developed with a different philosophy and treatment approach, which are at times contradictory. This has led to a tendency for clients with dual diagnosis being treated by a serial model: that is by a single service, concentrating on only one aspect of the person's difficulties, and then referring on to another service resulting in negative treatment outcomes. Occasionally, people with dual diagnosis will be treated with a parallel model: that is treated by both a mental health agency and a substance misuse agency, without any collaboration or consultation across the agencies. Multi-agency working, utilising an integrated or liaison model, provides a more comprehensive service for people with dual diagnosis and resultant better treatment outcomes. Evaluations of the integrated approach suggest that this treatment model is more effective than either the serial or the parallel models of treatment.

The guide also identified the need for training for all staff that are in regular contact with people with dual diagnosis. As the study by Walsh & Frankland (2005) suggested, staff are not adequately trained to assess or treat service users with a dual diagnosis. The guide identifies the need to develop training across all agencies involved with dual diagnosis. The aims are to increase communication and collaboration between services, to agree on local definitions of dual diagnosis and to develop joint policies and procedures around the care and management of people with dual diagnosis. Supervision of staff who regularly work with comorbidity was also highlighted by the 'Best Practice Guide' due to the stressful and demanding nature of dual diagnosis potentially leading to burnout and a high staff turnover (Levenson et al 2003). Kipping (2005) also noted that the range of tasks and specialist knowledge in dual diagnosis made recruitment and retention in dual diagnosis roles problematic.

The Sainsbury Centre for Mental Health compiled a framework of essential capabilities for mental health workers based upon the NSF for Mental Health. 'The Capable Practitioner' defined 'capability' as having five specific components that provide the framework for more specific skills and attributes (SCMH 2001).

'The Capable Practitioner' competencies have been formulated in a hierarchy providing structure to the learning and development of the mental health workforce. All mental health workers should demonstrate 'Ethical Practice' competencies by practising with the values and attitudes necessary for working with people with mental health issues, for example, practising in an open, honest and non-judgemental manner. As mental health workers gain more experience and responsibility they are expected to demonstrate capability in the

'Knowledge of Mental Health', including mental health policy and the issues concerning mental illness. The 'Process of Care' component describes the competencies required to work within a multidisciplinary mental health system and includes skills such as communication, care planning and completing assessments. The 'Intervention' component highlights the competencies pertinent to delivering treatment to people with mental health problems, such as providing psychological or social interventions. The final component, 'Application', is concerned with specialist services. Practitioners working in these specialist services should be able to demonstrate competency in all the other components detailed in Ethical Practice, Knowledge of Mental Health, Process of Care and Intervention sections.

Although patients with dual diagnosis may require interventions from all the services identified in the Capable Practitioner, practitioners that work with patients with dual diagnosis require a particular set of knowledge and skills enabling them to work effectively with service users who are dually diagnosed. The knowledge set pertains to specific areas concerning substance misuse, mental illness and interactions between prescribed medication and substances of abuse. The skills set includes specific assessment skills and evidence-based interventions, such as motivational and cognitive behavioural strategies, to effectively engage and treat dual diagnosis. A similar set of skills were recommended for dual diagnosis practitioners in 'The Good Practice Guide'. These evidence-based interventions have been identified as useful in the treatment of substance misuse issues for people with mental health problems, however, these have yet to be thoroughly researched in the UK (DH 2002).

The NSF for mental health – five years on

The 'National Service Framework for Mental Health – Five years on' (Appleby 2004) compiled the progress since the NSF for Mental Health was published in 1999. By comparing the evidence base of the period prior to 1999 to the research compiled after 1999 it is possible to deduce the impact of the National Service Framework.

The first and most ambitious target of the NSF for mental health was regarding mental health promotion and combating discrimination. Mental health promotion was particularly concerned with promoting positive mental health. Prevalence rates of mental health disorders were compared between data collected in 1993 (Meltzer et al 1995) and data collected in 2000 (Singleton et al 2001). Comparative analysis revealed that there had been no change in the prevalence rates of neurotic or psychotic disorders in the general adult population over the seven years. It can be argued that the 2000 data was collected very shortly after the publication of the NSF for mental health and therefore the mental health services may not have had sufficient time to respond to the recommendations of the NSF for mental health.

Despite the stable prevalence of neurotic and psychotic disorders, prevalence rates for substance use have significantly increased over the seven-year period (HO British Crime Survey 2003/2004). Use of Class A drugs had increased during the period between 1996 and 2004. Most significantly, the use of cocaine and Ecstasy by people aged 25 to 59 had increased. There had also been an increase in the use of cannabis. The prevalence rates for substance use disorders had doubled within this same period (Appleby 2004). This increase in drug use does not appear to be translated into an equal increase in psychiatric disorders.

Combating discrimination and promoting social inclusion for people with mental health problems was the second target set by the NSF for mental health. Many organisations work to promote inclusion for people with mental health problems but wider reaching campaigns are less common. A national campaign to promote information regarding mental health and reduce exclusion and discrimination was launched by the Department of Health in March 2001 and ran until March 2004 entitled 'Mindout for Mental Health'. The effect of the campaign on public attitude was not evaluated.

Thornicroft (2006) has recently published his book on the discrimination of people with a mental illness with recommendations on how to reduce it.

Another area identified by the NSF was to develop effective mental health promotion for individuals with alcohol and drug problems. Drug use has been predominantly viewed as a societal problem where the solutions generated tend to focus on increasing awareness of the negative effects of substance use and the criminalisation of those that use drugs. There have been strategies developed in order to increase the awareness of high fat diets, for regular exercise, for the dangers of high salt and for the risks associated with smoking. The health problems associated with alcohol and drug use are not strategically considered. This is most likely due to drug use being viewed as a choice, and therefore self-inflicted, rather than a dependency with additional health issues compounding the problems.

The next aim of the NSF for mental health is the assessment of alcohol intake in primary care coupled with advice to help reduce problematic drinking.

There is some evidence to suggest that screening and brief intervention help to reduce problematic drinking (Babor & Higgins-Biddle 2000). The use of advice giving can easily be translated into confrontation of problematic drinking, which has been shown to result in poor treatment outcomes (Miller & Rollnick 2002). Early screening of alcohol intake combined with psychoeducation may reduce problematic drinking and the difficulties associated with it. Screening and brief intervention is unlikely to have an impact on a person with comorbid mental health and substance use issues due to the severity and complexity of the client's difficulties.

It has been recognised that people with dual diagnosis need access to a range of services round the clock. Very often the only services available to a person with dual diagnosis at the time they are in crisis are accident and emergency services and these services are not always well equipped to adequately manage these clients. The person may present with overdose or self harm. Due to pressures and constraints of accident and emergency services these clients are often treated for the presenting problem and discharged without further investigation. Contrary to the common sense viewpoint, there is a clear link between hurting oneself and getting medical attention, even if the medical attention is inadequate. A more appropriate strategy would be to ensure through-care of patients into appropriate treatment. This would require the training of A&E

staff in the identification of comorbidity and awareness of the appropriate treatment pathways.

Assertive outreach, crisis intervention, early intervention and home treatment teams have all been identified as positive approaches to target and engage hard to reach clients, such as those with a dual diagnosis. The majority of these teams have received no training in the management of substance misuse or dual diagnosis. Similarly, the NSF recommended training for all staff in dual diagnosis and strategies for long-term engagement with clients. A number of training programmes have been developed for staff who work with clients with dual diagnosis ranging from short awareness-raising training through to academic programmes up to masters level. These training programmes are not accessible to all staff working with clients with dual diagnosis.

Looking forward

The 'National Service Framework for Mental Health – Five Years On' (Appleby 2004) recognised that, despite the progress that had been made in mental health services in the five years since the NSF, there were some areas of provision that require significant input. Amongst those highlighted was dual diagnosis:

> *'One of the most pressing problems facing mental health services day to day is dual diagnosis, and we now see the broad coordinated response that it demands.'*
>
> (Appleby 2004, p73)

'Five Years On' highlighted five key areas for work in the area of dual diagnosis. The first is the importance of assertive outreach teams and dedicated services for dual diagnosis. Assertive outreach services have been identified as able to achieve engagement with hard-to-reach populations that are resistant to approaching traditional services, such as those people with issues of dual diagnosis (Rassool 2006). Dedicated services for dual diagnosis were identified as a further key area by Appleby (2004), but additionally by services users who are dually diagnosed (Drake & Wallach 2000). Service users want to access a single service provider that addresses all of their needs rather than having to visit multiple agencies and multiple workers, who individually only address one aspect of their treatment. This relates to the next of the key areas identified in 'Five Years On' – better integration of drug services and mental health services.

A number of different treatment models exist to highlight the ways in which drug services and mental health services work together – see the 'Dual Diagnosis Good Practice Guide' (DH 2002) for more information. Although lacking evidence for the effectiveness in the UK, evidence from the USA supports the integration of drug services and mental health services (Drake et al 2001). The current thinking is that clients with dual diagnosis should be mainstreamed through existing mental health services with support given from drug services. Mainstreaming however, requires the support of many other agencies to ensure a comprehensive care package is delivered. This requires that all agencies that work with dual diagnosis develop effective partnership working.

No single agency is equipped to manage clients with comorbid mental health and substance use issues. The nature and complexity of the issues faced by clients with a dual diagnosis requires a package of care delivered by a multi-agency team. Progress often occurs at the local level, but there have been no national strategies developed to see more comprehensive inter-agency working. Equally, the development of stronger links between mental health services and substance misuse services has been identified as a priority. Differences in treatment philosophy and service delivery have continued to hinder organisational collaboration between mental health and substance use services. There have been some examples of good collaborative practice highlighted (DH 2002) but generally, mental health and substance use services remain uncomfortable allies. There is a great deal of work to be done in fostering partnerships between these services.

The aim of improved training for those professionals working with dual diagnosis is one that has been carried over from the NSF for Mental Health (DH 1999). Kipping (2005) completed a mapping exercise of dual diagnosis provision, as mapped to the Best Practice Guide, of the 32 London boroughs. She found that relatively few of the 22 boroughs that responded had a dual diagnosis strategy in place. Each of the 22 boroughs however, reported having dual diagnosis practitioners in place, highlighting a recognised need for dual diagnosis services. One of the main findings of the study was the lack of strategic support for the development of dual diagnosis services. Kipping (2005) recommended that broader support from a wider audience was required for any significant change to occur in dual diagnosis provision.

The final target for 'NSF – Five Years On' was to ensure the safety of clients with mental health issues by keeping drugs off in-patient units. The Department of Health has published 'The Dual Diagnosis in Mental Health In-patient and Day Hospital Settings' guidance manual (DH 2006a), which builds on the work of the 'Dual Diagnosis Best Practice Guide' (DH 2002). This manual provides in-patient staff with guidance on how to work appropriately with people experiencing comorbid mental health and substance use issues. Many staff working in in-patient mental health wards are admitting high numbers of patients with issues of dual diagnosis and experience difficulties in finding appropriate strategies to manage their care provision.

A number of recent developments in dual diagnosis highlight positive progress within the field. The Department of Health has also published 'The Cannabis Toolkit' (DH 2006b) to provide patients and practitioners with more information about the risks to mental health associated with the use of cannabis. The Government reclassified cannabis under the Misuse of Drugs Act in January 2004, from a Class B drug to a Class C drug. The change in law resulted in some misunderstandings about the legal status and the possible risks of cannabis use. Many young people believed that the change in the law made cannabis a legal drug, resulting in an increase in cannabis use. Since 2004, the British Crime Survey has identified possession of cannabis offences separately to possession of other controlled drugs. Since 2004, possession of cannabis has accounted for approximately two-thirds of the total possession of controlled drug offences and has been consistently on the increase (Nicholas et al 2007).

There are also increasing concerns about the relationship between cannabis use and the development of mental health issues. In a systematic review of the evidence, Semple et al (2005) reported that early use of cannabis increased the risk of psychosis by approximately 2.9 times. They concluded that cannabis use in adolescence may be one of a range of factors that influence genetically predisposed individuals towards the development of a psychotic disorder. 'The Cannabis Toolkit' (DH 2006b) was designed to provide practitioners and patients with information about the complex relationship between cannabis and mental illness.

The launch of 'The Cannabis Toolkit' (DH 2006b) coincided with the launch of a television and poster campaign 'Talk to FRANK' raising awareness of the dangers of cannabis use. 'Talk to FRANK', formerly the National Drugs Helpline, was launched in May 2007. It is a drug advice service targeting young people at risk from drug use providing information, advice and support for young people, parents and carers. The 2004–2006 FRANK review highlighted high numbers of people using the helpline and website for information and advice. The majority of helpline callers rated the service very highly reporting that the advisors were well informed (FRANKreview, 2004/06).

A 'Dual Diagnosis Capability Framework' (CAWI 2006) has been published by the Centre for Clinical and Academic Workforce Innovation, University of Lincoln, which brings together occupational standards across the various disciplines within dual diagnosis. This framework provides a set of core capabilities for practitioners to map their own learning against. The framework contains three levels: basic, for all staff who work with clients with a dual diagnosis; intermediate, for generalist practitioners who regularly have clients with a dual diagnosis in their care; and advanced, for specialist dual diagnosis practitioners. This framework introduces some uniformity and clarity into dual diagnosis service provision.

Turning Point (2007) has produced 'Dual Diagnosis: Good Practice Handbook', which maps how dual diagnosis services are delivered and highlights examples of good practice. The published document will further build on the Good Practice Guide (2002) and will model aspects of good service practice. It is hoped that this new Good Practice document will help improve care pathways and better support individuals with dual diagnosis.

A DVD video called 'Relative Values' has been launched by the Care Services Improvement Partnership (CSIP) documenting the experiences of people who care for clients with dual diagnosis. These documents and resources provide guidance at the service level. It is hoped that this guidance will effect change for the people who use dual diagnosis services.

A major barrier to implementing the recommendations of the National Service Framework for mental health is the current financial constraints of mental health services. Despite dual diagnosis being recognised as a priority for mental health services on a policy level, it is often not high on the agenda on the service level. Dual diagnosis is often viewed as a specialist service and therefore optional. Dual diagnosis practitioners are often paid higher salaries than generic staff, so when budgets force cuts upon services it is the specialist services that get hit.

Dual diagnosis maintains a high profile on the national agenda. The Care Services Improvement Partnership (CSIP) Mental Health Themed Review 2006 focuses on dual diagnosis. The aim of the review is to ascertain what information is available about services for people who have dual diagnosis needs. The Local Implementation Teams (LIT) have been charged with assessing their position on a number of criteria highlighted in the National Service Framework for mental health. Due to be published in 2008, this review should provide a good understanding of where things are and an idea of how things need to progress forward.

It is clear that there is still a great deal of work to be done in providing dual diagnosis clients with appropriate and effective care. One fundamental problem is the lack of research evidence on which to base service development. There has been a general lack of large-scale treatment trials examining the effectiveness of treatment for dual diagnosis. There is some evidence to support the use of integrated approaches that utilise motivational enhancement strategies and cognitive behavioural approaches (Watkins et al 2000, Barrowclough et al 2001, James et al 2004) but not all studies support this approach as being effective for clients with a dual diagnosis (Baker et al 2002). Proponents of harm minimisation state that this approach improves engagement and treatment retention but there is little evidence to suggest that this strategy works long term (Teeson & Gallagher 1999). Equally, little evidence suggests that any particular approach works. There are several areas of research that may have significant impact on how dual diagnosis should be treated. The MIDAS (Motivational Interventions for Drugs & Alcohol misuse in Schizophrenia) trial is aiming to evaluate cognitive-behavioural interventions for clients who are dually diagnosed, additionally RIOTT (Randomised Injecting Opioid Treatment Trial) is investigating the use of injectable heroin for treatment resistant clients, which may have implications for the treatment of clients with a dual diagnosis who have a history of opiate use.

Summary

This chapter has considered the service model for dual diagnosis in relation to the recommendations highlighted in the National Service Framework for mental health. It is clear that the NSF has made progress for services for people who are dually diagnosed. Most of the gains however, have been indirect, focusing on general improvements in mental health services. Direct attempts to improve services for people with a dual diagnosis have been slow in coming. Mental health services have a long way to go in providing appropriate care for those patients with a dual diagnosis. Equally primary health care, social services, housing and substance use agencies have a considerable role to play in developing effective treatment strategies for clients with dual diagnosis. Despite a slow response, dual diagnosis remains high on the agenda. The research evidence is emerging and services are recognising the need for dual diagnosis training and specialist practitioners. There are a number of guidance documents providing frameworks to shape dual diagnosis services around and the Dual Diagnosis Capability Framework which provides detailed competencies for workers to achieve. The Best Practice Mapping Project and Themed Review will give a broader picture of the services that exist and innovative ways of managing dual diagnosis more effectively. There are numerous challenges that exist in finding solutions for this client group but these are challenges that must be faced. The problem of comorbidity is not one that will vanish if ignored. Fortunately, evidence reveals that these problems are coming into focus.

References

Appleby L 2004 National Service Framework for Mental Health – Five Years on. Department of Health Publications, ref 265907 (also available at: http://www.dh.gov.uk/assetRoot/04/09/91/22/04099122.pdf)

Baker A, Lewin T, Reichler H et al 2002 Motivational interviewing among psychiatric in-patients with substance use disorders. Acta Psychiatrica Scandinavica 106:233–240

Babor T F, Higgins-Biddle J C 2000 Alcohol screening and brief intervention: dissemination strategies for medical practice and public health. Addiction 95(5):677–686

Barrowclough C, Haddock G, Tarrier N et al 2001 Randomized controlled trial of motivational interviewing, cognitive behavior therapy, and family intervention for patients with comorbid schizophrenia and substance use disorders. American Journal of Psychiatry 158:1706–1713

Cantwell R 2003 Substance use and schizophrenia: effects on symptoms, social functioning and service use. British Journal of Psychiatry 182:324–329

Department of Health 1999 National Service Framework for Mental Health: Modern Standards and Service Models. DH (available at http://www.dh.gov.uk/assetRoot/04/07/72/09/04077209.pdf)

Department of Health 2006a The Dual Diagnosis in Mental Health In-patient and Day Hospital Settings: Guidance on the assessment and management of patients in mental health in-patient and day hospital settings who have mental ill-health and substance use problems. DH, ref 276177

Department of Health 2006b How cannabis can affect people with mental health problems: information for patients and practitioners. DH, ref 266823PACK

Department of Health 2002 Mental Health Policy Implementation Guide: Dual Diagnosis Good Practice Guide. DH, ref 27767 (also available at http://www.dh.gov.uk/PublicationsAndStatistics/Publications/PublicationsPolicyAndGuidance/PublicationsPolicyAndGuidanceArticle/fs/en?CONTENT_ID=4009058&chk=sCQrQr)

Drake R E, Essock SM, Shaner A et al 2001 Implementing dual diagnosis services for clients with severe mental illness. Psychiatric Services 52:469–476

Drake R E, Wallach M A 2000 Dual diagnosis: 15 years of progress. Psychiatric Services 51(9):1126–1129

Clinical and Academic Workforce Innovation 2006 Dual diagnosis capability framework University of Lincoln, Lincoln (http://www.lincoln.ac.uk/ccawi/)

Duke P J, Pantelis C, McPhillips M A, Barnes T R 2001 Comorbid non-alcohol substance misuse among people with schizophrenia: epidemiological study in central London. British Journal of Psychiatry 179:509–513

Farrell M, Howes S, Bebbington P et al 2001 Nicotine, alcohol and drug dependence and psychiatry comorbidity: results of a national household survey. British Journal of Psychiatry 179:432–437

FRANKreview 2004–2006 http://www.drugs.gov.uk/publication-search/frank/FRANKReview2004-2006?view=Binary

Gournay K, Sandford T, Johnson G, Thornicroft G 1997 Dual diagnosis of severe mental health problems and substance abuse/dependence: a major priority for mental health nursing. Journal of Psychiatric and Mental Health Nursing 4:89–95

Graham H L., Maslin J, Copello A et al 2001 Drug and alcohol problems amongst individuals with severe mental health problems in an inner city area of the UK. Social Psychiatry and Psychiatric Epidemiology 36:448–455

Home Office 2003–2004 SN 5324. British Crime Survey, 2003–2004

Hunt G E, Bergen J, Bashir M 2002 Medication compliance and comorbid substance use in schizophrenia: impact on community survival 4 years after a relapse. Schizophrenia Research 54:253–264

James W, Preston N J, Koh G, Spencer C, Ki Sely S R, Castle D J 2004 A group intervention which assists patients with dual diagnosis reduce their drug use: a randomized controlled trial. Psychological Medicine 34:983–990

Kamali M, Kelly L, Gervin M, Browne S, Larkin C, O'Callaghan E 2000 The Prevalence of comorbid substance misuse and its influence of suicidal ideation among in-patients with schizophrenia. Hospital and Community Psychiatry 42:195–197

Kipping C 2005 Dual diagnosis: findings from mapping exercise. London Development Centre for Mental Health, London

Levenson R, Greatley A, Robinson J 2003 London's state of mind. King's Fund, London

Meltzer H, Gill B, Pettricrew M 1995 OPCS Surveys of Psychiatric Morbidity in Great Britain: Report No.1 The prevalence of psychiatric morbidity among adults age 16–64 living in private households in Great Britain. HMSO, London

Menezes P R, Johnson S, Thornicroft G et al 1996 Drug and alcohol problems among people with severe mental illnesses in south London. British Journal of Psychiatry 168:612–619

MIDAS (Motivational Interventions for Drugs & Alcohol misuse in Schizophrenia) http://www.midastrial.man.ac.uk/

Miller W R, Rollnick S 2002. Motivational interviewing: preparing people for change. Guilford Publications, London

Nicholas S, Kershaw C, Walker A (eds) 2007 Crime in England & Wales 2006/2007. Home Office, London (http://www.homeoffice.gov.uk/rds/pdfs07/hosb1107.pdf)

Olfson M, Mechanic D, Hansell S, Boyer C A, Walkup J, Weiden P J 2000 Predicting medication noncompliance after hospital discharge among patients with schizophrenia. Psychiatric Services 51:216–222

Rassool G H 2006 Understanding dual diagnosis: an overview. In: Rassool G H (ed) Dual diagnosis nursing. Blackwell Publishing, Oxford

Regier D A, Farmer M E, Rae D S et al 1990 Comorbidity of mental disorders with alcohol and other drugs of abuse. Journal of the American Medical Association 264:2511–2518

Ries R K, Russo J, Wingerson D et al 2000 Shorter hospital stays and more rapid improvement among patients with schizophrenia and substance disorders. Psychiatric Services 51:210–215

Randomised Injecting Opioid Treatment Trial (RIOTT): Evaluation of injectable methadone and heroin treatment in the UK http://www.iop.kcl.ac.uk/iopweb/departments/home/default.aspx?locator=355&project=10114

Sainsbury Centre for Mental Health 2001 The capable practitioner. Sainsbury Centre for Mental Health, London (available at: http://www.cpcab.co.uk/assets/zippedexedocs/The%20Capable%20Practitioner.pdf)

Semple D M, McIntosh A M, Lawrie S M 2005 Cannabis as a risk factor for psychosis: systematic review. Journal of Psychopharmacology 19(2):187–194

Singleton N, Bumpstead R, O'Brian M, Less A, Meltzer H 2001 Psychiatric morbidity among adults living in private households, 2000. HMSO, London

Talk to Frank http://www.drugs.gov.uk/publication-search/frank/FRANKReview2004-2006?view=Binary

Teeson M, Gallagher J 1999 Evaluation of a treatment programme for serious mental illness and substance use in an inner city area. Journal of Mental Health 8(1):19–28

Thornicroft G 2006 Shunned: discrimination against people with mental illness. Oxford University Press, Oxford

Turning Point 2007 Dual diagnosis: good practice handbook. (http://www.turning-point.co.uk/NR/rdonlyres/20B55142-816B-497F-B04D-3E0A37FC994D/771/DualDiagnosis GoodPracticeHandbook.pdf) Turning Point, London

Walsh Y, Frankland A 2005 Baseline survey (unpublished manuscript). NELMHT, London

Watkins T, Lewellen A, Barrett M. 2000 Dual Diagnosis: an integrated approach to treatment. Sage, Thousand Oaks, CA

Weaver T, Madden P, Charles V et al (COSMIC) 2003 Comorbidity of substance misuse and mental illness in community mental health and substance misuse services. British Journal of Psychiatry 183:304–313

Wright S, Gournay K, Glorney E. Thornicroft G 2000 Dual diagnosis in the suburbs: prevalence, need and in-patient service use. Social Psychiatry and Psychiatric Epidemiology 35:297–304

8

Personality disorder in community settings

K. Dent-Brown • G. Parry • I. Kerr

Introduction: historical and policy context

Unlike some of the mental health problems discussed elsewhere in this book, there is at present no National Service Framework (NSF) for personality disorder. This reflects a degree of discomfort with the concept of personality disorder not only within the National Health Service of the UK, but across mental health professions and systems world wide.

Historically personality disorder was a diagnosis of last resort within the UK psychiatric system, arrived at for one of two reasons. One possibility was that a patient, perhaps with a mixed presentation and an uncertain diagnosis, had been given a succession of tentative diagnoses and trial treatments. Once all of these had been tried and nothing had proved effective, all that was left was a diagnosis of personality disorder because all other psychiatric illnesses were, by definition, treatable and personality disorder in those days was, by definition, not. A second, even more deplorable, reason was that the patient was one of those described by Lewis & Appleby (1988) in their paper 'Personality disorder: the patients psychiatrists dislike'. Their suggestion was that the diagnosis was made on the basis of prejudice and dislike rather than on clinical presentation, and they suggested that 'PD . . . appears to be an enduring pejorative judgement rather than a clinical diagnosis. It is proposed that the concept be abandoned' (Lewis & Appleby 1988, p44).

The diagnosis persists two decades later, but the burden of pessimism does not. Despite the relics of stigma, there is cause for optimism for two reasons. First, there has been what Sperry (1995) describes as a paradigm shift in the treatment of personality disorder, analogous to that seen in the 1950s in schizophrenia after the introduction of neuroleptic drugs. Second, the original conception of personality disorder as a relatively stable, semi-permanent condition – almost a developmental disability – has been challenged by recent research findings suggesting that this is far from the case.

Research evidence base

Epidemiology

The prevalence of personality disorder, and the balance of disorders seen, varies greatly depending on whether a community-wide method is adopted, or a method concentrating on presentations to health care service. The former method was adopted by the UK Office for National Statistics in their large study of psychiatric morbidity (Singleton et al 2003). They approached almost 13,000 households in England, Scotland and Wales and interviewed over 8,000 adults at a first stage and 638 at a more detailed second stage.

They found an overall rate for any personality disorder of 4.4%, with disorders occurring more frequently in men (5.4%) than in women (3.4%). The most commonly occurring diagnosis was Obsessive Compulsive Personality Disorder (1.9%) which was twice as common among men as among women. Avoidant, Schizoid, Paranoid and Borderline Personality Disorders were all present at a rate of 0.7 or 0.8%. The other four DSM-IV personality disorders (Dependent, Schizotypal, Histrionic and Narcissistic) were each present at a rate of 0.1% or less of the general adult population. One surprise from this study for clinicians is the finding that in the community, Borderline Personality Disorder (BPD) is more common among men (1%) than among women (0.4%) which is the reverse of the picture seen in mental health services.

In primary care settings the observed prevalence increases as might be expected, to a range of 5–30% of all patients (Casey & Tyrer 1990). The higher figure was achieved following a structured research interview similar to that used by Singleton et al described above, suggesting that clinicians may underestimate the scale of the disorder. Casey & Tyrer found that Cluster C personality disorders (Obsessive Compulsive, Avoidant and Dependent) were the most common. In secondary care, epidemiological studies tend to be smaller, more varied in their sampling and assessment strategies and therefore harder to summarise. However Moran (2003) reports that many studies show an overall prevalence rate of over 50%. He summarises studies from six countries showing a range of 36–81% among psychiatric outpatients and inpatients. Moran reports that:

> 'In psychiatric settings, people with Cluster B disorders [Borderline, Narcissistic, Histrionic and Antisocial] ... attract the most attention. People with Cluster B disorders share the characteristic of poor impulse control and often present to hospital services in crisis.'

He further notes that 'Borderline PD is generally the most prevalent (and certainly the most researched) category in psychiatric settings'. Widiger & Weissman (1991) suggested that in the psychiatric in-patient setting Borderline PD is three times as common among women as among men, reversing the proportions found in community samples.

The natural history of personality disorder

Recent evidence from long-term studies suggests that personality disorder is not the enduring, stable phenomenon it was once thought to be. Grilo et al (2004) found that in 633 participants with a range of personality disorders, more than half no longer met the criteria for diagnosis after a period of 2 years. For Borderline PD, a longer study found that the rate of remission continues. Zanarini et al (2003) found that among 362 inpatients with a diagnosis of Borderline PD, rates of remission over 2, 4 and 6 years were 35%, 49% and 69% respectively. Only 6% of those with a remission experienced a relapse. If this 'half-life' of about 4 years is to be trusted, perhaps as many as 95% of people will no longer meet diagnostic criteria after 15 years; a far cry from the pessimistic 'dustbin diagnosis' of two or three decades ago.

Research on treatment

Although Borderline Personality Disorder (BPD) is relatively uncommon in community settings, it remains the most researched diagnosis in clinical settings. This is likely to be because of its greater prevalence in secondary care, and the extra management problems perceived by mental health teams and in-patient ward staff.

Arising from the greater research productivity in BPD, the Cochrane Collaboration has published systematic reviews of pharmacological and psychological treatment for personality disorder focussing on BPD (Binks et al 2006a,b) and the NHS Health Technology Assessment programme has published a systematic review and cost-effectiveness analysis (Brazier et al 2006). Since these were published, results of more randomised clinical trials have become available, which are incorporated in a forthcoming NICE guideline on BPD.

Psychological treatments for which randomised controlled trials evidence is available fall into two broad areas:

- cognitive or behavioural approaches such as Dialectical Behaviour Therapy (DBT) (Linehan et al 1991), Cognitive Behaviour Therapy (Davidson 2000) and Schema-Focussed Therapy (Giesen-Bloo et al 2006)
- psychoanalytically influenced treatments such as Mentalization Based Therapy (Bateman & Fonagy 1999), Transference Focussed Therapy (Clarkin et al 2007), and psychodynamic treatments (Marziali & Munroe-Blum 1998).

Non-randomised studies have investigated therapeutic communities (Chiesa & Fonagy 2000) and integrative approaches such as Cognitive Analytic Therapy (Ryle & Golynkina 2000), although randomised trials of CAT are forthcoming.

DBT is a complex multi-stage intervention involving individual therapy, group psycho-education and telephone support. It has been the focus of much attention during the 15 years since the first articles were published. The first studies were carried out by the technique's originators, and reported significant improvements in episodes of self-harm, suicide attempts and drug abuse. Subsequent studies by independent researchers have not always replicated DBT's superiority over other forms of treatment and although some of the early enthusiasm has moderated it remains a widely adopted approach world-wide. The method was specifically developed to help people reduce self-harming behaviours and has not been tested to the same extent for those people with borderline problems who do not injure themselves. The method combines classical behavioural techniques (aimed at the extinction of maladaptive behaviour) with techniques based on eastern meditative practice such as mindfulness (aimed at increasing awareness and tolerance of internal cognitive and emotional states).

Bateman & Fonagy (1999, 2001) have investigated a 'partial hospitalisation' approach using a psychoanalytically-based day hospital treatment with patients who would otherwise have been admitted to an in-patient unit. Their results suggest that a more sophisticated case management method such as this led to enduring changes in mood and interpersonal functioning. These effects continued to increase after the 18-month treatment for at least a further 18 months until follow-up, which was encouraging. The method was later formalised as 'mentalisation based therapy' (Bateman & Fonagy 2004) and research is being conducted into its delivery in outpatient settings.

Although there are clear differences between the 'brand name' therapies, psychological treatments for personality disorder have many factors in common, possibly even more than for other mental health problems, through adaptation to the needs of service users. These include a high level of structure, consistency, theoretical coherence, taking account of relationship problems (including the difficulty in engaging positively with the therapist), and adopting a flexible and individualised approach to care. Indeed, it is possible to outline a whole treatment approach along the lines of such general principles (Livesley 2007) and this is the method recommended by NIMHE (2003b).

Psychological treatments have been seen as the preferred approach to BPD, but drug treatments have also been investigated. Binks et al (2006a) report that well designed randomised controlled trials are few but that antidepressants may be useful, particularly in moderating symptoms such as explosive anger. Tyrer & Bateman (2004) concur, adding that there may be a place for antipsychotics and mood stabilisers in certain circumstances. They warn however that their effects are more impressive in the short term than over longer periods. There are also dangers in polypharmacy when people misuse prescription drugs in a desperate attempt to manage unbearable feelings. Drug treatments are therefore best seen as an adjunct for symptomatic relief, requiring careful monitoring, rather than an alternative to psychological approaches.

There are not only risks of harm from pharmaceutical treatments. Fonagy & Bateman (2006, p2) point out that in the case of psychosocial treatments: '...we all too readily assume that at worst such treatments are inert. However, there may be particular disorders where psychotherapy represents a significant risk to the patient.' There are theoretical reasons for believing that this may particularly be the case in BPD. For example, many therapies assume that the attachment to the therapist is a vital feature of a therapeutic relationship, but in the formulation of BPD it is axiomatic that close attachments are very problematic for people with the diagnosis. Chiesa et al (2003) report that in a controlled (but non-randomised) study there was a subgroup of patients with severe BPD for whom longer in-patient treatment was associated with a poorer treatment outcome; a reverse of the usual 'dose–effect' model and a finding supportive of the theoretical prediction of an iatrogenic effect.

Recommendations

The NSF for Mental Health (National Health Service 1999, p136) draws a distinction between mental illnesses and personality disorder; the NSF does not regard the latter as a subgroup of the former. Personality disorder is therefore in rather a limbo; its inclusion in the NSF implies that it is, uniquely, the only mental health problem that is not also a mental illness. The NSF document makes some references to severe personality disorders involving antisocial behaviour and risk to others, which have a clear forensic implication and lie outside the scope of this chapter on community settings. The only specific mention of personality disorder puts it in a minority context (albeit among some other rather large minorities) when it says:

> 'The needs of minority groups should be carefully considered, including women, young people, people from Black and minority ethnic communities, people with substance misuse problems as well as mental illness, personality disorder, or with a combination of learning disability and mental illness.'
>
> (National Health Service 1999, p66)

It was stated earlier that there is no NSF for personality disorder. While it is true that there is no independent document with this title, it is the case that the Department of Health used the seven standards from the NSF to formulate an informal description of what standards should look like (DH 2005, p14).

Subsequent to publication of the original mental health NSF, the Department of Health published a document which made more explicit reference to personality disorder. The evidence-based clinical practice guideline entitled 'Treatment choice in psychological therapies and counselling' (Parry 2001), which pre-dated the establishment of NICE, considered six areas of mental health problems, including personality disorder and repetitive self-harm as one of the domains. The guideline noted the small but growing body of evidence for effective treatments for personality disorder, and recommended that (Parry 2001, p38):

> 'In addition to therapy types, features of service systems are likely to be important in long term management, in terms of structured programmes using active methods to enhance engagement, which are well integrated with other services, and have a clear therapeutic focus. The expert consensus was that people in these difficulties are not appropriately seen by novice therapists or in very brief therapies.'

Although the DH guideline is now past its 'use by' date, no further evidence-based guidance on personality disorder treatment has yet been published. NICE has now commissioned a guideline on management of BPD, which is due for publication in 2008 or 2009.

A review article which complements the DH guideline (Bateman & Tyrer 2004) described three models of service provision currently observed in practice:

- First there are 'sole practitioners', individual clinicians, usually psychiatrists, who attempt to combine diagnosis, prescription of medication, psychotherapy and case management into one job.
- Second there is a 'divided function' model, with the above tasks being divided between two or more practitioners from the same or different community teams. This has the advantage of reducing the load on any individual practitioner, at the cost of immediately increasing the difficulties of communication and consistency.
- Third there is the 'specialist team' model, which implies that the patient is seen not by members of a generalist community mental health team, but by members of a dedicated team specialising in personality disorder.

Bateman & Tyrer proposed that the specialist team model was the best, allowing the best chance for providing the following general features of successful management (Bateman & Tyrer 2004, p429–431):

- assessment
- engagement
- consistency (ensuring the same approach from all team members)
- constancy (reducing turnover of team members)
- adequate in-patient support
- risk assessment
- optimum practitioner characteristics (recognising that not all CMHT members want, or are able to, work with this client group).

No longer a diagnosis of exclusion

The clinical practice guideline described above (Parry 2001) offered advice to clinicians, not recommendations to commissioners or managers. Only in 2003 did these appear in the form of the Policy Implementation Guideline (PIG) 'Personality disorder: no longer a diagnosis of exclusion' (NIMHE 2003b). The rubric on the inside cover of the document stated that the document:

'Aims to ensure that people with PD, who experience significant distress or difficulty as a result of their disorder are seen as being part of the legitimate business of mental health services.'

The Introduction stated the present situation succinctly (NIMHE 2003b, p4):

'As things stand today, people with a primary diagnosis of personality disorder are frequently unable to access the care they need from secondary mental health services. A few Trusts have dedicated personality disorder services but these are the exception rather than the rule. In many services people with personality disorder are treated at the margins – through A&E,

through inappropriate admissions to inpatient psychiatric wards, on the caseloads of community team staff who are likely to prioritise the needs of other clients and may lack the skills to work with them.'

The Guide concentrated on services, not 'brand name' treatments and noted that the best practice for community personality disorder services included:

• the development of a specialist multidisciplinary personality disorder team to target those with significant distress or difficulty who present with complex problems

• the development of specialist day patient services in areas with high concentrations of morbidity.

The Guide also made reference to the need for pre-registration training of health professionals and others to include personality disorder issues, and for the need for effective post-registration training to be provided by Trusts and other organisations.

Following the publication of the Policy Implementation Guide, the Department of Health issued a competitive call through NIMHE to commission a series of 11 pilot sites to develop community-focussed personality disorder services. At least one site was commissioned in each region of England and a total of £10.9 million over two years was devoted to the pilot services. The first services were launched in early 2004 and the rest came on stream over the next 12 months.

The services that were commissioned were very varied, having nothing in common except adherence to the general principles outlined in the bullet points above. It seems to have been DH policy to encourage a wide variety of service models, in order to test a range of possibilities before deciding on which design/s to recommend more widely.

Recommendations on training and workforce development

In parallel with the 11 pilot sites to develop services, there was an investment of £2 million made from April 2004 to develop training and learning opportunities in personality disorder. The Personality Disorder Training Initiative (PDTI) allocated money to each of the eight Regional Development Centres (RDCs) in England in order to analyse training needs and commission training which was to be sustainable, measurable, and to involve service users in planning and delivery. The conceptual base for the PDTI had been set out in the Personality Disorder Capabilities Framework published by NIMHE (2003a, p6). A key assumption was that efforts to implement the framework might '...interrupt the cycle of rejection that is deeply implicated in the development of personality disorders and which is compounded by the negative and rejecting attitudes and practices of many agencies'.

The Capabilities Framework underpinning the PDTI elicited 10 underlying principles, such as (NIMHE 2003a, p22):

• training should be based on respect for the human rights of service users and their carers

• training should encourage patient/client autonomy and the development of individual responsibility

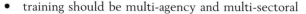

- training should be multi-agency and multi-sectoral
- training should be based on ... research evidence, where it exists.

Evidence of implementation

Not long after the launch of the 11 NIMHE pilot sites, the DH (2004) issued a letter to health commissioners reporting on the start of the pilot and promising a further £18 million to be available to Primary Care Trusts (PCTs) during 2004–6. This money was to allow a wider development of personality disorder services, but was made available to PCTs as part of their baseline allocation and was not ring-fenced. Commissioners were encouraged (but not required) to put these monies towards the continuation of the NIMHE pilot sites after their two-year pump-priming, and were further asked to develop 'whole system' services with other agencies. This was particularly important because individual RDCs are large and pilot sites were sometimes quite small. For example, the North East, Yorkshire and Humberside RDC stretches from the Scottish border to the English midlands (population 7.5 million), yet the site selected for the NIMHE pilot was restricted to Leeds (population 715,000).

However, this period coincided with one of intense financial pressures within the NHS, including high levels of deficit among commissioning PCTs and, for the first time, large scale redundancies among NHS staff. As a result many local clinicians and services, waiting for the promised £18 million to develop services, found that because the money was part of the baseline given to PCTs it was not protected in any way. Rather than being invested in the development of new services many PCTs had to use it to avert or lessen financial crisis.

At the time of writing this situation remains fluid and it is not clear what response PCTs will make to this, nor whether the development of personality disorder services will survive the adverse financial situation presently affecting PCTs.

One influence on the outcome may be the evaluation of the 11 NIMHE pilot sites. The pilot sites were formally evaluated by research led by Dr Mike Crawford of Imperial College London, commissioned via the NHS Service Delivery and Organisation research programme. The results refine the recommendations in the Policy Implementation Guide 'No longer a diagnosis of exclusion' (Crawford et al 2007). For example, the range of services piloted was very diverse and not all of the pilots included what the Policy Implementation Guide described as essential components; namely a day hospital and a specialist personality disorder team. One issue here may be that such services are relatively high cost, long term and hence low throughput. This means that their capacity to make inroads into the mental health at a population level is limited. This can be compared to the relatively 'low-tech' services, for example those with a high level of service user or self-help administered groups. While these may not meet the gold standard for treatment reproducibility and evidence-based interventions, their lower unit cost enables them to reach a much larger population than the small, long-term dedicated services – an important consideration bearing in mind the estimates for the population prevalence of personality disorder summarised earlier in this chapter.

The evaluation report found that despite major differences in the organisation and content of interventions delivered by the pilots, there was widespread agreement about key aspects of how such services should be delivered – for example, that services need to deliver psychological and social interventions, provide opportunities for peer support and help people across leisure activities, training and employment. They should provide long-term interventions, take on responsibility for co-ordinating care and consider accepting self-referrals. Teams providing dedicated PD services should have regular supervision, preferably with an external supervisor.

Little is known about outcomes of NHS care for people with PD, whether in dedicated or generic services. The Imperial College evaluation was unable to address cost effectiveness issues. Malone et al (2007) attempted to evaluate whether people with a personality disorder as well as a severe mental illness had substantially different response to CMHT management than those with a single diagnosis. Unfortunately, the evidence base was insufficient to answer this question.

All services face a challenge of how best to use limited resources in the face of the high prevalence of PD. Because many people are unwilling to engage with dedicated services, most people with PD will continue to be seen by generic services, and support for these staff will continue to be an essential component of the work of dedicated teams.

The issue of support for staff was highlighted in the 'Capabilities Framework' (NIMHE 2003a, p22). The conventional wisdom that this is an area of work in which staff burn out very quickly seems to be borne out in the pilot studies. Even in flagship services, with staff specially recruited and carefully supported, the levels of staff turnover remain high among those people who work exclusively with patients/clients with a personality disorder.

A recent initiative under the National Personality Disorder Development Programme has been a call to commission the development and implementation of a national knowledge and understanding framework for working with people with personality disorder, which promises to address these training and support needs more systematically.

Much of the future of these initiatives depends on whether the funding for the pilot sites continues once the piloting period is over. Preliminary indications are that just under half of the sites will be devolved to local commissioners in 2007–8, with the remainder devolved the following year. As noted above, with money for personality disorders not being ring-fenced within the budgets allocated centrally by the NHS it remains to be seen which of the pilot sites can roll their service model out across their RDC, which can simply survive and which ones wither on the vine. The decisive factor is likely to be the financial climate affecting PCTs rather than definitive research evidence supporting one method of intervention over another.

Implementation of training and workforce development

The Personality Disorder Training Initiative (PDTI) mentioned above was evaluated by a team from the University of Nottingham (Greatbatch et al 2005). The evaluation reported a very varied level of performance from the eight

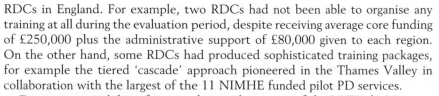

RDCs in England. For example, two RDCs had not been able to organise any training at all during the evaluation period, despite receiving average core funding of £250,000 plus the administrative support of £80,000 given to each region. On the other hand, some RDCs had produced sophisticated training packages, for example the tiered 'cascade' approach pioneered in the Thames Valley in collaboration with the largest of the 11 NIMHE funded pilot PD services.

Despite sustainability of training being a key target of the PDTI, the Nottingham report found that short-term delivery had been emphasised at the expense of long-term sustainability. Another criticism was that the requirement for training and support to managers and commissioners was largely ignored. Even in those regions that performed well, the evaluation report had some reservations. For example in one case '...a very effective regional strategy has ended up with reduced effectiveness because of the non-renewal of central funding at a critical time in the roll out of the strategy' (Greatbatch et al 2005, p43).

Progress, reasons for success/failure, challenges remaining

The final conclusions to be drawn from the personality disorder pilots still lie in the future, partly because of the need to wait for the formal evaluation and partly because the sustainability of the pilots after the initial funding period must be demonstrated. However officials from the DH are already suggesting what might be the essential characteristics of a tiered approach to PD. The tiers proposed range from consultation, support and education delivered at the widest and most local level up to national units for 'Dangerous and Severe Personality Disorder' catering for a very small number of high-risk clients in a secure hospital or prison setting.

The key recommendations for services at all tiers are:

- engagement/therapeutic alliance is key
- several approach and service models have been shown to work – the key is not in choosing the right approach, but in clarity and focus, the practicalities of delivery, service culture and (possibly) worker attributes
- case management of itself has a positive impact on individuals and systems
- peer group support can be effective with a positive impact on individuals and systems.

The implication is that services which have managed to maximise engagement and therapeutic alliance have been the most successful, and that this (rather than selecting the 'right' theoretical or service model) is the key to success. Some of the workforce implications are that staff members for PD services must be developed and cannot simply be recruited in from other posts. Effective training, support and supervision are essential for retention and safe, high quality practice. It is suggested that staff from a range of different backgrounds (and not simply traditional NHS professions) can make a positive contribution, and that worker attributes – rather than competencies – may be a crucial consideration.

It appears unlikely that major funding and initiatives will be forthcoming in the NHS, but some of the pilots have shown that minimal funding is not a bar to success. One difficulty for the future may be to draw together funding and commissioning arrangements for PD services which cross inter-agency boundaries to an unusual degree. For example, some of the pilot services include, as well as NHS and Social Services staff, personnel from housing, probation, drug and alcohol, voluntary and police services. It will be a challenge to persuade commissioners of each of these services that it is worth an investment by one agency to produce a larger cost saving for another. Close inter-agency commitment at the commissioning, as well as the service provision level, will therefore be essential, and this is not always a straightforward matter.

For further information see the National Personality Disorder website at www.personalitydisorder.org.uk/

References

Bateman A, Fonagy P 1999 Effectiveness of partial hospitalization in the treatment of borderline personality disorder: a randomized controlled trial. American Journal of Psychiatry 156:1563–1569

Bateman A, Fonagy P 2001 Treatment of borderline personality disorder with psychoanalytically oriented partial hospitalization: an 18-month follow-up. American Journal of Psychiatry 158(1):36–42

Bateman A, Fonagy P 2004 Psychotherapy for borderline personality disorder: mentalization based treatment. Oxford University Press, Oxford

Bateman A, Tyrer P 2004 Services for personality disorder: organisation for inclusion. Advances in Psychiatric Treatment 10:425–433

Binks C, Fenton M, McCarthy L, Lee T, Adams C, Duggan C 2006a Pharmacological interventions for people with borderline personality disorder. The Cochrane Database of Systematic Reviews 2006, Issue 1

Binks C, Fenton M, McCarthy L, Lee T, Adams C, Duggan C 2006b Psychological therapies for people with borderline personality disorder. The Cochrane Database of Systematic Reviews 2006, Issue 1

Brazier J, Tumur I, Holmes M et al 2006 Psychological therapies including dialectical behaviour therapy for borderline personality disorder: a systematic review and preliminary economic evaluation. Health Technology Assessment 10(35)

Casey P, Tyrer P 1990 Personality disorder and psychiatric illness in general practice. British Journal of Psychiatry 156(2):261–265

Chiesa M, Fonagy P 2000 Cassel personality disorder study – methodology and treatment effects. British Journal of Psychiatry 176:485–491

Chiesa M, Fonagy P, Holmes J 2003 When less is more: An exploration of psychoanalytically oriented hospital-based treatment for severe personality disorder. International Journal of Psychoanalysis 84:637–650

Clarkin J F, Levy K N, Lenzenweger M F, Kernberg O F 2007 Evaluating three treatments for borderline personality disorder: a multiwave study. American Journal of Psychiatry 164:922–928

Crawford M et al 2007 Learning the lessons: a multi-method evaluation of dedicated community-based services for people with personality disorder. Draft report to NIHR Service Delivery & Organisation Programme, May 2007. Imperial College, University of London

Davidson K 2000 Cognitive therapy for personality disorders: a guide for therapists. Butterworth-Heinemann, Oxford

Department of Health 2004 Developing and sustaining services for people with personality disorder. DH, London (accessed 9 August, 2006: www.dh.gov.uk/PublicationsAndStatistics/LettersAndCirculars/)

Department of Health 2005 Future commissioning of specialised personality disorder services. DH, London (accessed 9 August, 2006: www.dh.gov.uk/PublicationsAndStatistics/ LettersAndCirculars/)

Fonagy P, Bateman A 2006 Progress in the treatment of borderline personality disorder. British Journal of Psychiatry 188(1):1–3

Giesen-Bloo J, van Dyck R, Spinhoven P et al 2006 Outpatient psychotherapy for borderline personality disorder: randomized trial of schema-focused therapy vs transference-focused psychotherapy. Archives of General Psychiatry 63(6):649–658

Greatbatch D, Lewis P, Owen S, Tolley H, Wilmut J 2005 evaluation of the personality disorder training initiative. Centre for Developing and Evaluating Lifelong Learning (CDELL), University of Nottingham, Nottingham

Grilo C M, Shea M T, Sanislow C A et al 2004 Two-year stability and change of schizotypal, borderline, avoidant, and obsessive-cornpulsive personality disorders. Journal of Consulting and Clinical Psychology 72(5):767–775

Lewis G, Appleby L 1988 Personality disorder: the patients psychiatrists dislike. British Journal of Psychiatry 153(1):44–49

Linehan M, Armstrong H E, Suarez A, Allmon D, Heard H L 1991 Cognitive-behavioral treatment of chronically parasuicidal borderline patients. Archives of General Psychiatry 48:1060–1064

Livesley W J 2007 An integrated approach to the treatment of personality disorder. Journal of Mental Health 16(1):131–148

Malone D, Newron-Howes G, Simmonds S, Marriot S, Tyrer P. 2007 Community mental health teams (CMHTs) for people with severe mental illnesses and disordered personality (Review). The Cochrane Library, Issue 3

Marziali E, Munroe-Blum H 1998 Interpersonal group psychotherapy for borderline personality disorder. In Session – Psychotherapy in Practice 4(2):91–107

Moran P 2003 The Epidemiology of Personality Disorders. DII, London (www.dh.gov.uk/en/ Publicationsandstatistics/Publications/PublicationsPolicyAndGuidance/DH_4009546 – accessed 31 October 2007)

National Health Service 1999 National Service Framework for mental health: Modern standards & service models. HMSO, London

National Institute for Mental Health in England 2003a Breaking the cycle of rejection: The personality disorder capabilities framework. NIMHE, London

National Institute for Mental Health in England 2003b Personality disorder: No longer a diagnosis of exclusion. NIMHE, London

Parry G 2001 Treatment choice in psychological therapies and counselling: Evidence based clinical practice guideline. DH, London

Ryle A, Golynkina K 2000 Effectiveness of time-limited cognitive analytic therapy of borderline personality disorder: Factors associated with outcome. British Journal of Medical Psychology 73:197–210

Singleton N, Bumpstead R, O'Brien M, Lee A, Meltzer H 2003 Psychiatric morbidity among adults living in private households, 2000. International Review of Psychiatry 15(1–2):65–73

Sperry L 1995 Handbook of diagnosis and treatment of the DSM-IV personality disorders. Brunner/Mazel, Levittown, PA

Tyrer P, Bateman A 2004 Drug treatment for personality disorders. Advances in Psychiatric Treatment 10:389–398

Widiger T A, Weissman M M 1991 Epidemiology of borderline personality disorder. Hospital and Community Psychiatry 42(10):1015–1021

Zanarini M C, Frankenburg F R, Hennen J. Silk K R 2003 The longitudinal course of borderline psychopathology: 6-year prospective follow-up of the phenomenology of borderline personality disorder. American Journal of Psychiatry 160(2):274–283

9

Forensic service users

N. Humber • J. Senior • J. Shaw

Introduction

Forensic mental health services undertake the clinical assessment and treatment of individuals at the interface of the law, criminal justice system and mental health services. Secure mental health provision began in the early nineteenth century when it was recognised that simple imprisonment was not appropriate for mentally ill or 'insane' individuals who had committed a criminal offence. As an alternative, asylums for the 'humane' containment of such individuals were established. In 1856, the first high secure hospital, Broadmoor, opened, located in Berkshire. Subsequently, Rampton Hospital in Nottinghamshire opened in 1912 and Moss Side on Merseyside in 1933. Latterly the amalgamation of Moss Side and Park Lane Hospitals created Ashworth Hospital in 1990. The three high secure hospitals currently provide a total of approximately 970 beds.

In the latter half of the twentieth century, the future of secure mental health provision was the focus of government reports and parliamentary acts. With the move towards community based care and the progressive closure of large mental hospitals, the Glancy Working Party was established to review existing secure provision by assessing the needs of those patients already in hospital (DHSS 1974). The report recommended that 1,000 beds were required nationally in services holding 'difficult' patients needing increased, but not maximum, security. The following year the Butler Committee similarly examined provision for offenders with mental health problems in hospitals, prisons and the community, recommending that 2,000 secure beds (outwith the three high secure hospitals) were required to support their work (HO/DHSS 1975). The two reports formed the impetus behind the establishment of Medium Secure Forensic Psychiatric Units (MSUs; Coid et al 2001).

Whilst legislation and government guidance were framed around the fundamental principle that mentally disordered offenders needed specialist care from health and social services and should be diverted from the criminal justice system, large numbers of mentally ill offenders remained in custodial settings. In 1990, Home Office Circular 66/90 explicitly required consideration be given to ways of dealing with mentally disordered offenders other than straight-forward prosecution, for example cautioning, or diversion out of the criminal justice system into hospital or community care (HO/DH 1990). This approach was reiterated by the Reed Review of services for mentally disordered offenders (DH/HO 1992). Reed emphasised that mentally disordered offenders should, as far as possible, be cared for in the community rather than in-patient settings and that, if detention were required, it should be at a level of security no higher than needed; as close to home and family as possible; and aimed to maximise rehabilitation and chances of sustaining an independent life upon discharge.

Forensic mental health services have been cursed by very public failures. A number of homicides by people with mental illness and the subsequent inquiries commanded a high media profile in the latter part of the twentieth century (e.g. Ritchie et al 1994, Scotland et al 1998). Issues surrounding the ability of clinicians to effectively predict and manage risk attracted much public and political interest, sustaining intensive media attention on the complex and emotive issue of a safe society. Similarly, a number of reports into the high secure hospitals highlighted the complexity of providing care in these settings. Inquiries have focussed on allegations of deliberate cruelty by staff and unnecessarily draconian regimes and, conversely, corrupt regimes which lacked any control over patients' continued criminality (e.g. Blom-Cooper et al 1992, Fallon et al 1999).

The publication of the 'National Service Framework for Mental Health' in 1999 detailed how mental health services would be planned, delivered and monitored until 2009 (DH 1999). The seven separate standards outlined in the 'National Service Framework' have clear applicability to forensic mental health services and will be discussed below, where appropriate in the context of 'The National Service Framework for Mental Health – Five Years On' (Appleby 2004).

Standard 1: mental health promotion

Within our society, the twin stigmas of mental illness and criminality can pre-cipitate exclusion from society in general and the local community within which an individual lives. Mentally disordered offenders can experience victi-misation and suffering, as well as a host of unmet needs (Hodgins 1998). High rates of psychiatric morbidity are present within the criminal justice system (e.g. Gunn et al 1991, Birmingham et al 1996, Singleton et al 1998, Fazel & Danesh 2002).

As a result of their mental illness a person may become isolated and excluded from society and may therefore be reluctant to engage with services; this may lead to progressive deterioration linked with a serious index offence, warranting a long period of detention, either in prison or as a secure in-patient. The promo-tion of mental health is therefore crucial as a pro-active step in counteracting or preventing an individual's risk of criminality and possible escalation to commit-ting more serious offences. Needs are frequently complex, but there is evidence that, even in high-risk patients, offending can be prevented (e.g. Wilson et al 1995, Muller-Isberner 1996, Heilbrun & Peters 2000).

Prisoners are a particularly problematic group in terms of social exclusion, experiencing many health and social inequalities and disadvantages (DH 2002a). Rates of homelessness, unemployment and a lack of basic level education prior to prison are all high (Prison Reform Trust 2006). Mentally disordered offenders in prison have reported feeling vilified and marginalised as their mental illness may not be deemed serious enough to warrant involvement with forensic mental health services, yet is considered too complex for intervention from general community mental health services, thus leaving them effectively without help (Vaughan & Stevenson 2002).

The challenge faced by the NHS in promoting mental health in prisons is complex. Prisons contain a high proportion of vulnerable individuals, many of whom, whilst not floridly disordered, possess the characteristics associated with an increased risk of common mental health problems, suicide and self-harm (Singleton et al 1998). They find themselves in challenging environments where the apparently conflicting requirements of security, and care and rehabilitation, play out on a daily basis. They may be prone to the uncertainties inherent with being unconvicted or, upon conviction, they routinely face multiple moves taking them away from family support. Developing mental health promotion strategies in prisons requires a sustained programme approach, including a comprehensive suicide prevention strategy; the effective treatment of drug and alcohol misuse; anti-bullying schemes; peer support schemes; support to prisoners' families; parenting courses; 'well-man/woman' clinics; opportunities for education; and access to a variety of help agencies.

An over-arching aim would be for time in prison to be used as a valuable opportunity for mental health services to identify and engage with mentally disordered offenders, as well as promote general mental well-being for the prison population as a whole (Reed & Lyne 2000, DH 2002a). The Prison Service has acknowledged this, with the National Service Framework noting that (DH 1999):

> *'Mental health is a priority for the HM Prison Service's Directorate of Health Care ... The Directorate has issued detailed guidance on the value of promoting mental health in prisons through, for example, anti-bullying strategies, regular physical exercise and contact with families, friends and the outside community.'*

The National Service Framework also notes that community-based health and social services have a role in assessing the mental health needs of prisoners to prepare community support for them upon release, possibly at short, or no, notice. Currently, robust post-custody transitional period initiatives are being investigated (Shaw et al 2008). Services need to actively promote the engagement of discharged mentally ill prisoners into community mental health services. Post-release initiatives including 'meet at gate' transitional care arrangements require evaluation; criminal justice, healthcare and social service agencies need to work together to facilitate the success of such initiatives.

Standards 2 and 3: primary care and access to services

Most individuals with mental health problems are cared for at primary care level by their GP, with a minority needing access to secondary general mental health services, depending on the complexity of need and considerations of the level of risk they pose to themselves and to others. Mentally disordered offenders frequently present with complex treatment needs beyond the scope of primary care mental health services thus requiring intervention from secondary general mental health services or tertiary level forensic services.

There are currently no national protocols guiding the referral of mentally disordered offenders from primary care to secondary and tertiary level services, or from general to specialist forensic services. There is considerable variation in the type and volume of services available for mentally disordered offenders as services have developed in an ad-hoc way (Coid et al 2001). Surveys of existing community services have shown that they are inadequate in meeting the needs of mentally disordered offenders (Vaughan et al 2000). A more coordinated approach to the delivery of these services and increased integration between primary and secondary NHS mental health services, particularly for those with complex treatment needs, is required. Whilst new service models (Assertive Outreach, early intervention, crisis teams etc) have improved the provision of mental health care for many, they have, as yet, failed to positively impact upon the needs of mentally disordered offenders (Cree & Hodgins 2007).

Forensic services are relatively difficult to access for mentally disordered offenders unless they have committed a serious offence. As such, and in spite of nearly two decades of national policy promoting diversion from the criminal justice system into care services, individuals all too often continue to enter the criminal justice system with its primary emphasis on punishment and public protection, without being afforded access to the necessary treatment and rehabilitation. The first magistrates' court diversion scheme was established in London in 1989 (Joseph & Potter 1990), followed by a national expansion of local court-based initiatives in response to Home Office Circular 66/90 (HO/DH 1990). The National Service Framework requires that services identify and assess the mental health needs of individuals who come into contact with the criminal justice system. Interventions are to be offered on the premise that early access to health and social care should prevent further deterioration in a person's mental state, reduce the likelihood of offending and thus avoid unsuitable use of custody. However, research has demonstrated that diversion is labour and resource intensive; diversion from a custodial sentence can involve between 12 and 15 agencies from the offence through to court disposal and eventual treatment (Farrar 1996). It is unclear how many police diversion schemes are currently in operation and evidence has suggested a general decline in the provision of these schemes with resources being re-deployed elsewhere (NACRO 2005). Existing schemes are characterised by considerable variations in organisational delivery, quality, funding, effectiveness in terms of realising intended outcome for individuals, and efficacy of their links with health and social care services and other relevant agencies (Centre for Public Innovation 2005).

Concerted effort is required to improve diversion initiatives, requiring improved identification and assessment of offenders, improved liaison and referral pathways and increased diversion interventions into mental health services in and outside the criminal justice system. National protocols would be an important way of harmonising the approach to those with severe mental illness entering the initial stages of the criminal justice system. Good practice guidance should be developed which describes gold standard services which support the police, courts and others in their contact with mentally disordered offenders to divert from custody those inappropriately detained by criminal justice agencies. This has been addressed, in part, through the publication of the 'Offender Mental Health Care Pathway' document, which provides guidelines for those agencies which deliver services for offenders with mental health needs, outlining a broad framework for the end-to-end management of offenders with mental health needs (DH/NIMHE 2005).

Primary mental health care provision within prisons has been repeatedly criticised as inadequate and undeveloped, and consequently failing to meet the complex needs of the prison population (HAC 1997, SCMH 2006). The models of provision for primary mental health care vary considerably across the prison estate. Based on a concept of equivalence (such that government policy set out in the National Service Framework and the NHS Plan apply equally to prisoners), the document 'Changing the Outlook' outlined the areas in which prison mental health could be improved (DH 2001). These included access to mental health promotion; primary care services; wing-based services; day care; in-patient care service; through-care; and, when indicated, transfer to NHS facilities.

Strenuous effort and additional funding by government has seen some positive change in the provision of prison-based mental health services over recent years. However, these improvements have largely focussed on improving care and discharge planning for prisoners with severe and enduring mental illness through the introduction of mental health in-reach teams, providing the equivalent of secondary level community services. This initiative, although clearly laudable, has perhaps been at the expense of any weight being given to the pressing need to develop robust primary care services for the majority of prisoners whose mental health problems are less severe, and who would, in the community, be safely and appropriately cared for wholly within primary care services.

Williamson (2006) identified some of the challenges that community service providers face when providing primary care to former prisoners: high consultation rates; poor reliability in the self-report of symptoms and medical histories; poor treatment compliance; personal health neglect; and lifestyle behaviours detrimental to health.

There is an urgent need for models of primary mental health care in prison to be developed and trialled to address the complex needs of prisoners, ensuring continuity of care with primary care services in the community. Information systems between prison and NHS primary care services need to be developed (SCMH 2006). Clarity regarding the role of primary, secondary and tertiary mental health care services in prisons is required, so each level understands what is expected of them (Senior 2005). Integrated models of working are required between primary care and other agencies working with mentally disordered offenders, including information-sharing and regular liaison. Information-sharing protocols between standard and specialist services as well as external and internal healthcare agencies need to be developed to effectively share risk pertinent information.

Standards 4 and 5: services for individuals with severe and enduring mental illness

High rates of mental illness and comorbid substance abuse problems exist within the mentally disordered offender population, requiring concerted effort to provide comprehensive, effective and coordinated services. Forensic services are essentially capacity based, which means that there is difficulty in assessing the number of high and medium secure beds required, based on clinical presentation. It is widely recognised that providing specialised forensic care in secure conditions is expensive and a considerable proportion of NHS trusts' budgets is given to treating a relatively small number of patients.

The three specialist forensic high secure hospitals serving England and Wales provide in-patient treatment for individuals who present such a risk of immediate, serious harm to others and who cannot be safely cared for elsewhere. Over the last 30 years, the high secure bed numbers have more than halved, and a single, national facility for women requiring high security has been established at Rampton hospital. A target of reducing to 771 beds has been set, although this has not yet been achieved (Fender 2000). The reduction in numbers of patients resident in special hospitals has lead to a redistribution of patients to other facilities, frequently medium secure units. Fewer than 25% of patients are discharged directly from high secure care into the community and a further 12% return to prison on completion of their treatment (Davison 2004).

The provision of medium secure services across England and Wales has been slow and uncoordinated with resources struggling to meet the demands placed on them by the criminal justice system, high secure hospitals and general community mental health services (Coid et al 2001). It has been estimated that around 40% of prisoners held on healthcare wings would be more appropriately accommodated in NHS secure provision (HMPS 2004). Intended to compensate for the reduction in high secure beds, the National Service Framework outlined the need to increase medium secure provision by 300 beds and this figure has been achieved (Appleby 2004). There are approximately 2,800 medium secure beds in England, with around 40% being provided by the independent sector (RCP 2005). The continued expansion of medium secure beds and the need to target need-specific issues including those with personality disorders, women, young people and those with learning disabilities are some of the challenges to be addressed over the coming years (Hill 2006). There is an additional need to ensure that therapy provided in medium secure units such as anger management, problem solving and programmes to address substance misuse and sex offending are effective and evidence based (Hughes & Gladden 2003).

Community-based forensic mental health services are a relatively recent development in the UK, fuelled by organisational change in in-patient mental health services; an expansion in forensic medium secure facilities; changes in societal attitudes to, and tolerance of, risk; and changing practices in the risk management of offenders or high-risk individuals in the community (Mohan & Fahy 2006). Evidence has suggested that community mental health services may be effective in promoting greater acceptance of treatment, reducing hospital admission and avoiding deaths by suicide (Tyrer et al 2000). However, concerns that community services are overstretched, with excessively large caseloads, a heavy burden of administration and a lack of resources have prompted debate over whether individuals with more severe mental illness may be neglected if they are discharged to the care of generic, rather than specific forensic, community services (Harrison 2000). No overarching strategy for the care of mentally disordered offenders in the community is outlined in the National Service Framework and models of provision vary from area to area (Buchanan 2002).

Broadly, two types of community forensic mental health service model have developed. In some areas, they are *integrated* with the general community mental health team; in others they are completely separate or *'parallel'* to the general service (Snowden et al 1999, Mohan et al 2004). These two models differ in several service-related characteristics, including location, management, caseload, referrals, remits and liaison with criminal justice system agencies (Mohan et al 2004). A survey undertaken to identify the number of, workload type, and service models employed by community forensic mental health services identified the existence of 37 community forensic mental health teams (Judge et al 2004). Overall, the services showed a lack of innovation in the type of interventions being offered, with few teams offering more than that provided by standard general mental health services. Most forensic community teams offered risk assessment, but not specialised therapies to reduce offending behaviour. The remit of the teams, in terms of referral and management was frequently unclear. Services were found to have good communication links with the criminal justice system agencies, but poorer links with general community mental health services. The parallel model of care appeared to be the most widely employed in England and Wales, with approximately 80% of teams considering themselves to following this type of service provision (Judge et al 2004). In practice, parallel and integrated models are likely to operate on a continuum, and most services will combine features of both, with effective care for patients of both general and forensic community services requiring cooperation across a number of agencies (Shepherd 1993, Tighe et al 2002). Further examination of the adequacy and efficacy of different models of community based forensic services is needed (Mullen 2000, Judge et al 2004).

The prison population has reached record levels and criticism has been levelled against the care given to this increasing and vulnerable population. The National Service Framework identified the need for effective, specialist mental health services to provide secondary level mental health in-reach services to prisons for individuals with severe mental illness, including remand and assessment services with dedicated NHS secure beds. Improved care for seriously mentally ill prisoners requires liaison between services both within and outwith prisons, a fact recognised by HM Inspector of Prisons who acknowledged that (Home Office 2004):

'many in the prison system were suffering from mental illness and had been failed in the community ... care in the community for many people we see in the prison system doesn't exist at all.'

To improve secondary mental health services for prisoners, the mental health in-reach initiative is a fundamental component of the prison mental health modernisation agenda (DH 2001). Prison mental health in-reach teams are designed to provide services similar to those provided by community mental health teams to the wider population. The majority of prisons within the UK have developed these services, providing prisoners experiencing severe mental illness assessment, care planning, discharge planning and through-care. There has been a national commitment to the improvement of mental health care in prison settings and the NHS Plan target of having 300 additional prison mental health in-reach staff assessing and treating mental disorders by the end of April 2004 has been met (Appleby 2004).

Ongoing research into the introduction of in-reach services to prisons has highlighted certain challenges. Researchers have noted that so called 'mission creep' has arisen (Steel et al 2007). The original intention was to restrict in-reach services to treating people with severe and enduring mental illness (DH 2001). However, in view of the inadequate provision of primary care in prisons resulting in insufficient triage, in-reach teams report being overwhelmed by referrals for assessments for people with common mental health problems as well as those suffering severe illness. The result is frequently that teams find it difficult to remain focussed on their core task faced with such overwhelming levels of need (Brooker et al 2005, SCMH 2006, Steel et al 2007). The remit of in-reach team services in prisons frequently appears to be differentially perceived by the various professions and agencies within prisons, with disagreement and conflict as to what the core 'business' of the in-reach team should be. The result is that those teams that report undertaking the widest variety of tasks, for example referrals following incidents of self harm, are also those most likely to also report the highest perceived levels of staff burn-out and work overload (Brooker et al 2005). Secondly, prison in-reach services operate using idiosyncratic, localised models of care as official guidance has been deliberately non-prescriptive, with no implementation guidance provided for in-reach teams and those commissioning them (SCMH 2006).

It is commonly accepted that a prisoner with a severe mental illness should not remain in prison. However, it is also true that the transfer of acutely ill prisoners to NHS psychiatric facilities has frequently faced considerable delay. Legislation exists under the current Mental Health Act (1983) allowing for prisoners to be transferred to hospital for a period of assessment or treatment. Although the number of transfers from prison has risen over recent decades, a large number of prisoners remain in prison when transfer to hospital is clinically indicated (e.g. Gunn et al 1991, Birmingham et al 1996). The main problem surrounding transfers concerns delays in the process (e.g. Robertson et al 1994, Blaauw et al 2000). It is acknowledged that, in some cases, prisoners are given lower priority than those in the community regarding admission to mental health units (DH 2001); at times there is a shortage of suitable psychiatric beds (Birmingham 1999); disagreements over the required level of security (Mackay & Machin 2000); disputes over the catchment area of local hospitals (Robertson et al 1994); reluctance of hospitals to admit prisoner-patients (Blaauw et al 2000); and disagreements over severity of illness (Dell et al 1993). Studies of individual differences revealed longer waiting times for prisoners requiring high-security placements (Isherwood & Parrott 2002) and those diagnosed with personality disorder (Rutherford & Taylor 2004). Adverse effects of delays in transfer have been documented, including suicide and self-harm among waiting prisoners; and location in 'strip cell conditions' (Coid et al 2003).

An audit of the time taken to transfer prisoners out of prison into NHS psychiatric care, both before and after a prison in-reach service was developed, revealed an increase in the number of prisoners transferred, but a trend of increasing delay, which was dependent on the level of security needed (Isherwood & Parrott 2002). This suggests that improvements have been made in the recognition of cases suitable for transfer, but that the wider resources to support this improved service provision are lacking. In these circumstances, it remains doubtful as to how providing services in prisons equivalent in scope and quality to that provided in the wider community can be achieved. No part of a prison is recognised as a hospital under the Mental Health Act (1983) and circumstances in which treatment can be enforced against a prisoner's will are limited to situations of utmost emergency. Prisoners with severe mental illness who do not consent to treatment are thus, by legal necessity, frequently left unmedicated and prone to long-term deleterious effects, unless transferred.

Standard 6: caring for carers

The National Service Framework recognised that supporting the carers of individuals with mental health problems is an important element in providing a comprehensive mental health care package. All individuals who provide regular and substantial care for a person on the CPA should have an assessment of their caring, physical and mental health needs, on an at least annual basis, forming the basis of their own care plan. Within forensic groups, the practicalities of this can be problematic. Carers of individuals involved with legal or court proceedings share similar concerns with other carers, but may have additional ones including that they or other family members may have been victims of the offender, and the nature or severity of the offence may have caused them personal distress or social stigma. The specific practical needs related to caring for a mentally disordered offender need to be identified and addressed by mental health services. If the person is serving a custodial sentence, the encouragement and facilitation of as much contact as possible with carers or potential carers is particularly important.

Supporting carers of mentally disordered offenders may be made more problematic through increased levels of social chaos, with many offenders having no fixed abode and only sporadic or limited contact with family or friends. Upon release, prisoners may have no home to return to, no established roots within society, and no-one able to help to provide care and support.

Standard 7: suicide prevention

The first national suicide prevention strategy for England was launched in 2002, with aims to improve mental health care in general and to target specific high-risk groups such as prisoners (DH 2002b). The suicide rate in the general population has since fallen to its lowest recorded figure and there is evidence of a continued fall in the suicide rate in young men (DH 2006). However, a sustained reduction in suicide rates in prison has not been achieved. The prison suicide rate fell from 127 per 100,000 in 2004 to 90 per 100,000 in 2006 (HMPS 2007). The number of self-inflicted deaths does fluctuate and it remains to be seen whether this is indeed a healthy downward trend.

Currently, HM Prison Service has a comprehensive suicide prevention strategy in place. Over recent years, a number of risk reduction initiatives have been developed to improve the prevention of suicide and self-harm in prison. The Safer Custody Group is a dedicated unit within the Home Office formulating policy and guidance to help protect vulnerable prisoners. It takes the lead supporting prisons to implement policy on self-harm and suicide risk. A new system of managing at-risk prisoners called the Assessment, Care in Custody and Teamwork (ACCT) programme has been introduced. Any member of staff can initiate this process if they are concerned that a prisoner is at risk. Once monitored under this system, the prisoner is assessed and a plan of care formulated. The process is supervised by a case manager who ensures that ongoing interventions and reviews are completed. Practical skills and suicide awareness training are an integral part of the programme (HMPS 2005).

Following a number of deaths in local prisons, the 'Safer Locals Programme' was launched to implement and evaluate a series of measures aimed at reducing suicide in six local pilot prisons. A first-night centre and induction wing were two of a number of initiatives showing benefits for the care of prisoners on entry into prison, including reducing distress and improving feelings of safety (Liebling et al 2005).

The identification of mental health problems in prison is of particular importance in reducing risk of self-harm and suicide. Screening procedures in prison receptions have been reported to be ineffective. As a result, prisoners with mental health problems have often not been identified (Birmingham et al 1996, Parsons et al 2001). To futher improve screening procedures, an evaluation of the current screening tool is required.

In mental health services, the risk of suicide has been shown to be highest in the period immediately after hospital discharge (Appleby et al 1999) and research has suggested that, similarly, there are increased death rates among recently released prisoners (Graham 2003, Pratt et al 2006) and offenders in the community (Biles et al 1999, Sattar 2001). Efforts directed toward the prevention of suicide in this group are therefore particularly important and these research findings suggest that, as prisoners are released into the community, the NHS and other care providers need to overlap with criminal justice services to ensure the safe resettlement of ex-offenders. A shared responsibility to meet the complex needs of ex-prisoners ultimately lies with the prison, probation, health and social services to develop collaborative practices in providing services for this at-risk group and, although the National Service Framework stressed the importance of increased communication and liaison between agencies within health and social care and the criminal justice system for the prevention of suicide, it did not specify how this could best be achieved.

Critical review of the National Service Framework for forensic mental heath services

In general terms, the National Service Framework introduced seven standards, which gave a comprehensive vision for the development of mental health care in England and Wales for the next 10 years. It focused on the development and funding of multidisciplinary community mental health services, including the emergence of specialist community teams, such as early intervention, home treatment and assertive outreach. However, the framework failed to give specific mention to, or recommendations for meeting the complex and multi-faceted needs of mentally disordered offenders, possibly resulting in a lack of priority thus being afforded to funding and services for this group. Additionally, the National Service Framework does not seem to have significantly addressed the *number* of people with mental health problems in the increasing prison population although, inroads into improving *actual care* for those prisoners have been made. Similarly, forensic mental health services outwith prisons are not a specific focus of the National Service Framework, either at the time of its implementation, or in its review. Similarly, in reviewing the progress at five years, no specific mention of the services required by mentally disordered offenders has been made (Appleby 2004, 2007).

Although comprehensive, the guidance produced by the National Service Framework was not explicit or prescriptive about the service structures and models that may be required by forensic mental health services to deliver the seven standards. As the client group managed within these services can present particular challenges, and service provision can be particularly costly, detailed guidelines for practice would be valuable.

The increasing need for mental health care for a growing prison population and an increase in the number of medium secure beds has raised concerns that there is perceived to be a growing need to detain mentally disordered offenders, in either secure psychiatric care or prison (Priebe et al 2005). Alternatives to long-term hospitalisation and pro-active initiatives to enable reintegration into the community for forensic patients will require future service developments including: effective community forensic mental health services with access to community-based supported housing; greater liaison between the forensic mental health services and agencies within the criminal justice system; improved integration between hospital and community services; an examination of 'what works' for mentally disordered offenders in terms of treatment and reducing reoffending programmes; and clear exit criteria for patients in community forensic mental health teams to be transferred over to general mental health services when risks are sufficiently reduced.

Future developments in forensic mental health service provision

A number of new roles have developed for those working within forensic mental health services, based on current legislative and political changes, including forensic case management; liaison with the National Offender Management

Service (NOMS); involvement with Multi Agency Public Protection Arrangements (MAPPA) for specialist risk assessment and management; assessments, advice, and training for staff in general mental health and other related services; specialist psychological intervention; liaison with criminal justice agencies through court diversion and liaison schemes; and providing in-reach services to prison service establishments.

Significant changes in the future provision of forensic mental health services, both in prison and in the community, are predicted, with the continued development of prison in-reach teams; new arrangements for care pathways (DH/ NIMHE 2005); recommended changes to provision for women in prison (HO 2007); and policy changes to expedite transfers to hospital under the Mental Health Act (1983) in less than one week by 2008. These changes signal the continuation of a programme of diverse and complex mental health care improvements for mentally disordered offenders.

Future work is indicated around several important practice areas including matching mental health services to the needs of particular groups, such as Black and minority ethnic patients, women and young people; a greater focus on the principles of meaningful patient involvement and representation within services; ensuring the availability of a wide range of evidence based interventions and therapies; a greater focus on transitional periods to bridge gaps between healthcare, criminal justice and social services and between detention and the community; mental health promotion and a recognition of the effect of the custodial environment on a person's mental wellbeing; improvements in diversion and transfers from the criminal justice system where clinically indicated; coordinated models of care in which robust primary care services are available to support the work of secondary and tertiary mental health care; end-to-end offender management which ensures that agencies work with the individual for the entirety of their sentence; and effective communication and sharing of risk pertinent information.

The responsibility for addressing the complex needs of mentally disordered offenders is not solely rested on mental health services. Improved cooperation and coordination between all agencies within health and social services, and across the criminal justice system are required to effectively meet their complex needs.

Conclusion

Forensic mental health services have experienced extensive changes over the last few decades and rapid changes in provision have reflected the National Service Framework national directives aimed at improving the standards of mental health care. The development and evaluation of systems of care delivery in forensic mental health that aspire to encompass prisons, secure hospital facilities, and community services are currently evolving. The application of community care principles to mentally disordered offenders has amassed considerable interest and criticism and recent years have seen major reconfigurations of community-based psychiatric services.

If forensic mental health services are to deliver high quality care for their patients and deliver an increased sense of safety to the public, it is important for policy makers and service providers to compare and evaluate emerging service models for best-practice approaches to be developed.

The present day reform of forensic mental health services has only just begun. Health and social services and criminal justice agencies will have to work together to help improve the facilities available for mentally disordered offenders and create a culture that allows patients who fall in this remit comprehensive care for their complex, multifaceted needs.

References

Appleby L 2004 National Service Framework for Mental Health – Five years on. HMSO, London

Appleby L 2007 Breaking down barriers – the clinical case for change. Department of Health. HMSO, London

Appleby L, Shaw J, Amos T et al 1999 Suicide within 12 months of contact with mental health services: national clinical survey. British Medical Journal 318:1235–1239

Biles D, Harding R, Walker J 1999 The deaths of offenders serving community corrections orders. Trends and Issues in Crime and Criminal Justice, No. 107. Australian Institute of Criminology

Birmingham L 1999 Prison officers can recognise hidden psychiatric morbidity in prisoners. British Medical Journal 319:853

Birmingham L, Mason D, Grubin D 1996 Prevalence of mental disorder in remand prisoners: consecutive case study. British Medical Journal 313:1521–1524

Blaauw E, Roesch R, Kerkhof A 2000 Mental disorders in European prison systems: arrangements for mentally disordered prisoners in the prison systems of 13 European countries. International Journal of Law and Psychiatry 23:649–663

Blom-Cooper L, Brown M, Dolan R, Murphy E 1992 Report of the Committee of Inquiry into Complaints about Ashworth Hospital, Cmnd 2028, vols 1 and. HMSO, London

Brooker C, Ricketts T, Lemme F et al 2005 An evaluation of the prison in-reach collaborative. School of Health and Related Research, University of Sheffield, Sheffield

Buchanan A 2002 Who does what? The relationship between generic and forensic services. In: Buchanan A (ed) Care of the mentally disordered offender in the community. Oxford University Press, Oxford, p245–263

Centre for Public Innovation 2005 Review into the current practice of court liaison and diversion schemes. Update Report for Health and Offender Partnerships (Home Office/ Department of Health). Centre for Public Innovation, London

Coid J, Kahtan N, Gault S et al 2001 Medium secure forensic psychiatry services: comparison of seven English health regions. British Journal of Psychiatry 178:55–61

Coid J, Petruckvitch A, Bebbington P et al 2003 Psychiatric morbidity in prisoners and solitary cellular confinement. II. Special ('strip') cells. Journal of Forensic Psychiatry and Psychology 14:320–340

Cree A, Hodgins S 2007 Services for the treatment of mentally disordered offenders – from reaction to pro-action. Mental Health Review 12:7–15

Davison S 2004 Specialist forensic mental health services. Criminal Behaviour and Mental Health 14:19–24

Dell S, Robertson G, James K, Grounds A 1993 Remands and psychiatric assessments in Holloway Prison. I. The psychotic population. British Journal of Psychiatry 163:634–640

Department of Health and Social Security 1974 Report on Security in Special Hospitals (Glancy Report). HMSO, London

Department of Health 1999 Modern Standards and Service Models: National Service Framework for Mental Health. HMSO, London

Department of Health 2001 Changing the Outlook: A Strategy for Developing and Modernizing Mental Health Services in Prisons. DH, London

Department of Health 2002a Health Promoting Prisons: A Shared Approach. HMSO, London

Department of Health 2002b National Suicide Prevention Strategy for England. HMSO, London

Department of Health 2006 National Suicide Prevention Strategy. 3rd Annual Report. April 2006. Reference No: 2006/ 0144. DH, London

Department of Health and Home Office 1992 Review of Health and Social Services for Mentally Disordered Offenders and Others Requiring Similar Services (The Reed Report). Final summary report. Cm 2088. HMSO, London

Department of Health & National Institute for Mental Health in England 2005 Offender Mental Health Care Pathway. DH, London

Fallon P, Bluglass R, Edwards B, Daniels G 1999 Report of the committee of inquiry into the personality disorder unit, Ashworth Special Hospital. HMSO, London

Fazel S, Danesh, J 2002 Serious mental disorder in 23000 prisoners: a systematic review of 62 surveys. Lancet 359:545–550

Farrar M 1996 Probation in the community. Paper to the First Annual Colloquium of the Probation Studies Unit. University of Oxford, December 1996

Fender A 2000 Modelling strategic changes in high secure hospital services. London: High Secure Psychiatric Services Commissioning National Oversight Group

Graham A 2003 Post-prison mortality: unnatural death among people released from Victorian prisons between January 1990 and December 1999. Australian and New Zealand Journal of Criminology 36(1):94–108

Gunn J, Maden A, Swinton M 1991 Treatment needs of prisoners with psychiatric disorders. British Medical Journal 303:338–341

Harrison J 2000 Prioritising referrals to a community mental health team. British Journal of General Practice 50:194–198

Health Advisory Committee for the Prison Service 1997 The Provision of Mental Health Care in Prisons. HM Prison Service, London

Heilbrun K, Peters L 2000 The efficacy and effectiveness of community treatment programmes in preventing crime and violence among those with severe mental illness in the community. In: Hodgins S (ed) Violence among the mentally ill: effective treatments and management strategies. Kluwer, Dordrecht

HM Prison Service 2005 Safer Custody Group. The ACCT Approach. Caring for People at Risk in Prison. Home Office, London

HM Prison Service 2007 HM Prison Service Statistics, January 2007. Home Office, London

Hill S A 2006 The future of medium secure forensic psychiatry in Britain: a survey. Medicine, Science and the Law 46:245–247

Hodgins S 1998 Epidemiological investigations of the associations between major mental disorders and crime: methodological limitations and validity of the conclusions. Social Psychiatry and Epidemiology 33:29–37

Home Office 2004 Annual Report of HM Chief Inspector of Prisons for England and Wales 2002–2003. Home Office, London

Home Office 2007 The Corston Report: Baroness Jean Corston: A review of women with particular vulnerabilities in the criminal justice system. Home Office, London

Home Office and Department of Health and Social Security 1975 Report of the committee on mentally abnormal offenders (Butler Report) (Cmnd 6224). HMSO, London

Home Office and Department of Health 1990 Inter-Agency Working. Home Office Circular 66/90. Home Office, London

Hughes G, Gladden S 2003 A survey of clinical-forensic psychological services in secure mental health settings. Clinical Psychology, British Psychological Society 29:20–22

Isherwood S, Parrott J 2002 Audit of transfers under the Mental Health Act from prison – the impact of organisational change. Psychiatric Bulletin 26:368–370

Joseph P L A, Potter M 1990 Psychiatric assessment at the magistrates' court. British Journal of Psychiatry 164:722–724

Judge J, Harty M, Fahy T 2004 Survey of community forensic psychiatry services in England and Wales. Journal of Forensic Psychiatry and Psychology 15:244–253

Liebling A, Tait S, Durie L, Stiles A, Harvey J 2005 An evaluation of the safer locals programme: a summary of the main findings. Cambridge Institute of Criminology Prisons Research Centre, Cambridge

Mackay R D, Machin D 2000 The operation of Section 48 of the Mental Health Act 1983. British Journal of Criminology 40:727–745

Mohan R, Slade M, Fahy T 2004 Clinical characteristics of community forensic mental health services. Psychiatric Services 55:1294–1298

Mohan R, Fahy T 2006 Is there a need for community forensic mental health services? Journal of Forensic Psychiatry and Psychology 17(3):365–371

Mullen P E 2000 Forensic mental health. British Journal of Psychiatry 176:307–311

Muller-Isberner J R 1996 Forensic psychiatric aftercare following hospital order treatment. International Journal of Law and Psychiatry 19(1):81–86

NACRO 2005 Findings of the 2004 survey of Court Diversion/Criminal Justice Mental Health Liaison Schemes for mentally disordered offenders in England and Wales. NACRO, London

Parsons S, Walker L Grubin D 2001 Prevalence of mental disorder in female remand prisoners. Journal of Forensic Psychiatry 12:194–202

Pratt D, Piper M, Appleby L, Webb R, Shaw, J 2006 Suicide in recently released prisoners: a population-based cohort study. Lancet 368(9530):119–123

Priebe S, Badesconyi A, Fioritti A et al 2005 Reinstitutionalisation in mental health care: comparison of data on service provision from six European countries. British Medical Journal 33:123–126

Prison Reform Trust 2006 Prison Fact File. Bromley Briefing October 2006. Prison Reform Trust, London

Reed J, Lyne M 2000 Inpatient care of mentally ill people in prison: results of a year's programme of semi structured inspections. British Medical Journal 320:1031–1034

Ritchie J, Dick D, Lingham R 1994 Report of the Inquiry into the Care and Treatment of Christopher Clunis. North East Thames and South East Thames Regional Health Authorities, London

Robertson G, Dell S, James K, Grounds A 1994 Psychotic men remanded in custody to Brixton Prison. British Journal of Psychiatry 164:55–61

Royal College of Psychiatrists. 2005 Towards needs-based planning for medium security hospital provision. Royal College of Psychiatrists Forensic Faculty Seminar, London

Rutherford H, Taylor P J 2004 The transfer of women offenders with mental disorder from prison to hospital. Journal of Forensic Psychiatry and Psychology 15:108–123

Sainsbury Centre for Mental Health 2006 London's Prison Mental health Services: a review. Policy Paper 5. Sainsbury Centre for Mental Health, London

Sattar G 2001 Rates and causes of death among prisoners and offenders under community supervision. Home Office Research Study 231. Home Office Research, Development and Statistics Directorate, London

Scotland, Baroness, Kelly H, Devaux M 1998 The Report of the Luke Warm Luke Mental Health Inquiry (Vols I and II). Lambeth and Lewisham Health Authority, London

Senior J 2005 The development of prison mental health services based on a community mental health care model. Unpublished Doctoral Thesis submitted to The University of Manchester

Shaw JJ, Thornicroft G, Birmingham L et al 2007 An evaluation of mental health inreach in prisons. Report submitted to the National Institute of Health Research, London

Shepherd G 1993 Case management. In: Watson W, Grounds A (eds) The mentally disordered offender in an era of community care: new directions in provision. Cambridge University Press, Cambridge

Singleton N, Meltzer H, Gatward R et al 1998 Psychiatric morbidity among prisoners: Summary report. Office of National Statistics, London

Snowden P, McKenna J, Jasper A 1999 Management of conditionally discharged patients and others who present similar risks in the community: integrated or parallel? Journal of Forensic Psychiatry 10:583–596

Steel J, Thornicroft G, Birmingham L et al 2007 Prison mental health inreach services. British Journal of Psychiatry 190(5):373–374

Tighe J, Henderson C, Thornicroft G 2002 Mentally disordered offenders and models of community care provision. In: Buchanan A (ed) Care of the mentally disordered offender in the community. Oxford University Press, Oxford

Tyrer P, Coid J, Simmonds S et al 2000 Community mental health team management for those with severe mental illness and disordered personality. Cochrane Library, issue 3

Vaughan K, McConaghy N, Wolf C et al 2000 Community treatment orders: relationship to clinical care, medication compliance, behavioural disturbance and readmission. Australian and New Zealand Journal of Psychiatry 34:801–808

Vaughan P J, Stevenson S 2002 An opinion survey of mentally disordered offender service users. British Journal of Forensic Practice 4:11–20

Williamson M 2006 Improving the health and social outcomes of people recently released from prisons in the UK: a perspective from primary care. SCMH, London

Wilson D, Tien G, Eaves D 1995 Increasing the community tenure of mentally disordered offenders: an assertive case management programme. International Journal of Law and Psychiatry 18:61–69

CHAPTER

10

Assertive outreach

J. Freeman

Introduction

'Modernising Mental Health Services – Safe, Sound and Supportive' (DH 1998) endorsed the emerging concept of Assertive Outreach (AO), and subsequently the NHS Plan (DH 2000) identified a target number of 220 AO teams that were to be commissioned to meet the needs of an identified target group. Among service providers a consensus was emerging about the rationale for this new service model. Clinicians were excited about the approach, which appeared to herald a real opportunity to do some high quality work with a group of hitherto neglected service users. Enthusiasm for the approach was widespread, in spite of existing research on the effectiveness of the approach being equivocal – outside of the USA at least. Nearly 10 years later, the implementation of AO services represents a real success story and a significant contribution to the care and treatment of people with serious mental health problems. The achievement of policy makers and service providers in achieving full implementation of AO in England is something that is admired and respected throughout much of the world – perhaps most of all in the USA, where, as this chapter will demonstrate, much of this work originated, yet where full implementation of assertive community treatment (ACT) has never, and probably never will be fully realised.

ACT has most commonly been credited with having emerged during the 1970s by the pioneering team of Len Stein, Mary-Anne Test and Arnold Marx at the Mendota State Hospital in Dane County in Wisconsin (Stein & Santos 1998). Over a number of years the Special Treatment Unit (STU) of the hospital attempted a range of novel psychosocial interventions (Greenley 1995) with some success, however the team consistently found that many of their discharged clients appeared unable to manage any significant community tenure:

> '...although patients usually looked great at the time of discharge, many would be readmitted looking as if they had been living a horrible life in the community. It was as if no matter what was done with the patients in hospital, it did not seem to help them in the real world.'

> (Test in Hengeller & Santos 1997)

One member of staff was working in a highly unconventional manner however and was having considerably more success:

> *'She drove patients to their new residence in the community and then spent countless hours and days providing them with "hands on" support and assistance to help them live in the community … She worked next to her clients at the sheltered workshop until they felt comfortable. Barb telephoned clients often to problem solve and provide emotional support; she gave clients and their family and/or landperson her home telephone number to call evenings or weekends if a crisis arose. If there was an emergency she drove out and intervened.'*

(Test 1998)

In time the hospital base for the STU was closed and moved into the community to be based in a small office in downtown Madison, the patients' own neighbourhood becoming the 'therapy arena' (Marx et al 1973).

A number of factors were identified by the team (Stein & Test 1980) to promote successful community adjustment, including food, shelter, clothing and medical care, coping skills to meet the demands of community life and a supportive system that assertively helps the patient.

The project dramatically reduced hospitalisation, with few study patients readmitted (Stein & Test 1980), and the team was able to demonstrate that the model could be economically viable largely because the need for in-patient beds was reduced by this kind of community-focused working (Weisbrod et al 1980). A number of impressive claims were made about the model, including the virtual elimination of hospitalisation, reductions in stigma and dependency, an increase in independent living and productive functioning without reductions in quality of life or satisfaction. As well as this, no undue burdens on families were noted by the team (Stein & Test 1975).

By the early 1990s in the UK, significant problems were developing with the policy of 'care in the community'. A media frenzy following a number of homicides, including that of Jonathon Zito by Christopher Clunis, prompted an inquiry (Ritchie et al 1994) requested by the Chairs of North East and South East Thames Health Authorities. Published in February 1994, the report detailed a number of fundamental shortfalls in Clunis' care and treatment. Problems centred on poor communication between services, incomplete and inaccurate risk assessment, patchy discharge planning, and the absence of a seamless approach to care and treatment. The Ritchie Inquiry identified a target group whom they identified as the 'special supervision group' and predicted that if this group of persons was not cared for effectively then the policy of care in the community would become discredited. 'Keys to engagement' (Sainsbury Centre for Mental Health 1998) proposed a solution to many of these difficulties, i.e. the creation and widespread implementation of assertive outreach teams, and this was reinforced by the subsequent publication of the Government's Mental Health Strategy (DH 1998). Current policy it was argued insufficiently serviced the needs of this small group of very needy people in that there was no clear service model, no consistent strategy for managing risk and no timetable for service development.

Assertive outreach in this context was defined as:

'a flexible and creative client-centred approach to engaging service users in a practical delivery of a wide range of services to meet complex health and social needs and wants. It is a strategy which requires the service providers to take an active role, working with service users, to secure resources and choices in treatment, rehabilitation, psychosocial support, functional and practical help, and advocacy ... in equal priorities'

(Morgan 2000)

The Government had accepted that AO was a framework of care and treatment that would enable people experiencing severe mental illness living in the community to receive the range of mental health services they needed, ensuring prompt and effective help if a crisis did occur as well as timely access to an appropriate and safe mental health place or hospital bed. In this sense, AO was clearly a particular type of intensive case management.

Staff providing comprehensive AO care for clients would visit them at home, often intensively and over enduring periods, to build and maintain a therapeutic relationship and to provide – as well as facilitate – a wide range of services. Practical help is often needed focusing on basic and immediate day-to-day needs, for example to find adequate housing, income, and sustain basic daily living – shopping, cooking, and self-care. Clients of AO teams are frequently people felt to be hard to engage, in the main because of their negative experiences of statutory services. Through the NSF the Government committed themselves to a level of investment sufficient to ensure that AO teams would be developed throughout England (DH 1998).

Government recommendations

Through the Mental Health Strategy (MHS) (DH 1998) the Government committed to the delivery of effective community treatment. AO was earmarked as an active approach to treatment and care for those who are at risk of being readmitted to psychiatric hospital that involves the person fully. The MHS emphasised that AO could form an important component of safe care and treatment, and a safeguard was given that investment would be made to ensure that AO teams were developed where the need is greatest.

The NSF explicitly outlined the target group for AO services. The criteria focused on those people who were: working age adults with severe and persistent mental disorder; associated with a high level of disability; but who were not necessarily characterised by having spent long periods as a mental health in-patient. In this sense, the criteria mirrored the 'special supervision group' identified by the Ritchie Inquiry four years earlier. Nevertheless clients may have had a more recent history of high use of in-patient or intensive home based care and experienced difficulty in maintaining lasting and consenting contact with services. They were clients experiencing a range of complex needs including a history of violence or persistent offending, or risk of persistent self-harm or neglect. Notably AO clients may not have responded well to previous treatment. Clients may have been dually diagnosed with a serious substance misuse problem, and had repeated admissions under the Mental Health Act. An important feature of the AO team approach was the regular 'team' review of each client. This generally resembled a handover, in which all clients were discussed, albeit briefly, every day. Caseloads in each of these teams reflect the need to ensure intensive input and were projected at around ten clients per staff member.

In terms of achievements, the NSF was clear. Although 'Keys to Engagement' (Sainsbury Centre for Mental Health 1998) had never envisaged that AO would be a substitute for hospital admission, a reduced rate of emergency admission was one of a number of targets. Alongside this were improved care packages developed in partnership with other services and agencies, maintenance of contact with those in greatest clinical need, and a reduction in symptoms through specific interventions. Such was the standing of 'Keys to Engagement' that, in the absence of more authoritative guidance, these criteria were to form the core components of many fledging AO teams throughout the country. Independent sector and service user groups were mostly supportive (Morgan & Graley-Wetherell 2001). Clear guidance on the design and structure of teams became available (Burns & Guest 1999, Sainsbury Centre for Mental Health 1999), and this added to the body of debate about how teams should be commissioned, as well as providing information on fundamental issues such as target client group, likely resources required and operational definitions.

Within any population there are a small number of people with severe mental health problems with complex needs who have difficulty engaging with services and often require repeat admission to hospital. AO was increasingly viewed as an effective approach to the management of this group. By adopting AO local providers believed they could improve engagement among disenfranchised service users, reduce hospital admissions and – when hospitalisation is required – enable timely, proactive admission and reduce length of stay. For service users and their carers positive benefits included increased stability as well as improved social functioning. Perhaps most crucially, the approach was now clearly viewed as a cost effective one.

The pragmatic approach provided by 'Keys to Engagement' directly impacted on the nature of local service provision by enabling local teams to readily identify an evidence-based model which was effective and achievable. Resources earmarked by the Government in the form of the Modernisation Fund allowed Trusts to commission AO teams in their local areas. Such was the rapid pace of implementation that by 2000, the NHS National Plan (DH 2000) offered the target of an AO team in every area, and a total of 220 by 2003. The National Service Framework for Mental Health (DH 1999), published a year after the Mental Health Strategy, expedited the pace of change providing further support for the implementation of the model. Local Implementation Plans and Teams derived from the NSF required local areas to create teams to meet the needs that had been identified previously, and examples of centres of excellence were provided. This combined evidence served to create a huge groundswell of support for the AO model, and the turn of the century brought about rapid expansion of AO teams throughout England.

Clinicians welcomed the new initiative, and in spite of earlier concerns from some service users about the potentially coercive nature of AO many now welcomed the approach. It was hard to find service users indeed who were unappreciative of the support and care which they received from their AO team (Sainsbury for Mental Health 1998).

Assertive outreach's contribution to NSF implementation

AO's contribution to the implementation of the NSF has been considerable, and, in many ways, it may be considered to be the NSF's most notable success. Why has this been the case? Certainly, AO services predated the NSF – at least in part. The years between 1997 and 1999 saw a rapid expansion of teams throughout England and the NSF served as reinforcement as well as an encouragement to local providers who were eager to commission new AO teams. The proliferation of AO teams was also welcomed by clinicians who viewed the model as a long-overdue opportunity to undertake high quality work in the community with a previously neglected and highly deserving client group. This was the kind of approach that many community-based mental health professionals had wanted to be able to deliver for some years. This however conflicted with the overt message of the Mental Health Strategy (DH 1998) with its primary emphasis on public safety. The Government's clear priority was, and largely remains, public safety and the NSF was evidence writ large that they viewed AO as a mechanism to promote this driver.

Local services set about laying the organisational groundwork for the development of an implementation strategy and were required to commission a local implementation team (LIT) using a whole-system approach to service delivery. National action to underpin implementation focused around five areas – finance; workforce planning and education and training; research and development; clinical decision support systems; and information.

The National Institute for Clinical Excellence Guidelines for Schizophrenia (NICE 2002) added impetus to the delivery of AO by concluding that when compared with standard care, AO is more likely to improve satisfaction and contact with services, decrease the use of hospital, improve quality of life, and improve work and accommodation status for people experiencing serious mental health problems. Targets outlined in NICE Guidelines have added to the momentum that has enabled AO to be fully achieved in England. The targets of the NHS Plan proved realistic, and although there may have been some local issues with the rebranding of services, or paucity of resources, it is clear that the broad aim of AO services available for all who need them has been one of the more achievable targets of the NSFMH. The model has proven effective in other settings, e.g. homeless populations (Craig & Timms 2000), and persons diagnosed with personality disorder (Cupitt 1999). The nurse's contribution to the model was explored also (Standing Nursing and Midwifery Committee; DH 1999b). AO teams spread countrywide, yet it was not until

2001, when the DH published their first description of a recognisable concept of 'assertive outreach' (DH 2001), that reasonable claims could be made that a UK model of AO had emerged.

The implementation and AO and fidelity

AO teams set off to achieve the objectives outlined within the NSF although they lacked specific guidance on the implementation of the model. Nevertheless a momentum was formed and critical mass soon reached. Teams actively networked, and a grass-roots organisation, the National Forum for Assertive Outreach (NFAO), was created. The NFAO was aware that there was a research vacuum demonstrating effectiveness of the model in the UK and that already the model had received criticism (Thornicroft et al 1998). The spread of community services for people with mental health problems was already a diverse one with an array of providers from all sectors. The patchwork of services varied from one area to another, for example there tended to be more independent sector provision in urban areas than rural, and some agencies existed only in certain regions or cities.

The service specification for AO in the Mental Health Policy Implementation Guide (MHPIG) went some way towards remedying this challenge, setting out a clear structure for AO teams in sufficient detail for them to enable complex planning and implementation, in doing so providing a template that served as an exemplar of good practice (Table 10.1).

The MHPIG Service Specification provided the kind of detailed criteria that many local providers had needed to develop AO teams in their setting, and has had enduring influence. A study in the North-East of England (Schneider et al 2006) suggested that AO was successfully targeting people identified as being in need by the MHPIG (DH 2001) with as many as 95% of clients identified as 'psychotic' – with 30% having experienced three or more hospital admissions in the previous two years.

The MHPIG was welcomed by most. Some however resisted the constraining nature of the guidance either by virtue of its inappropriateness in their own area, e.g. in some rural, dispersed communities, or for the reason that a similar and equally effective service was already available. This contributed to arguments around the issue of fidelity. ACT services in the USA had earlier recognised the utility of the Dartmouth Assertive Community Treatment Scale (DACTS) (Teague et al 1998) in describing key elements of the ACT model. The argument surfaced in England when 'Keys to Engagement' (Sainsbury Centre for Mental Health 1998) used very much the same criteria to describe the model. Ever since, local services had argued about the appropriateness of unquestioningly adopting USA criteria to gauge the effectiveness of AO in England. Many local providers and clinicians in fact felt constrained by the fidelity tool arguing that it was culturally inappropriate to their setting. Some trusts had expressed fears that they would be deemed not to have met national targets because their work did not meet strict criteria for developing local services. The debate gained added urgency with fears that trusts would be marked down in Commission for Health Improvement (CHI) reviews, even though local services were a success.

Table 10.1

The policy implementation guidance for assertive outreach		
Key component	**Key elements**	**Comments**
Assessment	Comprehensive multidisciplinary screening and needs, physical health and risk assessment	Culturally competent assessment should focus on identifying the service user's strengths, goals and aspirations
Team approach	Staff know, and work with, all service users. Continuity of care provided by the team as a whole while the care coordinator has overall responsibility	Treatment should be given within a team framework
Age, culture and gender sensitive service	24-hour access to translation services and gender sensitive services should be provided	The high prevalence of diagnosed psychosis in certain cultural groups emphasises the importance of developing a culturally competent service
Regular review	Brief daily review meetings at which all service users are reviewed; weekly review meetings with consultant psychiatrist	Multidisciplinary, service user-focused review
Interventions		
Assertive engagement	High priority given to providing services and support to service users and family/carers in the initial stages of engagement	Focus on strengths and interests of service user and benefits that contact with the service can bring
Frequent contact	Capacity to respond rapidly and visit over 7 days	
Basics of daily living	Practical support emphasising daily living skills	'Hands on' involvement in improving service users' living conditions
Family/carers and significant others support and intervention	Care plan for carers including psycho-education and family work	Practical support should be provided as needed
Medication	Delivery and administration of medication to promote co-operation with treatment	Careful attention to avoiding/reducing side effects
Cognitive behavioural therapy	A range of techniques should be available within the team and used appropriately	Cognitive behavioural therapy can be of considerable benefit to service users
Treatment of comorbidity	Substance misuse, depression/suicidal thoughts and anxiety disorders	Specialist help for any of these conditions should be available

Table 10.1

(Continued)		
Key component	**Key elements**	**Comments**
Social systems interventions	Maintain and expand social networks and peer contact and reduce isolation	
Attention to service user's physical health	Physical health problems should be identified and addressed	Help should be given to the service user to access health services
Help in accessing local services, training and employment	Help to keep appointments and enable a pathway to training or employment	Referral to specialist services should be readily available
Relapse prevention	Individualised early warning signs plan developed and shared	Changes in thought, feelings and behaviours precede the onset of relapse
Crisis intervention	Intensive support in the community should be provided by the team during a crisis	Avoidance of hospitalisation and restrictive care wherever possible
In-patient and respite care	Avoidance of hospitalisation and provision of alternatives wherever possible	Service user/carer/family involved as much as possible
Discharge and transfers	As long as there is evidence of benefit, assertive outreach should continue indefinitely	Boundaries between different health care services need to be flexible to respond to different needs

In 'Counting Community Teams: Issues in Fidelity and Flexibility' (NIMHE 2003), mental health providers were given greater flexibility in meeting national targets. NIMHE (2003) acknowledged that service models, including AO, may need to be adapted to reflect such variations:

'It would clearly be unacceptable for services to gain agreement with DH policy officials to develop a service tailored to their local circumstances, only to have it criticised by the inspection agencies for failing to meet all the fidelity criteria in the policy implementation guide.'

A number of stringent criteria were set out by which such variations would be judged. Trusts were required to offer 'strong evidence' that their alternative services were delivering similar outcomes and that funding is 'roughly equivalent' to the implementation guide model. Existing services needed to be 'exceptionally well established and effective' and the proposed model must have the support of all key local stakeholders, including service users and carers. The rationale for developing an alternative service could not be a financial one,

Box 10.1
....

Fidelity criteria outlined in 'Counting Community Teams' (NIMHE 2003)

The following criteria were agreed by SHA Mental Health Leads:

(i)   A clear case has been made for not adhering to the model service specification in the MHPIG, e.g. an exceptionally well established and effective existing service which can be built upon; widely dispersed population in a rural area; particular needs of a particular ethnic minority community

AND

(ii) The proposed alternative service can demonstrate that it is in line with the principles for the relevant service in the PIG. In particular:

   it provides effective coverage of the target population, based on local needs analysis,

   it provides the full range of interventions set out in the PIG for that type of team,

   it allows for effective integration with other parts of the local mental health service

AND

(iii) Either there must be some strong evidence that the proposed model would deliver similar outcomes for service users, e.g. a published study; an example of good practice elsewhere.

OR in the case of an innovative model there must be robust proposals for the evaluation of outcomes.

AND

(iv) The proposed model must have the support of all key local stakeholders, including service users and carers, on the Local Implementation Team, (which should in itself conform to the standards set out in the recently issued NIMHE leaflet on 'The Capable LIT')

AND

(v)   The total resource input, including existing mental health funding, must be roughly equivalent to that which would have been required for the MHPIG model: it is not acceptable to propose an alternative model purely in order to avoid investment in mental health, which is essential for the development of services to meet need and achieve performance targets

indeed the total resource input was to be roughly equivalent to that which would have been required for the MHPIG model. The fidelity criteria outlined in the 'Counting Community Teams' is outlined in Box 10.1.

The debate around fidelity continues. The fidelity model for AO has usefulness, but it was developed in the USA in a very different context of community care. The fidelity model needs to be considered in the context of the particular social policy, cultural and legislative frameworks that exist in England. As AO continues to evolve, evidence emerges that may shape the future direction and nature of services. Not least the environment of mental health care changes (including new legislation and policy developments such as 'choice' and 'payment by results') may significantly affect the nature of AO. The DH has acknowledged that the MHPIG Service Specification for AO needs to be re-considered (DH 2005).

What has AO achieved?

There has been considerable progress since the NSF was published in 1999. The NHS Plan (DH 2000) envisaged 220 AO teams, building on the 170 teams proposed in the NSF. The target was met by the 2003 deadline and by

March 2004, 263 teams were in place (DH 2005). Training programmes aimed towards psychiatrists, non-medical practitioners and AO Team Leaders have been rolled out nationally, and a research programme has been nationally commissioned to evaluate the implementation and benefits of AO with the aim of shaping future service developments.

The NSF was backed by new money totalling £700 million over three years, compared to the 1999/2000 baseline. The NHS Plan committed a further £300 million of extra annual investment over the three years from 2000/01. It is nonetheless important that the Government commits to longer term funding for the NSFMH as currently the success of the mental health reform programme is threatened by financial constraints (Widenka 2006). The budget year of 2006–7 has seen new financial and accounting arrangements being introduced across the National Health Service. Trusts are being told to budget for a surplus – and not just break even. The new system of Payment by Results has provoked concerns among providers of mental health services. Yet concerns remain about accessibility – some Trusts may commission an AO team in order to meet targets but lack the ability or willingness to adequately resource it and in doing so fail to provide what is an essential component of a comprehensive service. It is particularly difficult for AO teams to operate in rural areas and efforts are being made to find alternative models which provide an equal level of service for rural communities (Fraser 2004).

There are high levels of satisfaction with services, particularly the service-user focus and coordination of activity across health and social care services. It appears to be the case that clients of AO services are overall more satisfied with their care and treatment than those clients of other services. There are also good examples of collaborative working with the voluntary sector, and although research remains equivocal in terms of some outcomes, e.g. number of days spent in hospital (Killaspy et al 2006), what seems clear is that persons receiving AO are more engaged in terms of contact with staff, and fewer clients were lost to services. Certainly one of the main messages emerging from the research is that AO is remarkably successful in engaging service users, and that loss of contact with clients is a relatively rare event. This is a considerable success given that the service users are among the most difficult to engage and maintain contact with (DH 2005). Teams should continue to prioritise those things which help with engagement, e.g. help with day-to-day activities, assistance with bills, and housing.

Conclusion

Although it is clear that there is a great deal of satisfaction and belief in AO amongst service users and staff and considerable success in engaging service users in care and treatment, more attention needs to be paid towards the clinical interventions that are provided. Whilst it is the case that engagement is a skilled approach that is rightly prioritised and implemented consistently, it is also the case that AO workers, from different professional backgrounds, can provide a range of evidence-based psychological interventions that are aimed towards people experiencing psychosis. The evidence base for a range of psychosocial interventions, for example Cognitive-Behavioural Therapy, is continuing to emerge and offers a genuine choice that service users and their families welcome in managing distressing psychotic symptoms. Such interventions have been supported by NICE Guidelines (NICE 2002), and local providers are expected to strive towards implementing these. Medication remains the most commonly used intervention and AO teams should be able to offer a range of strategies to promote service users' use of medication. Increasingly this may include nurse prescribing which has already gained a toe-hold in some mental health services. AO should continue as a central element of comprehensive community mental health care for people with severe mental illness.

This enthusiasm and success needs to be built on to make AO even more effective through the greater use of evidence-based clinical interventions. Significant funding towards increasing the availability of appropriately trained therapists would enable greater progress to be made in a cost-effective way (London School of Economics 2006) towards this goal. Thus, training in AO teams has emerged as an issue and remains a priority area for local providers (Schneider et al 2006).

The argument about the value of AO teams compared to Community Mental Health Teams (CMHTs) remains unresolved. If improved engagement and satisfaction among AO clients are its main outcomes, does this justify its implementation? Are CMHTs able to offer as high quality care and treatment in a sufficiently flexible way? It may be that the elements of AO that enhance engagement could be incorporated effectively into the work of CMHTs, but at present this is far from certain. So we need to learn more about the introduction of the new specialist community teams (among them AO), and how these fit with the generic CMHTs. Specifically whether this approach provides effective delivery of community-based mental health care (Boardman & Parsonage 2007) and does so in partnership with other services which have also experienced rapid change including in-patient units, day care and primary care.

AO continues to evolve, and one area where, in the future, there might be overlap is with personality disorder (PD) services (NIMHE 2003). The proposed Mental Health Bill is still a Government priority and pilot services for PD are being established across the eight NIMHE regions. The investment in these new services is expected to meet the target of 200 new specialist staff and six new outreach teams to begin the process of improving services for this challenging client group. AO was established to meet the needs of those with challenging and complex needs, and could develop meaningfully into the area of PD and indeed, offender mental health more generally.

References

Boardman J, Parsonage M 2007 Delivering the Government's Mental Health Policies Services, staffing and costs. The Sainsbury Centre for Mental Health, London (http://www.scmh.org.uk)

Burns T, Guest L 1999 Running an assertive community treatment team. Advances in Psychiatric Treatment 5:348–356

Craig T, Timms P 2000 Facing up to social exclusion: services for homeless mentally ill people. International Review of Psychiatry 12:206–211

Cupitt C 1999 All for one. Mental Health Care 2(11):386–388

Department of Health 1998 Modernising Mental Health Services: Safe, Sound and Supportive. HMSO, London

Department of Health 1999b Practice guidance: The Nurses' Contribution to Assertive Community Treatment. Standing Nursing and Midwifery Committee (SNMAC). HMSO, London

Department of Health 2000 NHS: The National Plan. HMSO, London

Department of Health 2001 Mental Health Policy Implementation Guide. HMSO, London

Department of Health 2005 National Institute for Mental Health in England, Care Services Improvement Partnership, Assertive Outreach in Mental Health in England. Report from a day seminar on research, policy and practice (http://www.nfao.co.uk/ResourceLibrary/AO%20seminar%20report.pdf)

Fraser M 2004 The National Service Framework for Mental Health – What progress five years on? MIND, London (http://www.mind.org.uk/NR/rdonlyres/D911226A-6ED5-47B4-9D35-E778714C41CF/2003/NSFfiveyearson.pdf)

Greenley J R 1995 Madison, Wisconsin, United States: creation and implementation of the program of assertive community treatment (PACT). In: Schulz R, Greenley J R (eds) Innovating in community mental health: international perspectives. Westport, CT

Hengeller A, Santos A B 1997 Innovative approaches for difficult to treat populations. APA Press, Washington, DC

Killaspy H et al 2006 The REACT study: randomised evaluation of assertive community treatment in North London. British Medical Journal 332:815–820

London School of Economics 2006 The depression report – a new deal for depression and anxiety disorders. The Centre for Economic Performance's Mental Health Policy Group (http://cep.lse.ac.uk/textonly/research/mentalhealth/depression_report_layard.pdf), LSE, London

Marx A J, Test M A, Stein L I 1973 Extra-hospital management of severe mental illness, feasibility and effects of social functioning. Archives of General Psychiatry 29: 505–511

Morgan S 2000 Risk-making or risk-taking? Open Mind 101, Jan/Feb (http://www.practicebasedevidence.com/risk/risk_open_mind.htm)

Morgan S, Graley-Wetherell R 2001 Active outreach an independent service user evaluation of a model of assertive outreach practice. The Sainsbury Centre for Mental Health, London

National Collaborating Centre for Mental Health http://www.nice.org.uk

National Institute for Clinical Excellence 2002 Schizophrenia: Core interventions in the treatment and management of schizophrenia in primary and secondary care. Clinical Guideline 1. NICE, London

National Institute for Mental Health in England 2003 Personality Disorder – no longer a diagnosis of exclusion – policy implementation guidance for the development of services for people with personality disorder. NIMHE, London (http://www.dh.gov.uk/en/Publicationsandstatistics/Publications/PublicationsPolicyAndGuidance/DH_4009546)

Ritchie J, Dick D, Lingham R 1994 The report of the inquiry into the care and treatment of Christopher Clunis. London, HMSO

Sainsbury Centre for Mental Health 1998 Keys to engagement: A review of care for people with serious mental illness who are hard to engage with services. The Sainsbury Centre for Mental Health, London

Sainsbury Centre for Mental Health 1999 Developing assertive outreach services: for vulnerable with severe & enduring mental illness who do not engage with traditional services. The Sainsbury Centre for Mental Health, London

Schneider J, Brandon T, Wooff D, Carpenter J, Paxton R 2006 Assertive outreach: policy and reality. Psychiatric Bulletin 30:89–94

Stein L I, Test M A 1975 Alternative to the hospital: a controlled study. American Journal of Psychiatry 132(5):517–522

Stein L I, Test M A 1980 Alternative to mental hospital treatment, 1. Conceptual model, treatment program, and clinical evaluation. Archives of General Psychiatry 37:392–397

Stein L I, Santos A B 1998 assertive community treatment of people with severe mental illness. Norton, New York

Teague G B, Bond G R, Drake R E 1998 Program fidelity in assertive community treatment: Development and use of a measure American Journal of Orthopsychiatry 68(2):216–232

Test M A 1998 The Origins of PACT. The Journal, Volume 9, Issue 1, 1998 (http://www. actassociation.org/origins)

Thornicroft G, Wykes T, Holloway F, Johnson S, Szmukler G 1998 From efficacy to effectiveness in community mental health services: the PRiSM Psychosis Study 10. British Journal of Psychiatry 172:423–427

Weisbrod B A, Test M A, Stein L I 1980 Alternative to mental hospital treatment II: Economic cost–benefit analysis. Archives of General Psychiatry 37:400–405

Widenka L 2006 A cut too far – a Rethink report into budget cuts affecting mental health services. Rethink, London (http://www.rethink.org)

Early interventions in psychosis

S. McGowan • Z. Iqbal • M. Birchwood

Introduction

Early Intervention in first-episode Psychosis (EIP) first appeared as a discrete service model in the mid-1980s in Australia, where it emerged as a reaction against conventional approaches to first-episode psychosis (FEP) and their pre-occupation with diagnosis, symptom management and models of care based on chronic disease management (Sanbrook & Harris 2003).

In the UK, EIP teams specialise in working with young people aged between 14 and 35 who are experiencing their first episode of psychosis. They provide a range of interventions, including anti-psychotic medications and psychosocial interventions tailored to the needs of young people with a view to facilitating recovery. They emphasise the need for early detection and engagement, proper attention to the impact of interrupted development and also take an optimistic view of the person's ability to recover.

The UK service model was extensively based on the North Birmingham experience and the advice of the IRIS group (Initiative to Reduce the Impact of Schizophrenia; www.iris-initiative.org.uk). Underpinning this model were two central principles:

- that the time between the emergence of symptoms and effective treatment should be as short as possible
- that interventions to promote recovery and maximise social functioning and resilience should be provided assertively in the first three years following the onset of psychosis.

Research had already demonstrated a link between the duration of untreated psychosis and outcome (Johnstone et al 1986), and the 'Critical Period' hypothesis (Birchwood et al 1997), based on longitudinal outcome studies, argued for targeting a high-resource intervention at the early phase of illness in order to optimise an individual's chances of making a good recovery and to reduce overall long-term disability. The hypothesis states that functioning at 3–5 years following an initial episode of psychosis strongly predicts functioning at 20 years;

therefore, interventions aimed at achieving optimal functioning within this timescale will be most effective in terms of sustained recovery, user and carer satisfaction and costs.

The proposed 'Assertive Outreach' model of team configuration and deployment described in the IRIS tool kit (www.iris-initiative.org.uk) and adopted subsequently in UK policy guidance derives from Assertive Community Treatment (ACT) in the United States. The National Institute for Health and Clinical Excellence (NICE) appraised the evidence for ACT in their schizophrenia guideline (NICE 2002) and concluded that when compared with standard care, ACT is more likely to improve satisfaction and contact with services, decrease the use of hospital, improve quality of life, and improve work and accommodation status for people with severe mental disorders.

Shortly after the publication of the Critical Period hypothesis, Early Intervention in relation to schizophrenia received its first 'official' reference in this country. 'Modernising Mental Health Services' (DH 1998), the predecessor to the National Service Framework for Mental Health (NSF; DH 1999), includes the following two paragraphs:

> 'Delays in access to assessment, effective treatment and care result in unnecessary distress, an increased risk of relapse and potential harm to the patient and others. For example, early intervention with the right drugs and structured psychological therapy also matters in patients with schizophrenia to prevent relapse, reduce the risk of suicide and ensure public safety.'
>
> 'Such action requires the maximum involvement of patients and service users, their friends and family. Professionals in primary care and in specialist services need the proper education and training to recognise early symptoms and risk, and to take appropriate action.'

However, Early Intervention for first episode psychosis received only the briefest of specific references in the National Service Framework itself. Within standards four and five, which deal with effective services for people with severe mental illness, is included the statement:

> 'Prompt assessment is essential for young people with the first signs of a psychotic illness, where there is growing evidence that early assessment and treatment can reduce levels of morbidity.'

It goes on to say:

> 'there is also evidence that delaying treatment with anti-psychotic medication leads to poorer long-term outcome for individuals with schizophrenic illness. Better public and professional understanding together with integrated mental health systems across primary and specialist services will promote earlier intervention.'

The year after the publication of the NSF, the Government published the NHS Plan, setting out its intention to establish 50 new early intervention services by 2004. However, meaningful detail about EIP and the Government's national ambitions did not become available until the publication of the Mental Health Policy Implementation Guide (MHPIG) in 2001.

From a historical perspective this might be viewed as disappointing, given the level of international interest in EIP and the research evidence that was emerging at this time. As early as 1986 the Northwick Park Study of First Episodes of Schizophrenia (Johnstone et al 1986) had demonstrated the long interval between the onset of psychosis and treatment, and showed the link between this delay and severe behavioural disturbance, disability and family difficulties. By the time of the NSF publication Patrick McGorry and the EPPIC (Early Psychosis Prevention and Intervention Centre; McGorry & Edwards 1998) service had already accumulated over 10 years of evidence for the effectiveness of EIP in Australia. In England Birchwood and colleagues had postulated the landmark 'Critical Period' hypothesis the year before Modernising Mental Health Services was published.

The Department of Health (DH) view was that back in 1999, the research base for Early Intervention was 'not as robust as would have been desired' (Appleby 2006). In fairness, a great deal more research evidence for EIP has emerged since this time and there is now a sturdy scientific rationale for earlier intervention. Much more is now known about the long-term trajectories of psychosis and their biological and psychosocial triggers. Delay in first treatment is linked strongly with poor outcomes (Norman & Malla 2001, Marshall et al 2005) and Harrison et al (2001) showed how the outcome at 2–3 years strongly predicts outcome 20 years later. More recently, a systematic appraisal of the evidence for EIP was undertaken for the Cochrane Database (2006). It found strong evidence for the link between a long duration of untreated psychosis (DUP) and poor outcomes. There is also encouraging evidence for the impact of EIP teams, for example in terms of reduced bed days and improved mental states. Looking ahead to the near future, national and large-scale evaluations of Early Intervention services are already being conducted, e.g. the First Episode Research Network (FERN; www.fernonline.org.uk) and National EDEN (DH/University of Birmingham).

The recommendations

Despite the relatively minimal direct reference to Early Intervention in Psychosis in the NSF, two of the seven standards (four and five) were devoted to services for people with severe mental illness. Also, on reflection, there was much of relevance to first episode psychosis in the document as a whole. Standard one deals with mental health promotion and the reduction of stigma surrounding mental health – objectives that relate to help seeking behaviour in individuals and families. Sections two and three are concerned with primary care and access to services and improvements here are central to the need for early signs of psychosis to be recognised/suspected, and the requirement for reduced duration of untreated psychosis. Section six covers caring for carers and EIP strongly advocates involvement, support, education and adjustment interventions for families and carers. Finally, section seven concerns suicide prevention, which is highly relevant given the substantial suicide risk that is present in the early phase of psychotic illness. Thus it can be seen that values and practices central to EIP can be found throughout the NSF.

Subsequently, the MHPIG prescribed in detail the teams that were required to provide EIP. It described whom the service was for, what it was intended to achieve, and what it did. It also specified management and operational procedures covering commissioning, project management and team structure. It detailed the staffing and skill mix required, training requirements and operational details such as hours of service. Importantly, it set timescales for the achievement of key stages of service development. In 2001/2 services were required to set up a project management team and advisory group, appoint a project manager and develop a local plan. In 2002/3 a first team was required, with ongoing development of the overall service in 2003/4.

Catering to a population of approximately one million people, it was anticipated that each new EIP service would comprise three or four teams, each managing 120–150 cases (service total of 450) after three years. Each team would have roughly 10 full-time care co-coordinators (each managing less than 15 clients), a half-time consultant psychiatrist, one full-time staff grade medic, support workers and administrative staff. This staff group would include the full range of skills required to provide the necessary care, and be able to work effectively with service partners both within mental health services and other key agencies such as primary care, education, employment and youth services. Table 11.1, published originally in 'A Window of Opportunity; a practical guide to developing Early Intervention in Psychosis services' (SCMH 2003a), summarises the core features of EIP as envisaged by the MHPIG.

Early intervention's contribution to NSF implementation

EIP has sought to address the full range of needs of young people with first episode psychosis, from its focus on primary prevention, health promotion and anti-stigma, through help seeking, access and assessment, to best-practice interventions and recovery. It has described a vision of mental health care that is based on humane values, scientific evidence, harm avoidance, person centred approaches and meaningful definitions of recovery. Ultimately it has argued for mental 'health' rather than 'illness' services; for services where good outcomes and social inclusion are the norm and where chronic disability is the outcome for only the smallest minority. As such, it has been suggested that EIP has provided a blueprint for all modern mental health services.

EIP has had three main drivers: evidence, policy and what amounts to a 'social movement' for the reform of services for people with serious mental illness.

The evidence base for EIP was covered briefly in the introduction to this chapter and as discussed, wasn't always regarded as completely irrefutable. The rationale for EIP is that recovery rates are better if psychotic symptoms are treated earlier rather than later, and that appropriate interventions early in the course of the illness can reduce psychosocial impact and secondary disability. Doubt remained as to whether these assertions had been empirically demonstrated. The nature of the studies necessary for demonstrating the effectiveness of complex service models drew criticism and fuelled the argument for randomised controlled trials to demonstrate the efficacy of the EIP concept.

Table 11.1

	Core features of an EIP service	
	Core feature	**Service design**
1	Early detection and assessment	Detecting psychosis at the earliest possible stage Comprehensive assessment, involving all professional groups, client, family and friends Working with diagnostic uncertainty
2	Pharmacological treatment	Management of symptoms should be in accordance with NICE guidelines Routine monitoring for side effects and prompt action taken to alleviate the unwanted effects of treatment
3	Care co-ordination	Key workers must be allocated rapidly and, where necessary, adopt assertive engagement approaches Care plans need to be focused on recovery with an emphasis on empowering the client Sustained involvement should continue for three years Caseloads for individual key workers should not exceed 15 pro rata
4	Co-morbidity	There needs to be specific and ongoing assessment and planning for anxiety disorders, depression, suicidality and alcohol/substance use and misuse
5	Basics	Proper attention must be given to housing, income/finance, physical health and practical support
6	Psychosocial interventions	Young people's personal and social development needs must be recognised and addressed Psycho-education should be provided to clients, families and carers Families should receive support and training Strategies for preventing relapse are required Cognitive behavioural therapy (CBT) should be available
7	Education and occupation	All clients should undertake vocational assessment Clients need to be supported into employment, education or other valued occupations within normal environments
8	Acute care	Wherever possible, acute and crisis care should be provided at home Care away from home should be provided in suitable, safe, age-appropriate environments, which are not unnecessarily restrictive The use of the Mental Health Act should be avoided wherever possible
9	Style	Embracing and promoting optimism about recovery Sensitive to individual needs relating to culture, gender, age etc Accessible, acceptable and engaging
10	Partnerships	The service needs to be designed and delivered in partnership with many agencies, including primary care, social services, schools and colleges, youth organisations and criminal justice services

Sample sizes were often small in earlier studies and proponents were criticised for making presumptuous links between studies examining the effectiveness of component features of EIP, such as CBT for psychosis, and the effectiveness of a whole system. In 2003, Anthony Pelosi, an outspoken critic of EIP and its research pedigree, called for a halt to the introduction of early intervention teams in the UK, to provide an opportunity for proper scientific evaluation of newly established teams in comparison with areas where teams had not been established (Pelosi & Birchwood 2003). Opponents of these views have argued that randomising represents an ethical dilemma, given the critical period hypothesis, and this has been a reason for the lack of such trials in the field. Nevertheless, the injection of finances and NHS resources into the development of early intervention services does necessitate evaluation and projects such as National Eden and FERN have attempted to provide ethical alternatives to this dilemma.

Whatever the arguments for and against the need for trial data, the implementation of the NSF has continued and evidence for the effectiveness of services has mounted. In December 2002, NICE published their clinical guideline on schizophrenia (NICE 2002), detailing core interventions in its treatment and management, with appraisal of the underpinning evidence. Although criticised for including a large quantity of 'good practice points' as well as research-based recommendations, the guideline found good evidence for the component treatments within EIP, i.e. the use of low dose atypical antipsychotic medication for first episodes, Cognitive Behavioural Therapy, family interventions, Assertive Community Treatment and home/non-hospital treatment models for the acute phase. At the time, the guideline found insufficient evidence for the EIP team model, but called for further research studies to evaluate this.

National policy has provided the second impetus for the development of EIP in the UK. The explicit requirements of the NHS Plan and the NSF were translated into performance targets with deadlines, and the strategic health authorities were charged with overseeing a process of allocating local targets and managing the performance of Primary Care Trust (PCT) commissioners and local service providers. In addition, government bodies such as the Modernisation Agency, the Commission for Health Improvement and, latterly, the Health Care Commission, have evaluated progress with the modernisation agenda.

Finally, the programmatic development of EIP in this country has also been counterbalanced by a 'bottom up' approach that has witnessed the emergence of a 'social movement' for mental health reform: a diverse group of proponents, including statutory and non-statutory agencies, clinicians, service users and carer groups who are impatient for service reform and, whilst on a smaller scale, find commonality with the civil rights movement, equal rights for women campaigners and Gay Pride.

Social movements are emotionally driven, often arising from perceived inequality and injustice. Bate has described social movements in relation to health care reform and highlights the emphasis that is placed on:

> *'self-managed change which is much more unplanned and spontaneous and which finds its energy from the commitments of those involved both to the ends they are collectively seeking to achieve and to each other.'*
>
> (Bate et al 2004)

It is argued that the kind of radical, transformational change called for by the NSF will not be achieved by top down, programmatic approaches alone, but must be complemented by a grass roots desire for bold, sustainable change.

Despite its diversity, this mental health social movement is connected by a shared view that that the suffering associated with the poor outcomes experienced by people with serious mental health problems is unnecessary, and largely a product of inadequate and ineffective services. Bodies that would be considered to belong to this movement include the charity 'Rethink', IRIS, Mad Pride, the Recovery movement and supporters of the 'Early Psychosis Declaration'.

The Early Psychosis Declaration (EPD) started life as the 'Newcastle Declaration'; an intentional plagiarism of the St Vincent's declaration for diabetes, drawn together by a small group of activists, including representatives from IRIS and Rethink in the north-east of England in 2002. It rapidly gained national and international support and has been refined along the way. In 2004 it was ratified by the International Early Psychosis Association (IEPA) and subsequently adopted by the World Health Organization. Summarised in Table 11.2, the EPD represents a

Table 11.2

Early Psychosis Declaration, vision and values

Vision

Fundamental objectives derived from this declaration are to:

1. Challenge stigmatising and discriminatory attitudes so that young people are not disadvantaged by their experiences and are truly included in their local communities

2. Generate optimism and expectations of positive outcomes and recovery so that all young people with psychosis and their families achieve ordinary lives

3. Raise wider societal awareness about psychosis and the importance of early intervention

4. Attract and encourage practitioners from a wide range of health, social, non-governmental agencies (e.g. charitable, voluntary and youth), educational and employment services to reflect on how they can better contribute to supporting young people with psychosis, their families and their friends

Values

Programmes for the detection and treatment of early psychosis should value:

1. Respect of the right to recovery and social inclusion and support to the importance of personal, social, educational and employment outcomes

2. Respect of the strengths and qualities of young people with a psychosis, their families and communities, encouraging ordinary lives and expectations

3. Services that actively partner young people, their families and friends to place them at the centre of care and service delivery, at the same time sensitive to age, phase of illness, gender, sexuality and cultural background

4. Use of cost-effective interventions

5. Respect of the right for family and friends to participate and feel fully involved

consensus view of the values and standards of those affiliated to the early intervention movement. Arguably, it also represents a sustainable framework for the continuous improvement of services for people experiencing first episode psychosis that will outlive the present policy driven agenda.

The declaration also includes a number of five-year measurable outcomes that an individual and their family can expect from services (Table 11.3).

At the time of writing, EIP's contribution to the overall implementation of the NSF remains largely incomplete. Despite the view that the EIP model might be

Table 11.3

Early psychosis declaration, 5-year outcomes	
Comprehensive programme	**Measured outcome**
Improving access, engagement and treatment Walk in responsive services usually provided in primary care settings should be equipped to deal effectively with early psychosis Service interfaces are designed to support quicker and more effective engagements of young people	The mean duration of untreated psychosis from the onset of psychosis (DuP) is less than three months The use of involuntary treatments in the first engagement is less than 25% Effective treatment will be provided after no more than 3 attempts to seek help
Raising community awareness About the importance and the opportunities for earlier detection and improved management of psychosis	All 15 year olds are equipped by mainstream education to understand and deal with psychosis Psychosis specific training is available to teachers and other relevant community agencies
Promoting recovery Services should enable rather than disable, ultimately aspiring to healing and recovery Means receiving encouragement and sufficient support to retain/regain full participation in society	Suicide rates within the first two years from diagnosis will be less than 1% Two years after diagnosis 90% of affected individuals have employment/education rates similar to their age/gender matched peers Two years after diagnosis 90% of affected individuals will report satisfaction with their employment, educational and social attainments Days out of role over the 2 years post-diagnosis no more than 25%
Family engagement and support Families have better access to information and education, social, economic, practical and emotional support	Services will give a meaningful response to families or key supporters within one week 90% of families will feel respected and valued as partners in care
Practitioner training All primary care sites are equipped to deal effectively with early psychosis Continued professional development is supported for all specialist staff working with young people with psychosis	Recognition, care and treatment of young people with psychosis is a routine part of training curricula of all primary care and social care practitioners Specific Early Intervention training programmes are resourced and evaluated

regarded as a blueprint for modern mental health services, centrally imposed performance management strategies have resulted in EIP being the last of the new community mental health models to be implemented. To date, the majority of EIP service developments are unfinished and, along with Crisis Resolution and Assertive Outreach, often exist as adjuncts to core mental health services (i.e. inpatient units, community mental health teams and psychiatric out-patient models), that remain as recognisable today as when the NSF was conceived. The remainder of this chapter will describe implementation progress, examine some of the reasons for the delays that have occurred and consider implications for the future.

Implementation to date and fidelity

The original targets set by the Department of Health for EIP were 50 first teams by December 2004 and a national total of 22,500 clients by December 2006. As we have seen, explicit objectives had been set in the MHPIG for commencing projects and conducting local needs assessment; however, the reality to date has been one of late and incomplete achievement.

A 2002 report to the strategic health authorities in the north east (McGowan & Macdonald 2002) found that in an audit of 14 localities, only half had appointed a project manager, one-third intended to conduct a local needs audit, that most were only consulting with 'familiar' partners and that all but two had failed to secure any service development investment.

A mapping exercise was conducted jointly by Rethink and NIMHE in 2004 (Pinfold et al 2007) and gathered information from 110 sites across England. It found that 81 teams had acquired funding, of which 63 had started to see clients, but only eight were 'well established' (of which only 3 met 10 out of 10 fidelity criteria). Almost half reported funding difficulties as the main barrier to continued service development. It concludes that 'inequity of access and the early, fragile nature of service development means that Early Intervention in England has reached a critical phase requiring consolidation'.

In 'The NSF for mental health – 5 years on' (Appleby 2004), the Department of Health reported that it had been able to count 41 of the 50 new EIP teams required by the original deadline date in 2004 and predicted full delivery by the 2006 target date. The document concluded that it was time to move the emphasis of service reform from new specialist community teams on to primary care and the broader community. Unfortunately, as we have seen, this figure did not tell the whole story. Many of the teams referred to were very new, very small and most lacked the confidence that they would receive the resources necessary to develop at the rate required to meet the 2006 client number target. Importantly, this counting exercise lacked the scrutiny necessary to determine whether those 40 self-declared teams could be genuinely regarded as EIP.

In spring 2006 the Centre for Public Mental Health Mapping (Durham University 2006) produced a report using data from the 2005/6 mental health service mapping exercise for England and information from the DH monitoring of Local Delivery Plans. It explores the extent to which the expectations of the original targets have been realised and found 128 EIP teams supported by 53 different NHS Trusts by the close of the mapping exercise (March 2006).

Eight of these were still under development and had not appointed any clinical staff. Only 60 (50%) reported meeting all fidelity criteria.

A progress review conducted in the Yorkshire and Humber patch of the NHS north-east region (McGowan 2006), consulted 14 EIP team leaders and reported progress in relation to activity targets and Durham mapping fidelity criteria. It found problems with narrow skill mixes and specific skills deficiencies (including CBT, prescribing, working with adolescents and dual diagnosis), a shortage of early detection and assessment capacity and services that were mainly limited to Monday–Friday, 9am–5pm hours of operation. Operational issues apart, the main problem found to be facing teams in the Yorkshire and Humber region was the uncertainty regarding immediate and future funding. Many teams were reporting delays with promised funding, reviews of plans and recruitment embargoes.

In its target year (2006/7), EIP was the Department of Health's number one mental heath priority. Unfortunately though, despite appearing in the Government's 'top ten' health priorities it fell outside the critical top six that were eligible for new central funding.

Progress to date

Nine years into the implementation timetable for the NSF, much still remains to be done if the Government's ambition for all young people with a first presentation of psychosis to receive the early and intensive support they need is to be realised. Earlier in this chapter we discussed the powerful drivers that have existed for EIP, yet despite these, so many teams currently find themselves 'a day late and a dollar short'. There would appear to be a multitude of reasons for this, including costs, complexity of the model and distrust of the evidence base. In addition, resistance to top-down change management, the rigidity of guidance and a perceived lack of will on the Government's part to see the process through have all played their part in retarding the process.

The apparent costliness of EIP services was understood to be the main cause of reluctance among commissioners and providers to develop services in England when the Sainsbury Centre published its guide to implementing EIP (SCMH 2003b). It argued that it is important that costs are understood in the context of the health economics evidence for best practice interventions in psychosis: schizophrenia had been calculated to cost the NHS in excess of £1 billion per year (Bosanquet 2000). Furthermore, 30% of the total cost of mental illness is attributed to lost output as a result of unemployment, sickness absence and premature mortality.

The SCMH argue that the costs of introducing EIP services may appear prohibitive but that these apparently more expensive approaches promise to save as much as it currently costs to meet the long-term needs of people with high levels of disability. It calculated that the cost of implementing EIP nationally amounted to only 1% of the total cost of schizophrenia. This is brought sharply into focus by the first UK study to specifically analyse the economic impact of EIP. This study has modelled the costs associated with EIP over a one-year and a three-year period and found that when compared to usual care, the cost for EIP amounts to an annual saving of 53%, which is maintained after three years.

With regard to complexity, EIP is viewed as a considerably more complicated service model and implementation challenge than either Assertive Outreach or Crisis Resolution. The model itself is intricate, essential planning information needs to be gathered and there are a multitude of interfaces with other services. A highly skilled workforce needs to be created, significant barriers may need to be overcome and engaging stakeholders meaningfully in the planning process is vital. Planners need to recognise this complexity and invest the necessary planning resources into long-term development.

Distrust of the evidence base has been considered earlier in the chapter, but with the evidence for effectiveness becoming more overwhelming year on year, this may cease to be a problem. There will, of course, always be sceptics and there exists a powerful force for conservatism in the NHS within management, professional groups and staff at all levels.

Prescribed, programmatic change-management will always face resistance – and that has been the case with EIP. That said, from the outset there was much enthusiasm for this persuasive, optimistic model from early adopters, and broad support from both statutory mental health services and consumer groups such as Rethink. EIP arrived at a time when service user and carer influence was burgeoning and a newly emerging psychosocially minded workforce was eager to apply its skills. The highly structured policy implementation guidance provided by the government shortly afterwards should have meant that establishing these teams in practice couldn't have been simpler.

The reality was somewhat different. EIP became the last of the three new community mental health teams to be implemented and, in addition, all of this was happening at the advent of new and inexperienced Primary Care Trust (PCT) based commissioning and at a time when many mental health services were reorganising – moving away from acute trusts and into either specialist mental health trusts or PCTs.

The need for reform was far from unanimously accepted. In fact, one way or another, EIP policy and guidance managed to offend nearly every interested party. Outcomes for people with first episode psychosis were bad because adult services were inaccessible and offered lacklustre, age-inappropriate follow-up; in-patient units traumatised and institutionalised; and psychiatrists and drug companies medicated unnecessarily and excessively. CAMHS services were doubly offended – their emphasis on development and working with families was shamelessly nicked, whilst they were implicitly criticised for not offering more to the small numbers of children with first episode psychosis. Some service user and carer groups were offended by ideas of early and assertive engagement, which they feared would lead to an increase in false positives and the number of young people unhelpfully stigmatised by a mental illness label. Finally, local commissioners and managers were offended by the prescriptive nature of policy guidance which they perceived as insensitive to local variation and needs and which left little room for creativity in service planning.

In fact, many resisted the rigidity of the NSF and, in response, the Government published flexibility guidance to address common concerns such as the applicability of the MHPIG to non-urban communities. In 'Counting Community Teams: Issues in Fidelity and Flexibility' (NIMHE 2003), the authors acknowledged that service models may need to be adapted to reflect variations in local need, for example dispersed rural populations, but set criteria by which this could be done and set limitations on the types of flexibility that would be acceptable. In essence, new models could be organised in ways that were pertinent to local need and related services, but had to ensure effective coverage of the target population and the full range of interventions as set out in the MHPIG for that type of team. It required that the proposed model must have the support of all key local stakeholders, including service users and carers and, importantly, that the total resource input must be equivalent to that which would have been required for the MHPIG model.

Finally, during 2004, it started to be suspected by some that the Government was losing its resolve to see through the implementation of the NSF, and in particular EIP. It was rumoured that the Government was 'softening' with regard to mental health targets and in summer 2005 the Health Care Commission published its annual star ratings of performance for NHS trusts in England, showing that 79% of mental health trusts had either 2 or 3 stars (this was the final year that performance would be rated using the star ratings system). EIP had not been included in the Government's list of 'key deliverables' and in its five year review of the NSF the Government had concluded that it was time to move the emphasis of service reform away from the new specialist community teams. With regard to performance management, the Health Care Commission stated that the challenge in mental health was to 'measure what really matters to patients and staff in the most meaningful way' and that target-driven improvement and modernisation methods were to be replaced by broader, social-outcome models.

The NIMHE/Rethink national EIP team raised serious concerns about this and in early 2006 the Government reframed targets and reiterated its commitment to EIP as a 'key deliverable'. It sought to retain/reinvigorate impetus for service development, whilst accepting that the national target for 22,500 clients by December 2006 was unachievable. The DH acknowledged that performance incentives for EIP had been lacking and, in recognition of the delays in commencing service development that had occurred at a local and commissioning level (and which had been influenced by the uncertainty described earlier), the DH launched a 'Recovery Plan' for EIP in February 2006 (Selbie 2006).

The EIP Recovery Plan confirmed that early intervention services remained a key mental health priority. It was a plan to get performance 'back on track' and consisted of three elements:

- A national objective for early intervention services to take on 7,500 new cases of psychosis during 2006–07, with the aim of building up to 22,500 cases by March 2009.
- Strategic Health Authorities and Primary Care Trusts to be provided with an allocated share of the 7,500 new cases, in line with their existing commitments.
- SHAs would agree with PCTs local delivery plans to make sure they met their share of new cases.

In order to ensure the success of recovery plan, the DH and the Health Care Commission committed to work closely with SHAs as well as commissioners and providers. To add weight to their commitment, the DH also proposed that the achievement of the recovery plan should be a prerequisite to foundation status applications for mental health trusts. At the time of writing, a great deal now depends on the success, or otherwise, of this plan.

Conclusion

In this chapter we have seen how EIP became one of the key requirements of the NSF despite uncertain evidence for its effectiveness at the time. After a somewhat faltering start, there has been considerable progress in establishing these new services and at the same time the research evidence has accumulated. Uniquely among the new mental health teams proposed by the NSF, EIP has spawned a social movement that has seen service users, families, clinicians and academics come together in the common cause of bringing to an end the discriminatory practice of 'late intervention', which has resulted in so much unnecessary disability and suffering.

More than half way through the lifespan of the NSF, EIP finds itself at a critical point. There are over 100 EIP teams in England now, but too many of these teams are at an early stage of development, too small and unable to deliver all of the necessary interventions. The NSF has been absolutely critical to the existence of such services in this country and deserves recognising as such. The full development of services for young people with first-episode psychosis will continue within and beyond the 10-year duration of the NSF, and we have seen how the Early Psychosis Declaration offers a framework for continuous improvement. Never the less, funding problems represent the greatest challenge to the successful implementation of EIP, and we look to the government to see through this extraordinary modernisation initiative that promises so much for some of the most vulnerable young people in our society.

References

Appleby L 2004 The National Service Framework for Mental Health — Five Years On. DH, London

Appleby L 2006 Quoted in Early Intervention in Psychosis in England – Report from a day seminar on research, policy and practice. CSIP, London

Bate P, Robert G, Bevan H 2004 The next phase of healthcare improvement: what can we learn from social movements? Quality and Safety in Health Care 13:62–66

Birchwood M, McGorry P, Jackson H 1997 Early intervention in schizophrenia. British Journal of Psychiatry 170:2–5

Bosanquet N 2000 Early intervention: the economic issues. In: Birchwood M, Fowler D, Jackson C (eds) Early intervention in psychosis. Wiley, Chichester

Cochrane Database of Systematic Reviews 2006 Issue 4 Quoted in Early Intervention in Psychosis in England – Report from a day seminar on research, policy and practice. CSIP, London

Department of Health 1998 Modernising Mental health Services: safe sound and supportive. DH, London

Department of Health 1999 National Service Framework for Mental Health. DH, London

Durham University Centre for Public Mental Health 2006 Adult Mental Health. Service Mapping: Reporting Autumn 2004 and Spring 2006 (www.amhmapping.org.uk/reports/)

Harrison G, Hopper K, Craig T et al 2001 Recovery from psychotic illness: a 15- and 25-year international follow-up study. British Journal of Psychiatry 178:506–517

Johnstone E C, Crow T J, Johnson A L, MacMillan J F 1986 The Northwick Park study of first episodes of schizophrenia 1. Presentation of the illness and problems relating to admission. British Journal of Psychiatry 148:115–120

McGorry P D, Edwards J 1998 The feasibility and effectiveness of early intervention in psychotic disorders: the Australian experience. International Clinical Psychopharmacology 13(suppl):47–52

Marshall M, Lewis S, Lockwood A, Drake R, Jones P, Croudace T 2005 Association between duration of untreated psychosis and outcome in cohorts of first-episode patients. Archives of General Psychiatry 62:975–983

McGowan S, Macdonald K 2002 An evaluation of Early Intervention planning activity in the NHS North East, Yorkshire and Humberside region. Unpublished report. Northern Centre for Mental Health, Durham

McGowan S 2006 Early Intervention in Psychosis development progress in Yorkshire and the Humber in relation to national targets. Unpublished report. CSIP, London

NICE 2002 Schizophrenia: Core interventions in the treatment and management of schizophrenia in primary and secondary care. NICE, London

NIMHE 2003 Counting community teams: issues in fidelity and flexibility. London: NIMHE

Norman R M, Malla A K 2001 Duration of untreated psychosis: a critical examination of the concept and its importance. Psychological Medicine 31:381–400

Pelosi A, Birchwood M 2003 Is early intervention for psychosis a waste of valuable resources? British Journal of Psychiatry 185:172

Pinfold V, Smith J, Shiers D 2007 Audit of early intervention in psychosis service development in England in 2005. Psychiatric Bulletin 31:7–10

Sainsbury Centre for Mental Health 2003a A window of opportunity; a practical guide to developing early intervention in psychosis services. Sainsbury Centre for Mental Health, London

Sainsbury Centre for Mental Health 2003b The economic and social costs of mental illness. Sainsbury Centre for Mental Health, London

Sanbrook M, Harris A 2003 Origins of early intervention in first-episode psychosis. Australasian Psychiatry 11:215–219.

Selbie D 2006 Local delivery plans – mental health early intervention services. Letter to SHA Chief Executives, SHA Directors of Performance, Directors of Social Services. DH, London

Acute in-patient care

A. Simpson

Introduction

When national guidelines on acute psychiatric care were published in 2002, there was an acknowledgement that 'too often acute in-patient services are not working to anyone's satisfaction' and that in-patient practice and service delivery arrangements had not received the same level of attention or guidance as newer community services (DH 2002a, p3). A series of reports and studies highlighting difficulties in acute care were enough to depress even the most optimistic amongst us. Problems included deficits in leadership, clinical skills and risk management (SNMAC 1999); lack of nurse–patient interaction and therapeutic activities (Ford et al 1998); a high level of chaos and crisis-driven care (SCMH 1998); over-occupancy of beds (Greengross et al 1996); a non-therapeutic, fearful climate with overworked staff (Mind 2004); noisy wards with overly restrictive rules, lack of privacy or information about treatment (Goodwin et al 1999); and a medicalised view of care and indifference to civil rights (Walton 2000). In a questionnaire survey completed by over 400 members of the mental health charity Mind, more than half the respondents said that acute wards were untherapeutic environments with a similar number saying that conditions were bleak and had a negative effect on their mental health (Baker 2000). These are all serious concerns and led the Mental Health Act Commission to wonder 'whether all in-patient mental health services provide their patients with acceptable levels of security, care, or a sense of being treated as someone who matters' (MHAC 2005, p19).

Over the last 20 years, the focus of attention for policy makers and researchers has been on the implementation and development of different models of community care and the appropriate service configuration, standards, management and training to make that successful. Most recently, interest has been on developing alternatives to in-patient care, such as home treatment and crisis intervention teams, discussed elsewhere in this book. With the collective gaze directed towards community services, in-patient facilities have faced a demoralising combination of retrenchment and drift with little research, discussion or development. There has been a determined effort to reduce bed numbers to an historical low, although an effective mental health service requires a range of facilities and no psychiatric service has been able to cope without acute in-patient beds (Thornicroft & Tansella 2004). The total number of psychiatric beds in England fell from 154,000 in 1954 to around 67,000 in the late 1980s, to 32,400 in 2003–04, of which just over 13,200 were acute care beds (Warner 2005), spread across roughly 550 acute psychiatric wards (Ryan et al 2002, SCMH 2005a).

National guidance on acute psychiatric provision defines the purpose broadly as to provide a 'high standard of humane treatment and care in a safe and therapeutic setting for service users in the most acute and vulnerable stage of their illness' (DH 2002a, p5). However, the philosophy, purpose and nature of the service provided are to be determined locally. This reluctance to outline the purpose and function of acute in-patient services perhaps reflects the uncertainty and disagreement about the current focus and future direction of such services (Bowers et al 2005a).

The recommendations of the National Service Framework

When the NSF for Mental Health was first published, its contents appeared largely focused on community services, with just Standard 5 making direct reference to in-patient care (DH 1999). 'Standard 5: Hospital and Crisis Accommodation' states that each service user who is assessed as requiring a period of care away from their home should have:

- Timely access to an appropriate hospital bed or alternative bed or place, which is:
  — in the least restrictive environment consistent with the need to protect them and the public
  — as close to home as possible
- A copy of a written after-care plan agreed on discharge, which sets out the care and rehabilitation to be provided, identifies the care coordinator, and specifies the action to be taken in crisis.

However, later publications made clear that acute in-patient care was considered a core and integral component of the NSF to which all standards were relevant:

'Improving adult acute in-patient care and its connections and integration with the other key elements of the whole system of care in its local context is a priority NSF implementation target.'

(DH 2002a, p3)

It is not possible to consider implementation of the NSF in relation to in-patient care without also considering the impact of subsequent policies and guidelines designed to improve acute services. Above all, the NHS Plan provided a backdrop across the health service, with plans for extra funding; more, better paid staff; cleaner wards; national standards; regular inspections; and a focus on putting the patient at the centre of service provision (DH 2000a). Then, in 2002, the DH issued guidance on adult in-patient care and minimum standards for psychiatric intensive care units (PICUs) (DH 2002a,b). These guidelines provided the National Institute for Mental Health (England) (NIMHE) with the task of restoring the therapeutic status of acute in-patient wards and redefining their role within a comprehensive system of care (Appleby 2004).

Critical review of the research evidence

Funding

Between 1999 and 2004, overall funding for mental health services increased from £4.3 billion to £5.8 billion in real terms (Bosanquet et al 2006). However, an analysis by the Sainsbury Centre for Mental Health reported that after allowing for increases in health service pay and prices, the increase in real terms amounted to less than half the increase allocated to other areas of the health service (SCMH 2006). In addition, the Audit Commission reported large variations in spend on mental health by primary care trusts (PCTs), from less than £75 per head per year to over £300 in 2004/05 (Audit Commission 2006). How does this impact on NSF standards in acute in-patient units?

Hospital bed close to home

The NSF requires admissions to take place as 'close to home as possible'. This follows recognition that, as a direct result of the demand for in-patient beds, large numbers of patients were being admitted to hospitals in NHS Trusts in other areas or, frequently, in the private sector (Simpson 2000a). As well as being much more expensive than 'in-house' arrangements, out-of-area treatments (OATs) create enormous difficulties in the provision of planned, coordinated care as the proximity of services and usual close working relationships between local community and in-patient staff are replaced by arm's length arrangements frequently marked by poor communication and different opinions as to the aftercare required (Simpson 2000b). Ryan et al (2004) conducted a study of 70 adult patients with severe mental illness placed in hospitals out of their home area and found that significant numbers of patients were not in receipt of the CPA (64.3%) or multidisciplinary review (62.9%) and clinical and treatment histories were absent in half of the cases. Involvement of patients (27.1%) and relatives (42.9%) in care planning was limited.

In line with NSF and NHS Plan targets, there has been an increased provision of 300 medium-secure beds (so that numbers increased between the late 1990s and 2002–03 from 1,750 to 2,060) and 200 extra long-term secure beds in the NHS (Appleby 2004). This investment aimed to reduce the need for Trusts to buy in expensive secure provision in the private sector for the most difficult to manage patients, aided the transfer of patients inappropriately placed in high secure hospitals and addressed NSF standards to ensure that people are admitted to the least restrictive environment as close to home as possible. But the picture concerning acute in-patient admissions is less clear. Surprisingly, given the costs involved, most services do not have figures for out-of-area referrals of acute in-patients. Appleby (2004) suggests there is anecdotal evidence that the introduction of crisis resolution and home treatment teams and stricter managerial regulation has reduced dependence on OATs in some areas, as has the use of 'half-way hotel' accommodation and community link workers (Greatorex 2002), but such initiatives need to become commonplace.

Care planning

The intolerable pressure of bed over-occupancy reported on acute units in the 1990s has continued. A national survey of adult psychiatric wards in England reported average bed occupancy rates of 100% (SCMH 2005a), at the very time when home treatment teams and crisis resolution services were expected to reduce the demand for in-patient beds. The continuation of such a level of occupancy prevents the provision of an effective, quality service and leaves staff managing crises rather than providing care (Quirk & Lelliott 2001). Such bed pressures also require staff to move acutely unwell patients between wards, to 'sleep over' and then return for their daily 'treatment', as though this is in some way divorced from the provision of a therapeutic milieu. Ward staff also have to use patients' beds when they are on leave and when demand is greatest, send people home before they, their family, informal carers and community support are prepared (Brennan et al 2006). Such procedures stretch any interpretation of the NSF standard that service users should have timely access to an appropriate hospital bed. It also challenges the capacity of staff to ensure that after-care arrangements and written care plans are in place when patients are discharged at short notice, a factor reported by occupational therapists working on acute wards, frustrated when their assessments of the person's ability to live independently are ignored because of the need to discharge patients quickly (Simpson et al 2005).

The failure to ensure all patients are provided with comprehensive, written care plans under the Care Programme Approach (CPA) was identified in inspections of mental health trusts conducted by the Commission for Health Improvement (CHI 2004). Implementation of the CPA remained problematic with large numbers of people not placed on the CPA or allocated a care plan and coordinator. In some trusts, CHI found continued clinical resistance to the CPA and the associated documentation. Although some trusts had reviewed CPA procedures, redesigned documentation and piloted electronic systems, practice in many trusts remained inconsistent and incomplete.

These findings were also reflected in a survey of care planning for people who are repeatedly admitted to hospital under the Mental Health Act (SCMH 2005b). This group includes those most in need of comprehensive, co-ordinated care planning – given that they were identified in the survey as being admitted to hospital because of concerns for their safety or the safety of others and for non-compliance with treatment. As part of their normal visiting programme, Mental Health Act Commissioners visited 119 wards in 57 units within 15 NHS Trusts, across all 8 NIMHE regions. Information was collected from the case notes of 277 service users, 151 of whom were also interviewed. Although the survey found pockets of good practice, the overall picture was poor. There was wide variation between groups of patients in the type and level of needs being assessed and addressed, with people from Black and Asian groups, women and older people faring less well. From both the review of case notes and interviews with patients it was clear that few patients were being given written care plans prior to discharge, that those plans frequently omitted key information such as the next review date, and CPA care coordinators were infrequently involved in either aftercare planning or immediate follow-up of discharged patients. A fifth of service users were re-admitted within 90 days.

Hospital environment

Several actions have been taken to improve the physical, environmental and therapeutic status of in-patient wards and the Government has made available significant new funds to initiate a programme of new building and the refurbishment of in-patient wards (Appleby 2004). In 2004, the Commission for Health Improvement (CHI) summarised the results of clinical governance reviews undertaken in half the mental health Trusts in England and other special investigations. They acknowledged that the inspections took place whilst many Trusts were being re-organised and the 10-year plan for improvements was still only halfway completed, but found enormous variations in quality of environment with the better services showing what is possible:

> *'Some of the new accommodation provides excellent facilities with single sex sleeping and bathroom facilities, gyms, multisensory rooms, libraries, gardens, music and computer rooms.'*
>
> (CHI 2004, p21)

But services in older buildings or where modernisation was yet to take place left much to be desired, with CHI describing the physical environment of many in-patient units as 'unacceptable', reflecting the historical legacy of the neglect of mental health services (CHI 2004, p9). Appleby (2004) reported that in 2003 the Patient Environment Action Team (PEAT) paid particular attention to mental health units, addressing standards of cleanliness and the quality of the environment and food. No mental health trust was assessed as less than acceptable and many were rated as good. This positive picture, however, has been challenged by more recent and arguably tougher inspections conducted by the Healthcare Commission (2005a), which visited 33 NHS mental health hospitals (60 wards and 20 outpatients) and 17 independent mental hospitals (21 wards and 2 outpatients). Facilities were placed in one of four bands with band one signifying a good level of cleanliness, band two generally good with some room for improvement, band three suggested systemic problems with the cleaning programme and band four signified serious concerns. The authors concluded that:

> *'Overall, standards were markedly poorer in mental health hospitals compared to acute hospitals (mental health hospitals made up all six hospitals in the bottom band four and 18 out of the 22 hospitals in bands three and four).'*
>
> (Healthcare Commission 2005a, p16)

In many ways mental health hospitals serve a different purpose to acute hospitals, with fewer concerns about pre- and postoperative infections. Mental health patients also sometimes make requests to not have their sleeping areas cleaned and the therapeutic concern is more one of treating patients with dignity and respect and of creating an environment in which patients can be looked after effectively. However, the Healthcare Commission concluded that there was still an expectation that mental health patients are cared for in a safe and clean environment and that some acute psychiatric wards in both NHS and independent hospitals were rated in band one, illustrating that achieving good standards of cleanliness was possible.

Therapeutic activities

Service users regularly report that being in an acute ward is, above all else, boring with little available to keep people occupied (Lelliott & Quirk 2004). CHI (2004) reported that the availability of therapeutic activities varied from trust to trust, with low staffing levels and the use of agency staff frequently affecting the range of activities available. Users commonly report that the range and quality of activities are limited, with few organised to keep them occupied in the evening and at weekends. The absence of occupational therapists in the staff team in particular reduces therapeutic activity on wards. One study that explored the work of occupational therapists on acute wards, reported that their input was highly valued by other members of the multidisciplinary team in relation to the overall assessment and treatment planning of users as well as in the provision of therapeutic groups and other activities. However, even where therapists were regularly available, the high level of acuity amongst patients and the pressure to discharge people swiftly posed particular challenges in the design and delivery of activities (Simpson et al 2005).

Many nurses working in acute settings are hugely frustrated at the way documentation and administrative tasks have become such a large part of their role. When combined with scheduled tasks such as medication rounds, meal times and doctors' rounds, to find some quality time to sit down and talk with users is very difficult. Yet most nurses would prefer to spend time engaging with the people they are looking after and go home with some feeling of job satisfaction. One initiative that seems to have caught the imagination of staff on mental health units is that of 'Protected Engagement Time' (Kent 2005). First introduced as part of a ward 'refocusing project' (Bowles & Howard 2003), it has subsequently been used to good effect in various parts of England and elsewhere where there has been a desire to improve the level of therapeutic interaction on wards.

When protected engagement time is introduced, nurses come out of their offices, divert the ward phone, ignore the photocopier, lock the ward door and spend time engaging with patients. Activities are planned and are a major focus for this period and on most wards, involvement of occupational and art therapists, psychiatrists and pharmacists is actively encouraged. It seems to work best for an hour or two during afternoons as morning shifts often bring too many demands and diversions, including blood tests, admissions, routine activities, ward rounds, and so on.

A series of ideas and initiatives, including protected engagement time, designed to improve the quality of the ward environment and the range of activities available on acute psychiatric wards have been collated into one document. 'Star Wards' provides practical ideas for improving the daily experiences and treatment outcomes of acute mental health in-patients and includes 75 ideas for making the most of patients' time. This commendable report and more recent suggestions can be downloaded free from the Star Wards website (Janner 2006).

Of course, providing therapeutic input and activities would be a lot easier if staffing levels on acute wards were at a reasonable level. The national survey of acute wards reported a national average vacancy rate for qualified nurses of 13% and 22% in London with staff working unpaid overtime on a quarter of all wards (SCMH 2005a). But given the extra demands now being placed on acute in-patient staff – to provide more intensive care for acutely ill and resistant patients, provide more activities and effective therapy, administer CPA documentation and liaise with community services – it has also been argued that staffing levels and skill mix need to be reconsidered in order to reflect the true cost of delivering care in this setting and to ensure that high quality, effective in-patient care and treatment takes place (McKee et al 2006).

Safety and security

In line with the NSF, admission to a psychiatric ward is often required to ensure the safety of the person being admitted and of others. Consequently, patient and staff safety is a critical issue for modern acute psychiatric services. The Ward Watch survey by mental health charity Mind reported that 27% of respondents rarely felt safe in hospital and half of recent or current in-patients reported being verbally or physically threatened during their stay (Mind 2004). The Royal College of Psychiatrists' National Audit of Violence, commissioned by the Healthcare Commission, found that a third of in-patients had experienced violent or threatening behaviour while in care. This figure rose to 41% for clinical staff and nearly 80% of nursing staff working in in-patient units (Healthcare Commission 2005b), although there is evidence that feeling threatened is a far more likely outcome than experiencing any kind of injury (Foster et al 2007).

The National Patient Safety Agency analysed nearly 45,000 mental health incidents reported to the National Reporting and Learning System from almost 80% of mental health/combined trusts in England and Wales (NPSA 2006). A staggering 83% of mental health patient safety incidents occurred in in-patient areas that received just 162,250 admissions out of more than a million people receiving mental health care across the NHS in 2003/4. After accidents, the three most commonly reported incidents were disruptive/aggressive incidents (10,467; 23%); self-harm (7,726; 17%); and absconding (3,827; 9%); totalling nearly half of all reports. Almost all reported incidents of aggression (9,591; 92%) occurred in in-patient settings and over half of all claims of clinical negligence refer to incidents of self-harm or violent/disruptive behaviour. As a result, the National Patient Safety Agency has identified acute psychiatric care as a priority area for attention.

The Commission for Health Improvement (CHI) has expressed concern at the way mental health trusts deal with safety issues and found problems with the quality of hospital environments, staffing levels and skills and systems for preventing and managing risk (CHI 2004). They reported that whilst trusts were generally good at reporting incidents, they were less successful at feeding back to staff and learning from episodes. Some staff lacked confidence in managing violence due to lack of training or shortage of the necessary skills and permanent staff often felt unsafe because bank and agency staff do not have the skills to support them when a violent incident occurs.

In-patient care of Black and Minority Ethnic patients (BME), especially in relation to disproportionate use of containment, is also an issue of growing concern, as highlighted by the Count Me In census (CHAI 2005). The census found that Black, African and Caribbean people are three times more likely to be hospitalised with mental health problems than the rest of the population, and that once in hospital, Black men are 50% more likely to be secluded and 29% more likely to be subject to physical control or restraint than white men. Plans to address this situation are outlined in the NHS Developing Race Equality strategy (DH 2004) (see Chapter 4).

Patients in mental health units and those recently discharged are also at high risk of suicide (Meehan et al 2006). The National Suicide Prevention Strategy for England includes actions targeting the reduction of suicide among people who are known to mental health services (DH 2002c) and there has been a steady reduction in completed suicide by in-patients. The latest figures from the Confidential Inquiry into Homicides and Suicides show that as a proportion of all patient suicides, in-patient suicides have fallen from 17% in 1997 to 11% in 2004 (Appleby et al 2006). Deaths by hanging or strangulation on the ward itself fell from 53 in 1997 to 26 in 2004. However, more than three in-patient suicides still take place each week and every suicide is a tragedy for the person and their family, and is often devastating for the staff directly and indirectly involved (Bowers et al 2006). Reporting of self-harm amongst psychiatric patients remains high and is a strong predictor of suicide (Appleby et al 2006). Results from a large study of self-harm on 136 acute psychiatric wards in England found that frequent checks on patients through intermittent observation, increased activities for patients on the ward and greater presence of qualified nursing staff were strongly associated with reduced levels of self-harm, including suicide (Bowers et al 2007).

Another area of concern is that of sexual harassment and assault. In 1998, the Mental Health Act commission found sexual harassment of women patients on over half the mixed wards surveyed, while only 34 of the 291 wards had written policies on sexual harassment and abuse (Ford et al 1998). The Department of Health pledged to abolish mixed sex wards and all mental health trusts were required to comply with guidance on single sex accommodation, which aimed to increase the safety of female patients especially through the introduction of women-only sleeping, bathroom and day facilities (DH 2000b). According to the 2004 star ratings, 98% of mental health trusts were complying with the guidance on women only facilities (Appleby 2004), but academics and campaigners suggested this was far from the experience of many mental health service users, with some mental health trusts making superficial changes to comply with the guidance (Copperman 2006).

The National Patient Safety Agency reported that there were 122 reported sexual incidents involving patients in mental health care settings in England between November 2003 and September 2005 (NPSA 2006). The NPSA suggested that such incidents were most likely under-reported and a survey by mental health charity, Mind, found that fewer than four in ten harassment or abuse incidents were reported to staff, with fear of reprisal and a lack of confidence that any action would be taken as the main reasons for this (Mind 2004). Such disclosures underscore the need to ensure that patient safety remains a key priority. But even if policy recommendations are fully implemented, it is unlikely that all risk of sexual harassment and assault can be removed in environments where disinhibited behaviours are common as a result of mental illness. It would appear that this is another area that would benefit from greater staff presence and interaction with patients.

Absconding by patients from acute psychiatric wards is a significant problem and the National Confidential Inquiry into Suicides and Homicides found that 27% of psychiatric in-patients who died by suicide had absconded from the ward at the time (Appleby et al 2006). While the majority of absconds pass with no harm being caused and patients return by themselves, they still cause the staff a considerable amount of anxiety. In addition, a great deal of work is required on the part of both psychiatric staff and the police, in order to complete reports, and occasionally assist the patient to return to hospital. The confidence of relatives and carers in the psychiatric services can also collapse when a patient leaves the ward without the knowledge and agreement of the clinical team. Research into the problems of absconding has led to the development of an evidence-based intervention and training package for acute ward staff that has been shown to reduce officially reported rates of absconding from partly locked or open wards by a quarter (Bowers et al 2003, 2005b). The package has been recommended for use by the Mental Health Act Commission (MHAC 2005).

Progress and challenges

Undoubtedly, more attention in terms of policies, guidance, training and research has been lavished on acute services in the wake of the alarming reports of the late 1990s. Yet, at the same time, genuine, frustrating pressures are faced by acute care managers, staff and service users as wards and beds are closed, occupancy rates remain unmanageably high, throughput is frantic and staffing levels are a concern. At the time of writing, this situation was being exacerbated as mental health trusts were forced to make cuts to services to help resolve wider NHS funding difficulties. Freezing vacancies and cutting in-patient units and beds were identified as the primary methods employed to make large savings (SCMH 2006).

The evidence suggests that the NSF standard that requires patients to be provided with a written after-care plan agreed on discharge remains elusive. Whilst there may well be pockets of good practice, it is a serious cause for concern that significant numbers of service users, including those people with the most severe and complex needs, are still not being provided with effective after-care planning. Despite being a key plank of mental health policy for 15 years now, compliance with the requirements of the CPA has long been problematic (Simpson et al 2003). It is likely to remain so as long as there is a refusal to acknowledge and address the structural tensions that undermine this policy, such as the constant demand for in-patient beds and the high caseloads of community staff and teams. Effective care planning has also been found wanting where people are admitted to hospitals out of their local area.

The combined impact of home treatment teams and heavy pressure from senior NHS management has most likely reduced the reliance on out of area treatments, with most people now admitted to hospitals close to home. However, this has been achieved by placing additional pressures on acute ward staff and their patients, forced to make beds available for people desperate to be admitted, often by moving or discharging others not quite ready for a return to community living – even with the support of home treatment teams. In addition, the early data on home treatment teams suggests that only certain demographic groups are being diverted from hospital admissions and that young, male, more disturbed patients and those compulsorily detained under the law are as likely to be admitted (Glover et al 2006). The impact on patients and staff of a more acutely unwell, treatment-resistant ward population has yet to be investigated but needs doing with some urgency. Equally, the tendency of Trusts to close beds and wards as home treatment teams take on more patients simply maintains the pressures on ward staff instead of enabling them to develop more sensitive, effective care.

The results of the national census on ethnicity in psychiatric services also suggest the need for more attention to be paid to the experiences of people from Black and Minority Ethnic communities. The Government's five-year action plan, 'Delivering Race Equality in Mental Health Care', calls for more responsive services delivered by a more culturally capable workforce and for training in cultural sensitivity for all those involved in planning or delivering services. Some have concerns that such approaches will fail to improve delivery of services as the design and patterns of service use are more important in determining use and acceptability of services.

The evidence concerning safety and security on acute wards remains contradictory and complex. Suicide rates appear to be reducing but can still be significantly improved with particular attention to absconding and post-discharge planning and aftercare. Aggressive and antisocial behaviour appears to be a constant problem for staff and patients and makes in-patient services unwelcoming places to be cared for and to work in. Similarly, the need to prevent sexually inappropriate behaviour and sexual assault pose daunting questions for the organisation and operation of our services.

The challenge remains to provide a place of safety and care whilst balancing the desires of service users and staff alike to avoid creating an authoritarian, prison-like environment where restrictions and regulations submerge the considerate, nurturing, humane interactions and interventions that are required to encourage recovery and the achievement of potential. Promising initiatives are emerging to increase the level of contact and therapeutic interaction between ward staff and patients and the wards continue to be staffed by many committed, skilled staff keen to make a difference in people's lives. However, the blocks and barriers to creating and maintaining positive change continue to be considerable and will require dedicated and substantial political and financial commitment to overcome.

Acknowledgements

Thanks to all members of the research team in the Department of Mental Health at City University for sharing and discussion of projects and ideas, although the choice of content and responsibility for the above remains the author's.

References

Appleby L 2004 The National Service Framework for Mental Health – Five Years On. London, Department of Health

Appleby L, Shaw J, Kapur N, Windfuhr K et al 2006 Avoidable deaths: five year report by the national confidential inquiry into suicide and homicide by people with mental illness (accesssed 21 August 2007: http://www.medicine.manchester.ac.uk/suicideprevention/nci/Useful/avoidable_deaths_full_report.pdf)

Audit Commission 2006 Managing finances in mental health. The Audit Commission, London

Baker S 2000 Environmentally friendly? Patients' views of conditions on psychiatric wards. Mind, London

Bosanquet N, de Zoete H, Haldenby A 2006 Mental health services in the NHS: using reform incentives. Reform, London

Bowers L, Alexander J, Gaskell C 2003 A controlled trial of an intervention to reduce absconding from acute psychiatric wards. Journal of Psychiatric and Mental Health Nursing 10:410–416

Bowers L, Simpson A, Alexander J 2005b Real world application of an intervention to reduce absconding. Journal of Psychiatric and Mental Health Nursing, 12, 598–602 (accessed 21 August 2007: www.citypsych.com/absconding_home.asp)

Bowers L, Simpson A, Alexander J et al 2005a The nature and purpose of acute psychiatric wards: the Tompkins acute ward study. Journal of Mental Health 14(6):625–635

Bowers L, Simpson A, Eyres S et al 2006 Serious untoward incidents and their aftermath in acute in-patient psychiatry: the Tompkins acute ward study. International Journal of Mental Health Nursing 15(4):226–234

Bowers L, Whittington R, Nolan P et al 2007 The city 128 study of observation and outcomes on acute psychiatric wards: report to the NHS SDO Programme. City University, London (accessed 21 August 2007: www.citypsych.com/docs/city128.pdf)

Bowles N, Howard R 2003 The refocusing model: a means of realising the National Acute In-patient Strategy. Mental Health Review 8(1):27–31

Brennan G, Flood C, Bowers L 2006 Constraints and blocks to change and improvement on acute psychiatric wards – lessons from the City Nurses project. Journal of Psychiatric and Mental Health Nursing 13(5):475–482

CHAI 2005 Count Me In: Results of a national census of in-patients in mental hospitals and facilities in England and Wales. Commission for Healthcare Audit and Inspection, London

CHI 2004 What CHI has found in mental health trusts: sector report. Commission for Health Improvement, London

Copperman, J 2006 The abuse that no one stops. London, Guardian Unlimited (accessed 21 August 2007: http://www.guardian.co.uk/uk_news/story/0,1827866,00.html)

Department of Health 1999 National Service Framework for Mental Health. DH, London

Department of Health 2000a The NHS Plan: A plan for investment. A plan for reform. DH, London

Department of Health 2000b Safety, privacy and dignity in mental health units. DH, London

Department of Health 2002a Mental Health Policy Implementation Guide: Adult Acute In-patient Care Provision. DH, London

Department of Health 2002b National Minimum Standards for General Adult Services in Psychiatric Intensive Care Units (PICU) and Low Secure Environments. DH, London

Department of Health 2002c National Suicide Prevention Strategy for England. DH, London

Department of Health 2004 Delivering Race Equality: A Framework for Action in Mental Health Services. DH, London

Ford R, Durcan G, Warner L 1998 One day survey by the Mental Health Act Commission of acute adult psychiatric in-patient wards in England and Wales. British Medical Journal 317:1279–1283

Foster C, Bowers L, Nijman H 2007 Aggressive behaviour on acute psychiatric wards: prevalence, severity and management. Journal of Advanced Nursing 58(2):140–149

Glover G, Arts G, Babu K S 2006 Crisis resolution/home treatment teams and psychiatric admission rates in England. British Journal of Psychiatry 189:441–445

Goodwin I, Holmes G, Newnes C, Waltho D 1999 A qualitative analysis of the view of in-patient mental health service users. Journal of Mental Health 8:43–54

Greatorex H 2002 A fresh strategy on in-patient beds. Mental Health Practice 5(6):8–10

Greengross P, Hollander D, Stanton R 1996 Pressure on adult acute psychiatric beds. Results of a national questionnaire survey. Psychiatric Bulletin 24:54–56

Healthcare Commission 2005a A snapshot of hospital cleanliness in England: Findings from the Healthcare Commission's rapid inspection programme. Commission for Healthcare Audit and Inspection, London

Healthcare Commission 2005b National Audit of Violence (2003–2005). Healthcare Commission, London

Janner M 2006 Star Wards: Practical ideas for improving the daily experiences and treatment outcomes of acute mental health in-patients. Bright, London (accessed 21 August 2007: www.starwards.org.uk)

Lelliott P, Quirk A 2004 What is life like on acute psychiatric wards? Current Opinion in Psychiatry 17:297–301

Kent M 2005 My mental health: protected therapeutic time. Mental Health Practice 8(8):22

McKee P, Harrison A, Smith G 2006 Nursing establishments within acute in-patient mental health units: the need for clarity. Mental Health Practice 9(8):18–21

Meehan J et al 2006 Suicide in mental health in-patients and within 3 months of discharge. British Journal of Psychiatry 188:129–134.

MHAC 2005 In place of fear? The eleventh biennial report of the Mental Health Act Commission. The Stationery Office, London

Mind 2004 Ward watch: Mind's campaign to improve hospital conditions for mental health patients: Report summary. Mind, London

NPSA 2006 With safety in mind: mental health services and patient safety. Patient Safety Observatory Report 2. National Patient Safety Agency, London

Quirk A, Lelliott P 2001 What do we know about life on acute psychiatric wards in the UK? A review of the research evidence. Social Science and Medicine 53:1565–1574

Ryan T, Hills B, Webb L 2002 Nurse staffing levels and budgeted expenditure in acute mental health wards: a benchmarking study. Journal of Psychiatric and Mental Health Nursing 11:73–81

Ryan T, Pearsall A, Hatfield B, Poole R 2004 Long term care for serious mental illness outside the NHS: a study of out of area placements. Journal of Mental Health 13(4):425–429

SCMH 1998 Acute problems: a survey of the quality of care in acute psychiatric wards. Sainsbury Centre for Mental Health, London

SCMH 2005a Acute Care 2004: a national survey of adult acute wards in England. Sainsbury Centre for Mental Health, London

SCMH 2005b The Care Programme Approach – Back on Track? Sainsbury Centre for Mental Health, London

SCMH 2006 Under Pressure: The finances of Mental Health Trusts in 2006. Sainsbury Centre for Mental Health, London

Simpson A 2000a Taking a pounding. Health Service Journal 110(5710):26–27

Simpson A 2000b Private care's win-win. Mental Health Nursing 20(8):6–9

Simpson A, Bowers L, Alexander J, Ridley C, Warren J 2005 Occupational therapy and multidisciplinary working on acute psychiatric wards: the Tompkins acute ward study. British Journal of Occupational Therapy 86(12):545–552

Simpson A, Miller C, Bowers L 2003 The history of the care programme approach in England: where did it go wrong? Journal of Mental Health 12(5):489–504

SNMAC 1999 Mental health nursing: Addressing acute concerns. London: Standing Nursing and Midwifery Advisory Committee, Department of Health

Thornicroft G, Tansella M 2004 Components of a modern mental health service: a pragmatic balance of community and hospital care. British Journal of Psychiatry 185:283–290

Walton P 2000 Psychiatric hospital care – a case of the more things change, the more they stay the same. Journal of Mental Health 9:77–88

Warner L 2005 Acute care in crisis. In: Bell A, Lindley P (eds) Beyond the water towers: the unfinished revolution in mental health services, 1985–2005. Sainsbury Centre for Mental Health, London, p37–48

Community Mental Health Teams

J. Boardman

Introduction

Teams have held great currency throughout the post-war transition of mental health services in England from the asylum system to the more comprehensive hospital and community based mental health services seen at the close of the twentieth century. In practice, teams and their approach have become ubiquitous and a consensus about their worth has developed but, in particular, the Community Mental Health Team (CMHT) has gained a prominent place in the delivery of community based mental health services and it is these teams that are discussed in this chapter. In relation to the National Service Framework for mental health (NSF-MH) the CMHT in England cannot be understood without considering its historical development and this will be outlined before considering the research evidence for its worth and its particular status in the NSF-MH.

Policy and the development of the Community Mental Health Team

Since 1948 developments in mental health services have featured the running down and closure of large mental hospitals, the development of extra-mural facilities and the increasing realisation of the importance of primary health care (Jones 1972, Rose 2001, Boardman 2005). Associated with these post-war developments has been one area on which those working in mental health services may agree a consensus – there is a need to replace large psychiatric hospitals with community provision for those people who would have traditionally been admitted to the asylums. The development of generic, community based, mental health teams for working age adults, with a multidisciplinary membership, often providing services to a geographically defined catchment area service, has been central to this community provision.

Community Mental Health Centres and Teams

The literature on the development of CMHTs has used two terms: Community Mental Health Team (CMHT) and Community Mental Health Centre (CMHC). In this chapter, the term CMHC will denote a building, CMHT will denote a multidisciplinary team which may be based in a CMHC.

In the USA, CMHCs were developed in the 1960s as a 'system for delivery of services' and were seen as a *network* (Sharfstein 1978, Fink & Weinstein 1979, Mollica 1980, Levene 1981). In the UK, CMHCs have more often been equated with buildings and the conception has never been as grandiose as in the USA although a UK CMHC movement has had its proponents (Jones 1979). In the literature CMHCs were associated with CMHTs and these terms, at times, have been used interchangeably.

Before the late 1980s, there was little information on the existence of CMHCs and CMHTs in the UK. There were reports from individual centres (e.g. Brough & Bouras 1982, McAusland 1985) but no national overview. In 1987 the first national conference on CMHCs was held (Boardman et al 1988) and in 1987/88 the first survey of CMHCs was undertaken. In 1987 the British CMHC was considered an innovation, an occasional departure from more traditional forms of psychiatric service. The only available list suggested that there were 20 in the country (Good Practices in Mental Health 1985). At that time the debate on their role and contribution concentrated on two areas: the potential neglect of people with long-term mental illness and the possible advantages of a new style of service exploring accessibility, multidisciplinary skills, and sensitivity to the needs of users and local communities.

In the 1987/88 survey, conducted in the UK, a CMHC was defined as that which provided adult services, was outside hospital, staffed by a multidisciplinary team and conducted at least some direct patient work from the centre but offered more than structured day care (Sayce et al 1991). The survey showed that there had been a rapid growth of CMHCs during 1980s. The numbers doubled every two years culminating in 81 centres opened by end 1987. A further 61 were planned with allocated funding, as well as 169 planned less firmly. A follow-up survey, conducted in 1989 (Sayce et al 1991), showed no let up in this trend: twice as many CMHCs were reported open at the end of 1988 as at end of 1987. At the time it was noted that if this trend were repeated nationally it would mean an average of more than one CMHC per district at end of 1989.

The national survey highlighted several problems of CMHCs, not least their possible drift from patients with severe mental illness. This survey was supported by evidence from a CMHC in Lewisham, south-east London, which had reported improved access but with a result of seeing an increasing number of patients with short-term disorders (Boardman & Bouras 1988). A more in-depth study of six comprehensive CMHCs by Patmore & Weaver (1991) raised further concerns. They found a large variation in the extent to which they served sufferers of severe mental illness and noted that access for the severely mentally ill was the main CMHC shortcoming.

In 1993 a survey of CMHTs in 183 districts in England revealed changes since 1988 (Onyett et al 1994). People with severe and long-term mental health problems now comprised an average 57% of teams' caseloads. The majority (96.3%) of CMHTs had catchment areas. Over 50% of CMHTs were based in CMHCs or resource centres and 57% offered first point of contact of all mental health referrals in a sector. Despite this there were no emergency services outside office hours, a finding reinforced by Johnson & Thornicroft (1995).

These studies indicated that generic CMHTs, by the early 1990s, were in the ascendancy, with the increase seen in the 1980s being continued into the 1990s. As CMHTs continued to develop in the 1990s the literature began to focus on the purpose and working of the multidisciplinary team (Galvin & McCarthy 1994, Onyett 1995, Mistral & Velleman 1997, Norman & Peck 1999). The possible neglect of people with severe and long-term mental illness and the targeting of services on this group of users were largely resolved and their priorities gained support from government policy (DH 1994, 1995). Doubts expressed about the efficacy of CMHTs (Galvin & McCarthy 1994) were countered by others (Onyett & Ford 1996, Onyett 1999, King 2001) who saw the benefits of CMHTs.

By the end of the 1990s, CMHTs were part of government policy (DH 1995, 1996) and became the most common model for the coordination of community mental health services for people with severe mental illness in the UK (Peck 1999). They became central to the delivery of the standards of the NSF-MH, but now supported by a planned development of a number of multidisciplinary specialist community teams which were outlined in the NSF-MH and the Mental Health Policy Implementation Guide (DH 1999, 2001a).

CMHTs are now ubiquitous and a core means of delivering secondary mental health care in England. From the 81 recorded by Sayce et al (1991) in 1987, they had grown to 826 by spring 2006 (Centre for Public Mental Health, University of Durham, 2006). In England there is now one team per 38,868 adult population with a total of 13,502 care staff.

Research/evidence base

A belief in the value of CMHTs, a consensus about their place in community mental health care and their position in government policy now places the CMHT at the centre of mental health services. But what research evidence backs the confidence placed in them? Summarising the research and evidence base for CMHTs is fraught with difficulty, not least because of the difficulty in defining the subject of the research, the CMHT.

In Simmonds et al's (2001) systematic review of CMHT management of people with severe mental illness (SMI), CMHT management was defined as:

> *'generic care (i.e. care not supplemented by ACT, intensive case management or any other specified model) from a community-based multidisciplinary team that provides a full range of interventions to adults aged 18–65 years with severe mental illness from a defined catchment area.'*

The studies examined in the review compared this form of management to 'standard care' which was 'usual care in the area concerned, provided that this care was not furnished by another community team'. In practice this was mainly hospital based out-patient care. Only five studies satisfied the inclusion criteria for the systematic review and these were from: Australia (Hoult et al 1981, Hoult & Reynoulds 1984), Canada (Fenton et al 1979) and London (Merson et al 1992, Burns et al 1993a,b, Tyrer et al 1995). Combining the results from these studies, the reviewers concluded that CMHT management was associated with fewer deaths from suicide and in suspicious circumstances, less dissatisfaction with care, fewer drop outs, shorter duration of in-patient treatment and lower costs of care. Whilst there were no reported gains in symptoms or social functioning, there were no outcomes for which the standard care was superior to the care delivered by a CMHT.

In the commentary to the review, Holloway (2001) expressed disappointment at the paucity of evidence for CMHTs, given their centrality in modern mental health care, but this disappointment may be tempered if a broader perspective is taken. The studies included in the review overlap with those included in other systematic reviews of community based care: crisis care (Joy et al 1998) and home-based care (Catty et al 2002) highlighting the overlap of a range of approaches to community-based mental health care including Assertive Community Treatment (ACT; Marshall & Lockwood 1998), Case Management (Marshall et al 1998), Home treatment (Catty et al 2002) and Crisis Care (Joy et al 1998) – all of which show some positive support for a 'community team' approach for people with SMI.

Notwithstanding the debates about the worth of particular approaches, for example ACT versus Care Management (Mueser et al 1998), the reviews generally conclude that these community based approaches prove to be superior on a range of indicators (to a greater or lesser extent) than 'treatment as usual' (usually hospital based care – in- or out-patient) and can reduce bed use and increase satisfaction without increasing overall costs. In addition, the studies that use community based mental health services as controls achieve less reduction in hospitalisation rates than studies where the controls were based on hospital care (Catty et al 2002), suggesting an overall greater worth of community based care. Other studies support and illustrate the superiority of community based team approaches over hospital care. The PRiSM study (Thornicroft et al 1998) and the UK 700 study (Burns 2002), whilst yielding no differences in the approaches tested, both showed satisfactory outcomes which were superior to hospital based models of care. These research studies are in agreement with other more polemically argued reviews suggesting that community care has not 'failed' (e.g. Thornicroft & Goldberg 1998).

Whilst these studies lend support to the general effectiveness of community based mental health teams, they do not directly address the matter of the efficacy of generic CMHTs as characterised at the beginning of this chapter. In addition, they focus on the CMHT care of people with SMI, ignoring that CMHTs often have another function – the assessment and management of people with more prevalent disorders referred by General Practitioners. This CMHT function is less widely researched and the evidence is less convincing. The setting up of sector-based CMHTs (Boardman et al 1987) and the presence of a multidisciplinary team in primary care (Jackson et al 1993) increases access to care. Two studies have shown some improved outcome in patients with anxiety and depression who use CMHTs compared to conventional outpatient clinics (Boardman et al 1986, Goldberg et al 1996).

Overall there appears to be support for the effectiveness of CMHTs over hospital based care for people with SMI, which is an endorsement of an approach based on multidisciplinary teams working in the community. The work of CMHTs with people with more prevalent disorders has been less frequently evaluated but access for these groups to assessment and treatment does appear to be improved. The key question now is how does the generic CMHT fit with the new Assertive Outreach, Crisis Resolution and Early Intervention teams. Does this approach provide effective and efficacious delivery of community based mental health care? How does this balance with the other services in the community, including the in-patient units, day care and other services, and primary care? The creation of these teams in line with the NSF-MH has not been evaluated and we may have missed an opportunity to monitor and assess the implementation of these teams, their effect on the delivery of local services for people with SMI and more prevalent forms of disorders.

Recommendations of mental health policy

CMHTs have been part of government policy since the mid-1990s (DH 1995, 1996). The Spectrum of Care (DH 1996) provided a description of CMHTs consistent with that used in this chapter and emphasised the importance of skills and roles of the professionals in the team:

> 'Community mental health teams cover defined population groups. This means each team is responsible for delivering and co-coordinating a specialised level of care. The teams include social workers; mental health nurses; psychologists; occupational therapists and psychiatrists.
> These professional groups will have skills specific to their particular profession, and will have other skills in common with others. They are expected to use skills in a flexible way, so that they can work together as teams to meet the full range os the people referred to them. If they need to treat a patient in hospital they should continue to provide care and support during the admission as well as at home after discharge.'
>
> (Spectrum of Care, p5)

The Spectrum of Care (DH 1996, p10) also offered a view on CMHCs, which has never been adopted policy:
'CMHCs offer bases for local teams to:

- assess health and social care needs
- carry out interviews
- run clubs
- provide adult education
- provide advice
- run other schemes.

The centres also provide valuable links with primary health care, and so allow the monitoring of significant, and sometimes chronic, physical health care problems.'

The NSF-MH (DH 1999, p47) gives the CMHT a role of central importance in the delivery of community mental health services:

> 'Community mental health teams provide the core of local specialised mental health services. Service users are more likely to stay in contact with community rather than hospital based services and are more likely to accept treatment. Studies suggest that these services help to reduce suicide rates.'

Their comprehensive function is acknowledged, but there appears to be some ambivalence as to their relationship to the other specialised community teams and the functions that they provide:

> 'Community mental health teams may provide the whole range of community based services themselves, or may be complemented by one or more teams providing specific functions. This latter model is common in inner city and urban areas. Whichever model is used, the mental health system will need to provide the range of intervention and integration across all specialist services.'
>
> 'Community mental health teams may work with other specialist teams covering early intervention; assertive outreach; home treatment; the needs of those with co-morbidity; black and minority ethnic communities; homeless people; or mentally disordered offenders. Rehabilitation teams focus specifically on the housing, income, occupational and social needs of people with serious disabilities resulting from their mental illness.'

The Mental Health Policy Implementation Guide (MHPIG) (DH 2001a) reiterates the central importance of CMHTs, but leaves open the possibility of CMHTs changing their role over time to work more closely with primary care:

> 'CMHTs, in some places known as Primary Care Liaison Teams, will continue to be a mainstream of the system. CMHTs have an important, indeed integral, role to play in supporting service users and families in community settings. They should provide the core around which newer service elements are developed. The responsibilities of CMHTs may change over time, however they retain an important role. They, alongside primary care will provide the key sources of referral to the newer teams. They will also continue to care for the majority of people with mental illness in the community.'
>
> (Mental Health Policy Implementation Guide, p6–7)

> 'In the future, especially as other services and teams come on stream, it may be helpful to scope new roles for CMHTs in relation to primary care.'
>
> (Mental Health Policy Implementation Guide, p66)

The Mental Health Policy Implementation Guide for Community Mental Health Teams (DH 2002a) reiterates the view that these teams are the mainstay of the system and the core around which newer services are developed. The CMHT was seen as providing functions for two groups of people:

1. *Most patients treated by the CMHT will have time limited disorders and be referred back to their GPs after a period of weeks or months (an average of 5–6 contacts; Burns et al 1993b) when their condition has improved*
2. *A substantial minority, however, will remain with the team for ongoing treatment, care and monitoring for periods of several years. They will include people needing ongoing specialists care...*

(Mental Health Policy Implementation Guide for Community Mental Health Teams, p4)

The Mental Health Policy Implementation Guide for Community Mental Health Teams gives more specific details on the functioning of these teams than has been seen before in government policy documents. The Department of Health suggest that CMHTs should offer people short-term contact services and continuing treatment, care and monitoring, and that their functions include:

- work with primary care to provide a single point of entry
- assessment
- a multidisciplinary team approach
- regular review, including multidisciplinary and multi-agency review
- a range of interventions
- liaison with other parts of the health system and other agencies
- provision of discharge and transfer arrangements.

The Mental Health Policy Implementation Guide for Community Mental Health Teams recommends that each CMHT serve a population of 10,000–60,000 depending on the local levels of morbidity and travelling distances. It suggests a staffing of 8 whole time equivalent (WTE) care co-ordinators each with a maximum caseload of 35 people (and suggests a maximum caseload for the team of 300–350). The suggested staff mix is:

- 3–4 CPNs ⎫
- 2–3 ASWs ⎬ Care coordinators
- 1–1.5 OTs ⎭
- 1–1.5 Clinical Psychologists
- 1 Consultant Psychiatrist
- 1–1.5 other medical staff
- 1–3 support workers
- 1–1.5 WTE secretaries
- Reception staff
- IT and audit support.

The staff listed in the Policy Guide is limited to the usual professional groups that presently work in many CMHTs up and down the country. However other

Department of Health policy documents suggest that additional staff will be required to achieve other policy objectives. These staff include:

1. *Pharmacists*. Whilst there was little mention of pharmacists in the NSF-MH, subsequent policy documents have indicated their important role in improving medicines management (DH 2000, 2004c, Audit Commission 2002). Within this role they are seen as forming partnerships with users and carers, play a role alongside other professionals in the team, support extended prescribing and contribute to the re-design of the workforce (DH 2005a,b) The need for training of clinicians in medicines management was identified in the David Bennett inquiry (DH 2005c). Pharmacists, supported by Pharmacy Technicians, may have a role in, for example, reviewing medication (CPA and clinics), medicines information, supporting and informing patients and their carers, staff support, advice and education, supply of medicines, liaison with GPs and community pharmacists about shared care prescribing.

2. *Dual diagnosis workers*. The 'Mental Health Policy Implementation Guide, Dual Diagnosis Good Practice Guide' (DH 2002b) recommends a policy of 'mainstreaming': that the care for people with dual diagnosis should be delivered within mental health services. One way of achieving this is to employ professionally affiliated Dual Diagnosis workers to work in CMHTs and the other specialised community teams. These workers would have the requisite training and experience in working with people with substance misuse and severe mental illness.

3. *Learning difficulties worker*. It is recognised that some people in contact with CMHTs will have learning difficulties or autism spectrum disorders (ASD). These staff may provide assessment for these groups of users, support to other team members and liaise with local learning difficulty services. This is in line with the strategy for people with learning difficulties (DH 2005d).

4. *Employment lead*. The addition of this professional to CMHTs is recommended in the recent guidance on vocational services for people with severe mental health problems (DH/DWP 2006). The role could be carried out by any mental health professional with the appropriate skills and experience, but may be suitable for those with an occupational therapy background.

5. *Psychology assistants*. These are additional staff to support the work of the clinical psychologist (British Psychological Society 2004).

6. *Support workers*. The creation of Support, Time and Recovery (STR) workers was recommended by the Workforce Action Team (WAT) (DH 2001b). The role of these workers is set out in the relevant Policy Implementation Guide (DH 2003).

7. *Support workers for those from BME communities*. The role of this group of workers is set out in the relevant Policy Implementation Guide (DH 2004b). The precise number of these workers for each team will depend on the size and make-up of the local BME community.

8. *Employment specialist worker*. The addition of this group of workers is recommended in the recent guidance on vocational services for people with severe mental health problems (DH/DWP 2006).

A recent Sainsbury Centre for Mental Health report (Boardman & Parsonage 2007) examined the staffing needs and costs of implementing government policy on mental health services for adults of working age by 2010. One section covered the resources required for CMHTs (for the overall costs see Chapter 20 by Parsonage). In line with the NSF-MH and the associated policy documents discussed above it was assumed that:

1. CMHTs need to cover two separate functions: assessment and continuing care.
2. Most assessments will be requested by primary care.
3. The referral rate from primary care is 15% of all people with mental health problems seen in primary care.
4. Users needing continuing care will be those with severe and enduring mental illness.
5. The case load per team is 325. This is based on a *maximum* case load size as opposed to an *ideal* size.

The figures were calculated for a catchment area of 250,000 total population (working age adult population of 165,525), which requires 4.5 CMHTs. It was calculated that 30.44 WTE staff were required for each CMHT, including the new staff members listed above and administration staff, giving 137 WTE staff for the 4.5 CMHTs required for an area of 250,000 people. These figures should be considered 'average' estimates and may need to be adjusted for the population needs of a local area. This means that 931 teams are required for England by 2010 with 28,340 total staff (24,519 care staff) and a caseload of 302,533 people with severe and enduring mental illness (out of estimated range of 102,809–513,840). In Spring 2006 the Durham AMH mapping data reported 826 teams (one per 38,868 adult population) with 13,502 care staff (Centre for Public Health, Durham University, 2006), suggesting that an additional 11,017 care staff are required for English CMHTs by 2010 if the implementation of the NSF-MH and associated government policy is to be achieved. In 2003 the CMHTs had a total caseload of 309,893 (mean of 373 per team) (Glover et al 2004), which compares favourably with our estimates.

Conclusions

There has been a rapid rise in CMHTs in England over the last 20–25 years and they have become central to community mental health care and delivery in England. They have become a core part of government policy, are generally accepted by practitioners and their continued use is backed by some research evidence.

Along with the success of CMHTs there are several current and remaining challenges. One challenge, inherent in the implementation of the NSF-MH, is their role in relation to the other emerging community modernisation teams (assertive outreach, crisis and early intervention teams) and the possible increase in fragmentation of services. Whilst the creation of these new teams has increased the spectrum of community mental health services, particularly for users with SMI, they remain untested in the context of day-to-day service provision and the funding of these services has varied geographically (Sainsbury Centre for Mental Health 2003, DH 2004a). The creation of these teams requires a rigorous national review before the final implementation date of 2010. Whilst a crucial opportunity has been missed in creating a continuous evaluation of the implementation and progress of these teams, it is not too late to provide a retrospective view of their implementation or a prospective evaluation over the next few years. If the creation of these new teams was considered a live experiment then an evaluation of their efficacy should be considered fundamental. The CMHTs and new teams should be placed in context of other mental health services for working age adults including inpatient units, specialist services (for example forensic and rehabilitation), primary care and services provided by the independent sector. The community teams may be considered to be the central hub of local secondary services, dealing with many of the population of people with SMI at some time; the question arises not only as to the cooperation and coordination between these services but also to the balance between them (Thornicroft & Tansella 2004).

The past concerns about the loss of focus on people with SMI has not been realised, rather the CMHT has emerged, both in policy and in practice, as a co-coordinator of care and services for those with SMI and a point of access and liaison for primary care and other community services. This focus survived the past threats from the development of General Practice fundholding, but the advent of practice-based commissioning may place additional pressures on CMHTs to develop services for people with common mental disorders who form the most prevalent group of people with mental health problems in general practice consulters. This is reinforced by other policy pressures involving welfare reform and the attempts to halt the rise of people with mental health problems who remain on welfare benefits (HM Government 2005, 2006a) and the push to improve access to psychological therapies (DH 2004a, Layard 2005, 2006). These competing pressures need to be resolved and accommodated. The need to provide services for the most vulnerable with long-term mental health problems remains, and this must be balanced with the need to improve services for people with anxiety and depression. This puts the onus on developing clear commissioning briefs for these groups of users, as well as thinking of more imaginative ways of delivering services (for example intermediate care teams – Sainsbury Centre for Mental Health, 2005) and the use of evidence based methods.

The central position of CMHTs always places them in the 'default position' for any new policy development. The five-year review of the NSF-MH (DH 2004a) set several priorities for the succeeding five years which impinge on CMHTs – including dual diagnosis, social exclusion, ethnic minorities, the care of long-term mental disorders and the availability of psychological therapies. In addition, it put mental health services in the context of overall developments in health and social services:

'We now need to plan for the next five years in a way that re-casts our NSF in line with the direction that the NHS as a whole is taking – towards patient choice, the care of long-term conditions and improved access to services'

(DH 2004a)

These priorities raise further challenges for CMHTs (working presumably with other available local services supplied by a range of providers) to work towards a 'whole community approach' (DH 2004a) including improving work and employment prospects for people with SMI (DH 2006a,b, DH/DWP 2006), improving the experience of BME users (DH 2005c), and implementing the NICE guidelines for schizophrenia and other disorders (e.g. NICE 2002, 2004a,b, 2006). Some immediate threat may come from the development of Foundation Trusts who may be less driven to involve professionals in core services such as CMHTs and devalue the expertise required to provide quality services at this level. Other challenges may come from the uncertainty as to whether voluntary sector providers have the capacity to compete in the delivery of the additional services required.

Several reports have offered a vision for future services (Rankin 2005, Sainsbury Centre for Mental Health 2006), but there is a vision of services implicit in much of central policy, particularly those aspects of policy that implicitly and explicitly promote social inclusion, citizenship and rights (Social Exclusion Unit 2004, HM Government 2006b). These principles are not merely abstract, but are central to the lives of current and potential service users. CMHTs are being asked to be a central pivot in the delivery of mental health services and play a large part in the policy ambitions. This raises questions as to whether we have the resources available to match the vision and what might be our longer-term strategy to achieve equitable distribution of these.

References

Audit Commission 2002 A spoonful of sugar – medicines management in NHS hospitals. Audit Commission Publications, Wetherby

Boardman, J. 2005 New services for old – An overview of mental health policy. In: Bell A, Lindley P (eds) Beyond the water towers. The unfinished revolution in mental health services 1985–2005. Sainsbury Centre for Mental Health, London

Boardman A P, Bouras N, Watson J P 1986 Evaluation of a community mental health centre. Acta Psychiatrica Belgica 86:402–406

Boardman A P, Bouras N, Cundy J 1987 The Mental Health Advice Centre in Lewisham. Service Usage: Trends from 1978 to 1984. National Unit for Psychiatric Research and Development, Research Report No. 3. NUPRD, London

Boardman A P, Bouras N 1988 The Mental Health Advice Centre in Lewisham. Health Trends 20:59–63

Boardman J, Parsonage M 2007 Delivering the Governments Mental Health Policies. Sainsbury Centre for Mental Health, London

Boardman A P, Sayce E, Craig T K J 1988 Community Mental Health Centres Conference. Bulletin of the Royal College of Psychiatrists 12:61–62

British Psychological Society 2004 Estimating the applied psychology demand in adult mental health. British Psychological Society, Leicester

Brough D I, Bouras N 1982 The development of the Mental Health Advice Centre in Lewisham Health District. Health Trends 14:65–69

Burns T 2002 The UK700 trial of Intensive Case Management: an overview and discussion. World Psychiatry 1:175–178

Burns T, Beadsmore A, Bhat A V, Oliver A, Mathers C. 1993a A controlled trial of home-based acute psychiatric services. i: Clinical and social outcome. British Journal of Psychiatry 163:49–54

Burns T, Raftery J, Beadsmore A, McGuigan S, Dickson M. 1993b A controlled trial of home-based acute psychiatric services. ii: Treatment patterns and costs. British Journal of Psychiatry 163:55–61

Catty J, Burns T, Knapp M et al 2002 Home treatment for mental health problems: a systematic review. Psychological Medicine 32:383–401

Centre for Public Mental Health, Durham University 2006 Adult mental health service mapping: reporting autumn 2004 and spring 2006 (available at http://www.amhmapping.org.uk/reports/)

Department of Health 1994 Hospital Discharge Workbook. A manual for hospital discharge practice. HMSO, London

Department of Health 1995 Building Bridges. A guide to arrangements for inter-agency working for the care and protection of the severely mentally ill. HMSO, London

Department of Health 1996 The Spectrum of Care. Local services for people with mental health problems. DH, London

Department of Health 1999 National Service Framework for Mental Health. Modern Standards and Service Models. DH, London

Department of Health 2000 Pharmacy in the future – implementing the NHS Plan. DH, London

Department of Health 2001a Mental Health Policy Implementation Guide. DH, London

Department of Health 2001b Mental Health National Service Framework (and NHS Plan): Workforce Planning, Education and Training. Underpinning Programme: Adult Mental Health Services. Final Report by the Workforce Action Team. DH, London

Department of Health 2002a Community Mental Health Teams: Policy Implementation Guide. DH, London

Department of Health 2002b Mental health policy implementation guide: Dual diagnosis good practice guide. DH, London

Department of Health 2003 Mental health policy implementation guide: Support, Time and Recovery (STR) workers. DH, London

Department of Health 2004a The National Service Framework for Mental Health – Five years on. DH, London

Department of Health 2004b Policy Implementation Guide. Community Development Workers for Black and Minority Ethnic Communities. Interim Guidance. DH, London

Department of Health 2004c Building a safer NHS for patients – improving medication safety. DH, London

Department of Health 2005a New Ways of Working for Psychiatrists. Enhancing effective, person centered services through new ways of working in multi-disciplinary and multi-agency contexts. Final Report July 2005 'but not the end of the story'. DH, London

Department of Health 2005b Improving mental health services by extending the role of nurses in prescribing and supplying medication. DH, London

Department of Health 2005c Delivering race equality in mental health care. An action plan for reform inside and outside services and the Government's response to the Independent Inquiry into the death of David Bennett. DH, London

Department of Health 2005d Valuing People: the story so far ... A new strategy for Learning Disability for the 21st Century – Long Report. DH, London

Department of Health 2006a From segregation to inclusion: commissioning guidance on day services for people with mental health problems. DH, London

Department of Health 2006b Supporting women into the mainstream. Commissioning women-only community day services. DH, London

Department of Health/Department for Work and Pensions 2006 Vocational Services for people with severe mental health problems: Commissioning guidance. DH, London

Fenton F R, Tessier L, Struening E L 1979 A comparative trial of home and hospital psychiatric care: one-year follow-up. Archives of General Psychiatry 36:1073–1079

Fink P J, Weinstein S P 1979 Whatever happened to psychiatry? The deprofessionalisation of Community Mental Health Centres. American Journal of Psychiatry 136:406–409

Galvin S W, McCarthy S. 1994 Multidisciplinary community teams: clinging to the wreckage. Journal of Mental Health 3:157–166

Glover G, Barnes D, Wistow R, Bradley S 2004 Mental Health Service Provision for Working age Adults in England 2003. University of Durham Centre for Public Mental Health (www. dur.ac.uk/service.mapping/amh/)

Goldberg D, Jackson G, Gater R, Campbell M, Jennett N 1996 The treatment of common mental disorders by a community team based in primary care: a cost-effectiveness study. Psychological Medicine 26:487–492

Good Practices in Mental Health 1985 Community Mental Health Centres and Teams – a contact list. Good Practices in Mental Health, London

HM Government 2005 Department for Work and Pensions Five Year Strategy. Opportunity and Security throughout life. CM 6447. The Stationery Office, London

HM Government 2006a A New Deal for Welfare: Empowering people to work. (Green Paper) CM6730. The Stationery Office, London

HM Government 2006b Reaching Out: An Action Plan on Social Exclusion. Cabinet Office, London

Holloway F 2001 Invited commentary on: community mental health team management in severe mental illness. British Journal of Psychiatry 178:503–505

Hoult J, Reynoulds I, Charbonneau-Powis M, Coles P, Briggs J 1981 A controlled study of psychiatric hospital versus community treatment – the effect on relatives. Australian and New Zealand Journal of Psychiatry 15:323–328

Hoult J, Reynoulds I 1984 Schizophrenia. A comparative trial of community orientated and hospital orientated psychiatric care. Acta Psychiatrica Scandinavica 69:359–372

Jackson G, Gater R, Goldberg D, Tantam D, Loftus L, Taylor H. 1993 A new community health team based in primary care. British Journal of Psychiatry 162:375–384

Johnson S, Thornicroft G 1995 Emergency Psychiatric Services in England and Wales. British Medical Journal 311:287–288

Jones K 1972 A history of the mental health services. Routledge and Kegan Paul, London

Jones K 1979 Integration or disintegration in the mental health services. Journal of the Royal Society of Medicine 72:640–648

Joy C B, Adams C E, Rice K 1998 Crisis intervention for those with severe mental illnesses (database of Systematic Reviews, 2006 www.cochrane.org/reviews)

King C. 2001 Severe mental illness: Managing the boundary of a CMHT. Journal of Mental Health 10:75–86

Layard R 2005 Mental Health: Britain's biggest social problem? Paper delivered to Cabinet Office (www.strategy.gov.uk/seminars/mental_health/index.asp)

Layard R 2006 The case for psychological treatment centres. British Medical Journal 332:1030–1032

Levene M 1981 The history and politics of community mental health. Oxford University Press, New York

McAusland T 1985 Planning and monitoring Community Mental Health Centres. Kings Fund Centre, London

Marshall M, Lockwood A 1998 Assertive community treatment for people with severe mental illness (database of Systematic Reviews, 2006 www.cochrane.org/reviews)

Marshall M, Lockwood A, Green R et al 1998 Case management for people with severe mental disorder (database of Systematic Reviews, 2006 www.cochrane.org/reviews)

Merson S, Tyrer P, Onyett S et al 1992 Early intervention in psychiatric emergencies: a controlled clinical trial. Lancet 339:1311–1314

Mistral W, Velleman R 1997 CMHTs: the professionals' choice? Journal of Mental Health 6:125–140

Mollica R F 1980 Community Mental Health centres. An American response to Kathleen Jones. Journal of the Royal Society of Medicine 73:863–870

Mueser K T, Bond G R. Drake R E, Resnick S G 1998 Models of community care for severe mental illness: a review of research on case management. Schizophrenia Bulletin 24:37–74

NICE 2002 Schizophrenia. Core interventions in the treatment and management of schizophrenia in primary and secondary care. NICE, London

NICE 2004a Anxiety: management of anxiety disorder (panic disorder, with or without agoraphobia and generalized anxiety disorder) in adults in primary, secondary and community care. NICE, London

NICE 2004b Depression; management of depression in primary and secondary care. NICE, London

NICE 2006 Bipolar disorder. The management of bipolar disorder in adults, children and adolescents, in primary and secondary care. NICE, London

Norman I J, Peck E 1999 Working together in adult community mental health services: An inter-professional dialogue. Journal of Mental Health 8:217–230

Onyett S 1995 Responsibility and accountability in community mental health teams. Psychiatric Bulletin 19:281–285

Onyett S 1999 Community mental health team working as a socially valued enterprise. Journal of Mental Health 8:245–251

Onyett S, Ford R 1996 Multidisciplinary community teams: where is the wreckage? Journal of Mental Health 5:47–55

Onyett S, Heppleston T, Bushnell D 1994 A national survey of community mental health teams. Team structure and process. Journal of Mental Health 3:175–194

Patmore C, Weaver T 1991 Community Mental Health Teams: Lessons for planners and managers. Good Practices in Mental Health, London

Peck E 1999 Tensions in mental health policy? Journal of Mental Health 8:213–214

Rankin J 2005 Mental health in the mainstream. Institute for Public Policy Research, London

Rose N 2001 Historical changes in mental health practice. In: Thornicroft G, Szmukler G (eds) Textbook of community psychiatry. Oxford University Press, Oxford

Sainsbury Centre for Mental Health 2003 Money for Mental Health. A review of public spending on mental health care. Sainsbury Centre for Mental Health, London

Sainsbury Centre for Mental Health 2005 The Neglected Majority. Developing intermediate mental health care in primary care. Sainsbury Centre for Mental Health, London

Sainsbury Centre for Mental Health 2006 The Future of Mental Health: a Vision for 2015. Sainsbury Centre for Mental Health, London

Sayce L, Craig T K J, Boardman A P 1991 The development of Community Mental Health Centres in the UK. Social Psychiatry and Psychiatric Epidemiology 26:14–20

Sharfstein S S. 1978 Will Community Mental Health Survive in the 1980s? American Journal of Psychiatry 135:1363–1365

Simmonds S, Coid J, Joseph P, Marriott S, Tyrer P 2001 Community mental health management in severe mental illness: a systematic review. British Journal of Psychiatry 178:497–502

Social Exclusion Unit 2004 Mental Health and Social Exclusion. Office of the Deputy Prime Minister, London.

Thornicroft G, Goldberg D 1998 Has Community Care Failed? Maudsley Discussion Paper No. 5. Institute of Psychiatry, London

Thornicroft G, Strathdee G, Phelan M et al 1998 Rationale and design. PRiSM Psychosis Study I. British Journal of Psychiatry 173:363–370

Thornicroft G, Tansella M 2004 Components of a modern mental health service: a pragmatic balance of community and hospital care. British Journal of Psychiatry 185:283–290

Tyrer P, Morgan J, Van Horn E et al 1995 A randomised controlled study of close monitoring of vulnerable psychiatric patients. Lancet 345:756–759

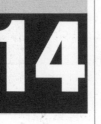

Mental health promotion

H. Guite • J. Bywaters

Introduction

'Mental health promotion has been described as "the art, science and politics of creating a mentally healthy society".'

(Friedli 2004)

Mental health promotion could potentially be all-encompassing: from the prevention of mental ill-health (such as family spacing and reduction in harsh or inconsistent discipline styles) to the promotion of positive mental health and well-being (such as improving our emotional intelligence or enhancing our physical environment) and the prevention of stigma for people with mental health problems.

In practice mental health promotion often includes suicide prevention and the promotion of mental health through the early management of common mental illnesses, even though these are secondary prevention initiatives. It is the breadth and scope of mental health promotion that can make it difficult to focus local strategies and identify who should be responsible for implementation of what mental health promotion interventions.

The inclusion of mental health promotion as the first standard in the National Service Framework (NSF) for mental health (Box 14.1) was both inspired and brave. Inspired because up to that point few people in local

---

Box 14.1

National Service Framework for mental health (DH 1999) Standard 1

Health and social services should:
- Promote mental health for all, working with individuals and communities
- Combat stigma and discrimination against individuals and groups with mental health problems, and promote their social inclusion

NHS services in 1999 had mental health promotion within their remit and brave because there was no template for how to make the task of 'promoting mental health for all', 'combating discrimination' and 'promoting social inclusion of those with mental health problems' manageable.

The development of mental health promotion policy

The first tranche of Mental Health Policy Implementation Guidance (DH 2001a) included a chapter outlining in general terms how to tackle mental health promotion at a local level but the much needed conceptual structure for mental health promotion was first introduced in 'Making it Happen' (DH 2001b). This document drew on the World Health Organization document 'Mental Health Promotion in Prisons' (WHO 1998) which identified that mental health promotion action was needed at individual, community and structural/policy levels. The DH guidance combined this framework with the idea of promoting protective factors and reducing risk factors (Commonwealth Department of Health and Aged Care 2000). 'Making it Happen' also provided practical guidance about mapping mental health promotion activity and gave examples of mental health promotion activity in different settings with different target groups.

In 2002 the National Suicide Prevention Strategy for England (DH 2002) was launched. This strategy outlined six goals:

- Goal 1. To reduce risk in key high risk groups
- Goal 2. To promote mental well-being in the wider population
- Goal 3. To reduce the availability and lethality of suicide methods
- Goal 4. To improve reporting of suicide behaviour in the media
- Goal 5. To promote research on suicide and suicide prevention
- Goal 6. To improve monitoring of progress towards the target to reduce suicides

Clearly Goal 2 in particular made explicit the link between mental health promotion and suicide prevention (see Box 14.2; DH 1999).

In 2003 a guide to mental health promotion evidence called 'Making it Effective' was published (Friedli 2003) that built on and complemented 'Making it Happen' (DH 2001b). In 2004 the public health White Paper 'Choosing Health' (DH 2004a) identified mental health as one of the government's six overarching priorities. It stated that:

'Transforming the NHS from a sickness to a health service is not just a matter of promoting physical health. Understanding how everyone in the NHS can promote mental well-being is equally important – and is as much of a cultural shift.'

It went on to reiterate the framework for tackling mental health promotion introduced in 'Making it Happen':

Box 14.2

....

National Service Framework for mental health (DH 1999) Standard 7

Local health and social care communities should prevent suicides by:

- Promoting mental health for all, working with individuals and communities (Std 1)
- Delivering high quality primary mental health care (Std 2)
- Ensuring that anyone with a mental health problem can contact local services via the primary care team, a helpline or an A&E department (Std 3)
- Ensuring that individuals with severe and enduring mental illness have a care plan which meets their needs, including access to services round the clock (Std 4)
- Providing safe hospital accommodation for individuals who need it (Std 5)
- Enabling individuals caring for someone with severe mental illness to receive the support which they need to continue to care (Std 6)

and in addition by:

- Supporting local prison staff in preventing suicides among prisoners
- Ensuring that staff are competent to assess the risk of suicide among individuals
- Developing local systems for suicide audit to learn lessons and take any necessary action

---

'a coherent approach to promoting mental health needs to work at three levels:

- *strengthening individuals: increasing emotional resilience through acting to promote self-esteem and develop life-skills such as communicating, negotiating, relationship and parenting skills*
- *strengthening communities: increasing social support, inclusion and participation helps to protect mental well-being. Tackling the stigma and discrimination associated with mental health will be critical to promoting this increased participation*
- *reducing structural barriers to good mental health: increasing access to opportunities like employment that protect mental well-being.'*

It reinforced Standard 1 of the NSF by saying: 'We will ensure that standard one of the NSF for Mental Health, which deals with mental health promotion, is fully implemented.' The Delivery Plan for Choosing Health (DH 2005) identified the key outcome: 'We will have delivered if we improve the mental health and well-being of the general population.'

Despite all this policy guidance and high-level support, feedback from front-line staff such as local leads for Standard 1 indicated that they felt they had been given 'mission impossible'. The competition for attention and resources against all the other priorities and targets was too intense. They identified a need to raise the profile of mental health promotion by producing some form of national framework. This led to the commissioning of a third document 'Making It Possible' launched in October 2005 (CSIP 2005a), which identified how mental health promotion activity and other government priorities could be mutually reinforcing; and outlined key areas for evidence-based mental health promotion work, many of which involved a public health approach to the wider socioeconomic and environmental determinants of health. These were:

- marketing mental health
- equality and inclusion
- tackling violence and abuse
- parents and early years
- schools
- employment
- workplace
- communities
- later life.

Picking up on the theme of marketing mental health the government white paper 'Our Health, Our Care, Our Say' (DH 2006) listed the 12 steps that we should all take to promote our mental well-being (Box 14.3) and made the following commitment:

> *'We will take steps to make these simple messages more widely known by ensuring that mental well-being is included in the social marketing strategy currently being developed to support Choosing Health.'*

The remainder of this chapter explores the evidence base for action, the recommendations of mental health policy, and a review of implementation. We end the chapter with an analysis of what has supported and hindered progress.

State of the evidence base

The more complex the intervention and the less control there is over the context within which it is implemented, the less likely it is that there will be

---

Box 14.3

Positive steps to improve mental health and well-being

- Keeping physically active
- Eating well
- If you do drink, drink in moderation
- Valuing yourself and others
- Talking about feelings
- Keeping in touch with friends and loved ones
- Caring for others
- Getting involved and making a contribution
- Learning new skills
- Doing something creative
- Taking a break
- Asking for help

Source: CSIP 2005a, DH 2006

randomised controlled trial evidence. This has resulted in few published reports of complex mental health promotion interventions and a preponderance of case reports of good practice with no control group or RCTs that report prevention but are in fact early treatment. Some have interpreted this as a lack of evidence but others would argue that complex interventions require a different approach to evaluation (Pawson & Tilley 1997). Pawson & Tilley have provided a rigorous framework for evaluating complex interventions. This includes measuring the most likely mechanisms by which an intervention will promote mental health, the context within which the intervention is being applied, the target groups and the outcomes analysed by group and context in order to establish what works for whom and where.

A meta-analysis of mental health promotion programmes (DH 2001b) showed that they are more likely to be effective if they:

- intervene at a range of different times in the life cycle, e.g. infancy and adolescence
- are integrated within different settings, e.g. schools and primary care
- are planned at different levels, e.g. local/regional/national
- target a combination of factors, e.g. coping skills and access to employment
- involve the social networks of those targeted
- intervene at different times and levels
- use a combination of methods.

Drawing mainly on a series of reviews of the evidence base for mental health promotion (Friedli 2003, WHO 2004, CSIP 2005a, Hosman et al 2005), boxes 14.4 and 5 summarise research in the area. Box 14.4 itemises topics for which a systematic review, meta-analysis or RCT evidence of effectiveness exists; Box 14.5 lists areas that require complex intervention and where there is evidence of good practice interventions.

It is important to note that, in addition to those interventions that work to promote mental health and reduce mental illness, there are interventions that have been found not to work, or may even be harmful. There are two such areas of note: suicide prevention and the prevention of post-traumatic stress disorder. These highlight the importance of rigorous evaluation of mental health promotion activities for both intended and unintended consequences.

Suicide prevention in schools that focuses on the symptoms of mental illness rather than the promotion of positive mental health may be harmful, particularly to vulnerable young men (Ploeg et al 1996, Lister-Sharp et al 1999). A risk factor for suicide in young people is poor problem-solving skills, and therefore mental health promotion in schools should include an element of problem-solving skills development. A Cochrane review (Rose et al 2002) found that debriefing people after traumatic incidents could in fact increase the risk of developing post-traumatic stress disorder. The reason for this may be that recounting and analysing a response to a stressful situation could act to 'seal' the emotional response in short-term memory.

There are also examples of interventions with only weak outcomes or no evidence of impact which should be noted so that resources are not wasted on ineffective interventions. A recent Cochrane review confirmed that provision of psychosocial interventions antenatally had no impact on the development

Box 14.4

Evidence from systematic reviews, meta-analyses or randomised controlled trials of interventions that promote mental health and well-being

Individual level
- Early years
  - Home based pre-school support including parenting support, education, work opportunities and social support (Horacek et al 1987, Olds et al 1997, Hodnett & Roberts 2000)
  - Nursery/day-care provision (Zorich et al 1998, 2000)
  - Parenting programmes: improvement of mental health (Barlow 1999, Barlow et al 2001)
  - Parenting programmes: improvement of antisocial behaviour (Scott et al 2001)
  - Detecting and treating depression with cognitive behavioural therapy in childhood (Harrington et al 1998)
- Young people
  - Social skills training (Erwin 1994)
- Adults
  - CBT for insomnia (Morin et al 1994, Murtagh & Greenwood 1995, Morin et al 1999)
  - Volunteering (Wheeler et al 1998)
  - Brief interventions for alcohol (Ashenden et al 1997)
  - Physical activity (Etnier et al 1997, Mutrie 2000)
  - Identification of women at high risk of post-natal depression and provision of intensive post-natal support (not antenatal support) (Dennis & Creedy 2004)
- Vulnerable groups
  - Home visiting the elderly to reduce isolation (Ciliska et al 1996)
  - Groups for retired people (Cattan 2002)
  - Travellers' community mothers' programme (Johnson et al 1993)

Community
- General public
  - Large scale stress workshops (Brown & Cochrane 1999)
- Schools
  - Health promoting schools where there has been: a change to the school ethos; the change has been implemented continuously for over a year; the emphasis is on mental health rather than mental illness; mental health has been discussed as part of the curriculum; families and communities are involved; staff morale and the environment are managed, and a problem-solving rather than a topic-based approach is taken (Lister-Sharp et al 1999, Thomas et al 1999, Weare 2000, Wells et al 2001)
  - For prevention of drug misuse the most effective approach has been a social competence model comprising self-management, problem-solving, communication, resisting negative social influences (Tobler & Stratton 1997)
  - A programme to tackle negative body image amongst teenagers (O'Dea & Abraham 1999)
- Workplace
  - Organisation-wide approaches that address: the effort–reward balance; two-way communication and staff involvement; increased social support from managers to their staff; increased job control and decision-making latitude; assessment of job demands; a culture where staff are valued; enhanced team working (Williams et al 1998) and where work–life balance is addressed (Donovan & Halpern 2002, review)

Source: Adapted from Friedli 2003, WHO 2004, Hosman et al 2005, CSIP 2005a and appended with systematic reviews or RCTs from 2003–2006.

Box 14.5

Other mental health promotion interventions which are likely to promote mental health but which do not yet have a good evidence base (based on expert opinions – see sources)

Individual

- Family planning
  - Family spacing and smaller family size
  - Reduction in teenage pregnancy
- Antenatal care to reduce complications in labour
- Relationship support

Community

- Arts and creativity as part of community development (Matarasso 1997)
- Improvements in the built and social environment, social capital and social support
  - Reduction in damp, reductions in crime and fear of crime, drug addicts using and dealing on the streets, improving the aesthetics of buildings (particularly large buildings), decrease people's sense of over-crowding, increase access to green open spaces, community facilities and entertainment facilities, more places for people to stop and chat and more events to get people together (Guite et al 2006)
  - Involving people in local decisions about their housing and neighbourhood (Halpern 1995)
- Information and empowerment about access to self help and services
- Support people to practise their chosen faith if that is want they want
- Adult education
- Community development (Donovan & Halpern 2002) to empower communities to manage problems arising in their communities themselves

Structural/policy

- Violence reduction
  - Making hitting children and harsh discipline styles unacceptable
  - Making domestic violence between partners and to elderly people within the home unacceptable
- Reduce the stigma of the mental illness
- Promote social inclusion of people with mental health problems
- Decrease unemployment

Source: Adapted from Friedli 2003, WHO 2004, Hosman et al 2005, CSIP 2005a and appended with systematic reviews or RCTs from 2003–2006

of post-natal depression, whilst identification of mothers 'at risk' with provision of intensive post-delivery support looks promising (Dennis & Creedy 2004).

One issue that has hampered research into effective mental health promotion interventions is the lack of consensus about appropriate outcome measures. A wide range of outcome measures have been used in the studies quoted here. They range from reductions in mental illness to improvements in quality of life. The Scottish Executive has funded a programme to develop a set of indicators for mental health promotion (progress can be followed on http://www.healthscotland.com/understanding/population/mental-health-indicators.aspx). This work will help to identify the secondary gains from effective mental health promotion for education in children, employment, crime, health behaviours and physical health.

Programme management of mental health promotion

'Making It Happen' (DH 2001b) first specified the targets (Box 14.6) against which the Department of Health would be assessing the performance of local health economies.

Evidence about implementation of Standard 1

There is evidence about the implementation of the NSF mental health promotion Standard 1 available from four sources:

- the year-on-year LIT self-assessments for 4 years from 2002 to 2005
- finance mapping information for five years from 2001/2 to 2005/6
- the Durham service mapping of mental health promotion conducted in 2001
- the results of the mental health promotion themed review in 2002.

Local Implementation Teams self-assessment

Table 14.1 shows the evidence relating to mental health promotion implementation from LIT self-assessments. It is important to note that the criteria for success become gradually more challenging, and that service reconfiguration resulted in substantial re-organisation of the LIT architecture over the period under review. It is therefore not possible to make direct comparisons from year to year.

Finance mapping

The difficulty in identifying precisely what activity was and was not included in 'mental health promotion' rendered it almost impossible to identify with confidence the associated financial investment. The best available data are shown in Table 14.2.

Box 14.6

Making It Happen (DH 2001b): Performance management targets

- By March 2002, develop and agree evidence-based mental health promotion strategy based on local needs assessment
- By March 2002, build into local mental health promotion strategy action to promote mental health in specific settings, based on local needs
- By March 2002, build into local mental health promotion strategy action to reduce discrimination
- By March 2002, the written care plan for those on enhanced Care Programme Approach (CPA) must show plans to secure suitable employment or other occupational activity, adequate housing and their appropriate entitlement to welfare benefits
- By March 2002, implement strategy to promote employment of people with mental health problems within health and social services

Table 14.1

Criteria for Local Implementation Teams (LITs) self-assessment of Standard 1 implementation and % of LITs reporting compliance 2002–2005				
Year	**Criteria**	**% LITs Red**	**% LITs Amber**	**% LITs Green**
2002	*Red*: as at September 2002, a MHP strategy is not being implemented *Amber*. no amber option *Green*: as at September 2002, a mental health promotion strategy is being implemented	12	n/a	88
2003	*Red*: as at September 2003, a mental health promotion strategy is not being implemented *Amber*. a mental health strategy is being implemented, but with little or no measurement of its impact or effectiveness *Green*: as at September 2003, a mental health promotion strategy is being implemented with good systems for measuring its impact and effectiveness	9	50	41
2004a	*Red*: there is no dedicated Standard 1 lead *Amber*. there is a LIT Standard 1 lead, who coordinates strategic and operational activity within the public health/health promotion department *Green*: the Standard 1 lead is an active member of the LIT and has adequate dedicated time for coordination and leadership	5	28	67
2004b	*Red*: the Standard 1 strategy does not include early years, children, young people, adults and older adults *Amber*. the Standard 1 strategy and action plan identifies joint working and priorities for all ages *Green*: the Standard 1 strategy and action plan identifies joint working and priorities for all ages, with close working arrangements between the adult and older people's LITs and the CAMHS strategy group	10	53	38
2005	*Red*: the Standard 1 strategy and action plan does not identify joint working and priorities for all ages *Amber*. the Standard 1 strategy and action plan identifies joint working and priorities for all ages, with close working arrangements between the adult and older people's LITs and the CAMHS strategy group *Green*: the Standard 1 strategy and action plan identifies joint working and priorities for all ages, with close working arrangements between the adult and older people's LITs and the CAMHS strategy group. There is an evaluation process with clear indicators to measure the impact and effectiveness of the action plan	8	53	39

Source: Adapted from Mental Health Strategies: Autumn Service Monitoring – self-assessment results Reports for 2002, 2003, 2004 and 2005.

Table 14.2

Planned real terms investment (£ million) in direct service categories over time (at 2005/06 pay and price levels)					
Service category	2001/02 £ millions	2002/03 £ millions	2003/04 £ millions	2004/05 £ millions	2005/06 £ millions
Mental health promotion	6	3	3	2	3
Total direct service categories	2960	3119	3439	3785	3748
% spend on mental health promotion	0.203%	0.096%	0.087%	0.053%	0.080%
Change in % spent on MHP against 2001/02 baseline	–	−53%	−57%	−74%	−61%

Source: Financial data: Mental Health Strategies: The 2005/06 National Survey of Investment in Mental Health Services. Author's calculations.

These data would suggest that, over the five years 2001/2 to 2005/6, investment in mental health promotion halved in real terms, and as a proportion of total investment fell by 61% from 0.2% of all mental health investment to 0.08%, but the limitations of the data and the associated caveats should be borne in mind.

Service mapping

An attempt was made in 2001 to include mental health promotion activity within the (then) Durham Service Mapping process. Three initial questions were asked to identify local infrastructure for mental health promotion. These were:

- Do you have a designated Standard 1 lead?
- Do you have an organisation responsible for the development of a mental health promotion strategy?
- Do you have a multi-agency group responsible for the development of a mental health promotion strategy?

Further questions were asked about interventions for individuals at risk, including both specific target groups and vulnerable groups. These were listed in detail, as were possible types of intervention and various settings, seeking to map mental health promotion activity across the country against the models outlined in 'Making It Happen' (DH 2001b).

Sadly, the returns simply demonstrated the extraordinary difficulty of mapping activity of this kind (Glover G, personal communication). For example:

- respondents frequently confused the concepts of settings and target groups
- the terms 'vulnerable groups' and 'individuals at risk' were not clearly differentiated
- respondents frequently reported the aims of a project (e.g. 'improving self-image' and/or 'providing support') rather than describing the actual intervention provided
- the questions asked did not allow for any indication of the size of a project, either in terms of inputs (e.g. number of staff employed) or impact (e.g. number of clients served)
- many of the projects reported as 'mental health promotion' were really offering interventions for people with mental health problems, e.g. counselling services, early psychosis services, community mental health teams, Social Services Department emergency duty teams, outpatient clinics, assertive outreach teams
- some respondents included nationally available resources accessible by their residents, such as Samaritans or the National Healthy Schools Initiative, while others focused purely on local projects.

Consequently it was decided that no meaningful data could be reported in the service mapping data for 2001, and this set of questions was not included in subsequent years.

Themed review 2002

Mental health promotion was the focus of the Themed Review within the Autumn Assessment process for 2002. While the format for reporting was not precisely specified, which, in retrospect, made comparative analysis of the reports very difficult, it was nevertheless possible to draw some broad conclusions:

- The majority of LITs had already identified a Standard 1 lead, in line with national guidance.
- Each LIT had carried out a full needs assessment of their area in consultation with a wide range of key stakeholders from the statutory and voluntary sector, users and carers.
- Key settings and target groups had been identified, though questions were raised about whether the special needs of rural communities were being adequately addressed, especially in the light of the outbreak of foot and mouth disease which was creating a great deal of stress at the time.
- Most, if not all, LITs had identified children and young people as a key target group and schools as a key setting. It was not so clear that they also recognised places of higher education as an important setting.
- LITs clearly demonstrated in their themed reviews their rationale for selected interventions: many used 'Making It Happen', in line with the national guidance they were receiving at the time.
- There was evidence of a lot of good work on tackling discrimination and promoting social inclusion, and many areas were engaging with local media.

- There was also evidence that the majority of LITs recognised the importance of employment, though it was not clear that this was being addressed everywhere.
- Most LITs were clearly linking mental health promotion efforts with other initiatives such as Neighbourhood Renewal, Healthy Schools, and Supporting People, though some were still in the developmental stage of forming local partnerships.
- While the importance of evaluation was clearly recognised, many LITs were still in the process of agreeing targets and processes for monitoring.

Review of progress to date

Starting from a very low base in 1999, when mental health promotion was scarcely recognised as an entity, considerable progress has been made. By 2004, 95% of LITS at least had an identifiable Standard 1 lead. By 2005 92% of LIT mental health promotion strategies addressed all age groups, and 39% reported that they had an evaluation process in place with clear indicators of impact and effectiveness.

Factors promoting the implementation of mental health promotion strategies

Internationally, the climate is becoming increasingly favourable to mental health promotion. A new emphasis on happiness and life satisfaction has begun to focus minds on the importance of mental well-being as an alternative to gross domestic product as a sign of prosperity in a country (Layard 2005) and the New Economics Foundation has sparked a debate about what implications this would have for policy (NEF 2005).

The WHO Report on Promoting Mental Health (WHO 2004) states clearly that 'the social and economic costs of poor mental health are high and the evidence suggests that they will continue to grow without community and government action'.

In January 2005, the Mental Health Declaration for Europe (WHO 2005a) and the associated Mental Health Action Plan for Europe (WHO 2005b) were signed by the English Minister of Health on behalf of the UK in Helsinki. It included these words:

'We, the Ministers of Health of member states in the European region of the World Health Organisation ... acknowledge that mental health and mental well-being are fundamental to the quality of life and productivity of individuals, families, communities and nations, enabling people to experience life as meaningful and to be creative and active citizens. We believe that the primary aim of mental health activity is to enhance people's well-being and functioning by focusing on their strengths and resources, reinforcing resilience and enhancing protective external factors ... We endorse the statement that there is no health without mental health.'

More recently, the European (EU) Commission issued a Green Paper consultation on whether there should be an EU Strategy for Mental Health, and in 2006 the European Parliament responded by adopting a resolution on 'Improving the Mental Health of the Population: towards a strategy on mental health for the EU'. While this resolution is not binding, the EU Commission must take the views of the European Parliament into account.

Within the UK and the Republic of Ireland, there has been increasing collaboration between the national administrations. The Four Nations Debate on Public Mental Health held in Edinburgh in October 2004 was valued by delegates for the quality of the debate, the contributions from a wide range of different disciplines, receiving a first-hand account of what was happening across the UK and Ireland, and the rare opportunity to give public mental health a strong profile (Henderson 2005). Since then, two Five Nations conferences have been held (Mental Health Promotion: Going from Strength to Strength – Dublin, April 2005; Mental Health Promotion: Progress Through Partnerships – London, May 2006). All three conferences were opened by a government minister from the host nation, which again signals a level of commitment to the issues.

The Scottish Executive in particular has invested heavily in their National Programme for mental health promotion, and the other home nations which have contributed less financially have benefited from involvement of their experts in contributing to aspects of the Scottish work, such as the Scottish Mental Health Indicators project (Parkinson 2006).

The National Institute for Mental Health in England (now part of the Care Services Improvement Partnership) funded a post in each of its eight Regional Development Centres to link with the regional public health groups to take forward the public mental health agenda, including providing support to the Standard 1 leads in their region's LITs. These regional leads formed a national network. They were also ex officio members of the new National Advisory Group for Mental Health Promotion which identified the need for 'Making It Possible', and for the regular quarterly newsletter 'Mental Health Promotion Update' (NIMHE 2005, 2006, 2007). Examples of local initiatives are highlighted in the newsletter and on the NIMHE website.

Another supportive factor has been the increasing interest in mental health shown by the Faculty of Public Health, which in 2005 signed a Memorandum of Understanding with NIMHE to collaborate on public mental health issues. The Faculty's Mental Health Working Group has influenced the content of the new examination curriculum for aspiring public health specialists and raised the profile of mental health with the membership.

The growing importance of Local Area Agreements in some areas has facilitated the inclusion of mental health promotion with the real possibility of inter-agency working. For example Greenwich has included mental health as a 'golden thread' linking areas of the local area agreement. Health trainers are being trained to provide signposting and initial support to people with mental health problems, front line staff from the PCT and the LA are being trained in mental health awareness training, and library staff are getting involved in the provision of self-help materials.

Factors hampering the implementation of mental health promotion strategies

The difficulties confronting those seeking to deliver on NSF Standard 1 (and 7) and on the aspirations outlined in 'Choosing Health' and 'Our Health, Our Care, Our Say' were identified as far back as the themed review in 2002. For some the key issue was the need for outcomes and evidence:

'There are difficulties identifying clear measurable outcomes and evidence based practice within mental health promotion and this can result in the activity slipping down the agenda.'

(Portsmouth LIT 2001)

Others mentioned lack of resources and capacity:

'The lack of any additional allocation from the centre specifically to support implementation of mental health promotion aspects of the NSF may limit the ability of the local group to achieve significant improvements.'

(Redcar LIT 2001)

These issues continue to impede progress. With the NHS trying desperately to balance its books, and the deficits in acute trusts impacting even on Mental Health Trusts and PCTs which have been financially prudent, mental health promotion is all too often seen as a soft target. Table 14.2 shows the fall in real and relative terms of investment in mental health promotion in England.

Another factor hampering progress was highlighted in the Durham service mapping. There is still confusion between Standard 1 (mental health promotion) and Standards 2 and 3 (treatment and access to primary care mental health services). The strategies in some areas have not moved beyond services into the root causes of mental health problems. The new government initiative to increase patient choice by widening access to psychological therapies is often mentioned in response to the question 'What is the government doing about mental health promotion?', as are the equally important efforts to promote recovery by enabling more people with mental health problems to return to work.

Indeed, the very welcome attention to this and other aspects of social exclusion has sometimes pushed primary mental health promotion off the agenda: for example, the only voluntary agency dedicated to mental health promotion, Mentality, closed in 2006.

Challenges that remain and how to meet them

The National Director for Mental Health concluded, in his review of the NSF 'Five Years On' (DH 2004b), that while there had been impressive achievement on Standards 4, 5 and 7, and reasonably good progress on Standards 2 and 3, 'less has been achieved on mental health promotion and social inclusion

(Standard 1)'. It is difficult to disagree with his assessment, though this should not be blamed on those staff who have struggled valiantly to deliver in this area.

The South East Region, which has conducted a detailed stock-take of mental health promotion activity, has concluded that 'very little is being done to promote mental health or to prevent suicides. Urgent action is needed to remedy this situation.' It found that the 'limited work being undertaken or planned for the standards of Mental Health Promotion and Suicide Prevention' across the region was 'being led by a handful of dedicated persons with virtually no budgets'. It concluded that 'the present levels of activity are unlikely to achieve these standards, as required in the white paper Choosing Health' (CSIP 2005b).

Those of us who believe that mental health underpins the whole of human well-being need to start identifying the economic as well as the humanitarian arguments for investing in mental health promotion, and to assemble the evidence that reducing investment in this work is a false economy.

We also need to seek allies among those whose main area of responsibility is not mental health, and show how promoting well-being can help them to deliver on other health targets.

Finally, we need to look beyond the traditional health sector altogether, and show how improving the mental health and well-being of the population will bring much wider benefits to our society.

References

Ashenden R, Silagy C, Weller D 1997 A systematic review of effectiveness of promoting lifestyle change in general practice. Family Practice 14:160–175

Barlow J 1999 Systematic review of the effectiveness of parent-training programmes in improving behaviour problems in children aged 3–10 years (second edition). Oxford Health Services Research Unit, Department of Public Health, University of Oxford

Barlow J, Coren E, Stewart-Brown S 2001 Systematic review of the effectiveness of parenting programmes in improving maternal psychosocial health. Oxford Health Services Research Unit, University of Oxford

Brown J S L, Cochrane R 1999 A comparison of people who are referred to a psychology service and those who self-refer to large-scale stress workshops open to the general public. Journal of Mental Health 8(3):297–306

Cattan M 2002 Supporting older people to overcome social isolation and loneliness. Help the Aged, London

Ciliska D, Hayward S, Thomas H et al 1996 A systematic overview of the effectiveness of home visiting as a delivery strategy for public health nursing interventions. Canadian Journal of Public Health 87(3):193–198

CSIP 2005a Making it Possible: Improving Mental Health and Well-being in England. NIMHE, CSIP, Leeds

CSIP 2005b South East Development Centre Mental Health Promotion audit. CSIP.

Commonwealth Department of Health and Aged Care 2000 Promotion, prevention and early intervention for mental health – a monograph. Mental health and special programs branch. Commonwealth Department of Health and Aged Care, Canberra

Dennis C-L, Creedy D 2004 Psychosocial and psychological interventions for preventing postpartum depression. Cochrane Database of Systematic Reviews 2004, Issue 4. Art. No.: CD001134. DOI: 10.1002/14651858.CD001134.pub2

Department of Health 1999 National Service Framework for Mental Health. DH, London

Department of Health 2001a The Mental Health Policy Implementation Guide (http://www. dh.gov.uk/assetRoot/04/05/89/60/04058960.pdf)

Department of Health 2001b Making it Happen: A guide to delivering mental health promotion. Ref 24509. DH, London

Department of Health 2002 National Suicide Prevention Strategy for England. DH, London

Department of Health 2004a Choosing Health. DH, London

Department of Health 2004b NSF for mental health. Five years on. DH, London

Department of Health 2005 Delivery Plan for Choosing Health. DH, London

Department of Health 2006 Our health, Our care, Our say. A new direction for community services. TSO, London

Donovan N, Halpern D with Richard Sargeant 2002 Life satisfaction: the state of knowledge and implications for government. Prime Minister's Strategy Unit, London (http://www. strategy.gov.uk/downloads/seminars/ls/paper.pdf)

Erwin P G 1994 Effectiveness of social skills training with children: a meta-analytic study. Counselling Psychology Quarterly 7(3):305–310

Etnier J L, Salazar W, Landers D M et al 1997 The influence of physical fitness and exercise upon cognitive functioning: a meta-analysis. Journal of Sport and Exercise Psychology 19:249–277

Friedli L 2003 Making it effective. A guide to evidence based mental health promotion. Radical mentalities (http://www.scmh.org.uk/80256FBD004F6342/vWeb/pcKHAL6UEETK)

Friedli L 2004 Editorial. Journal of Mental Health Promotion 3:2–6

Guite H F, Clark C, Ackrill G 2006 The impact of the physical and urban environment on mental well-being. Public Health 120(12):1117–1126

Halpern D 1995 Mental health and the built environment. Taylor & Francis, London

Harrington R, Whittaker J, Shoebridge P et al 1998 Systematic review of efficacy of cognitive behaviour therapies in childhood and adolescent depressive disorder. British Medical Journal 316:1559–1563

Henderson G 2005 Guest Editorial. Journal of Public Mental Health 4(1)

Hodnett E D, Roberts I. 2000 Home based social support for socially disadvantaged mothers. Cochrane Review. The Cochrane Library, issue 3

Horacek H J, Ramey C T, Campbell F A et al 1987 Predicting school failure and assessing early intervention with high risk children. Journal of the American Academy of Child and Adolescent Psychiatry 175:217–223

Hosman C, Jane- Llopis E, Saxena A 2005 Prevention of mental disorders Effective interventions and policy options. Oxford University Press, Oxford

Johnson Z, Howell F, Molloy B 1993 The community mothers programme: randomised controlled trial of non-professional intervention in parenting. British Medical Journal 306:1449–1452

Layard R 2005 Happiness: lessons from a new science. Penguin, Allen Lane

Lister-Sharp D, Chapman S, Stewart-Brown S et al 1999 Health Promoting schools and health promotion in schools: two systematic reviews. Health Technology Assessment. No 22, London

Matarasso F 1997 Use or ornament? The social impact of participation in the arts. Comedia, London

Morin C M, Culbert J P, Schwartz M S 1994 Non-pharmacological interventions for insomnia: a meta-analysis of treatment efficacy. American Journal of Psychiatry 151:1172–1180

Morin C M, Colecchi C, Stone J et al 1999 Behavioural and pharmacological therapies for late-life insomnia: a randomised controlled trial. Journal of the American Medical Association 281:991–999

Murtagh D R, Greenwood K M 1995 Identifying effective psychological treatments for insomnia: a meta-analysis. Journal of Consulting and Clinical Psychology 63:79–89

Mutrie N 2000 The relationship between physical activity and clinically defined depression. In: Biddle S J H, Fox K R, Boucher S (eds) The case for exercise in the promotion of mental health and well-being. Routledge, London, p46–62

NEF 2005 Manifesto for wellbeing. New Economics Foundation, London

NIMHE 2005–7 Mental health promotion updates. Quarterly newsletters. National Institute for Mental Health in England, Leeds

O'Dea J, Abraham S 1999 Improving body image, eating attitudes and behaviours of young male and female adolescents: a new educational approach which focuses on self-esteem. Journal of Abnormal Psychology 99:3–15

Olds D L, Eckenrode J, Henderson C R et al 1997 Long term effects of home visitation on maternal life course and child abuse and neglect: fifteen year follow up of a randomized trial. Journal of the American Medical Association 278(8):637–643

Parkinson J 2006 Establishing national mental health and well-being indicators for Scotland. Journal of Public Mental Health 5(1)

Pawson R, Tilley N 1997 Realistic evaluation. Sage, London

Ploeg J, Ciliska D, Dobbins M et al 1996. A systematic overview of the effectiveness of public health nursing interventions: an overview of adolescent suicide prevention programmes. Quality of Nursing Worklife Research Unit, McMaster University, University of Toronto, Toronto

Rose S, Bisson J, Churchill R et al 2002 Psychological debriefing for preventing post traumatic stress disorder (PTSD) (Cochrane Review). The Cochrane Database of Systematic Reviews 2002, Issue 2. Art. No.: CD000560. DOI:10.1002/14651858.CD000560

Scott S, Spender Q, Doolan M 2001 Multi-centre controlled trial of parenting groups for childhood antisocial behaviour in clinical practice. British Medical Journal 323:194–198

Thomas H, Siracusa L, Ross G et al 1999 Effectiveness of school-based interventions in reducing adolescent risk behaviour: a systematic review of reviews. Prepared by the Effective Public Health Practice Project. Public Health Branch, Ontario Ministry of Health, Ontario

Tobler N S, Stratton H H 1997 Effectiveness of school-based drug prevention programs: a meta-analysis of the research. Journal of Primary Prevention 18(1):71–128

Weare K 2000 Developing mental, emotional and social health: a whole school approach. Routledge, London

Wells J, Barlow J, Stewart-Brown S 2001 A systematic review of universal approaches to mental health promotion in schools. Health Services Research Unit, Institute of Health Sciences, Oxford

Wheeler F A, Gore K M, Greenblatt B 1998 The beneficial effects of volunteering for older volunteers and the people they serve: a meta-analysis. International Journal of Ageing and Human Development 47:69–79

WHO 1998 Mental Health Promotion in Prisons. Report on a WHO meeting. WHO Regional Office for Europe, The Hague

WHO 2004 Prevention of mental disorders: effective interventions and policy options: summary report. Prevention research centre of the Universities of Nijmegen and Maastricht. WHO, Geneva

WHO 2005a WHO Mental Health Declaration for Europe. WHO, Helsinki

WHO 2005b Mental Health Action Plan for Europe. WHO, Helsinki

Williams S, Michie S, Pattini S 1998 Improving the health of the NHS workforce: report of the partnership on the health of the NHS workforce. The Nuffield Trust, Leeds

Zorich B, Roberts I, Oakley A 1998 The health and welfare effects of day care: a systematic review of randomised controlled trials. Social Science and Medicine 47(3):317–727

Zorich B, Roberts I, Oakley A 2000 Daycare for pre-school children: Cochrane Review. The Cochrane Library: Issue 3

Primary care

D. Ekers • T. Ricketts

Introduction

Enhancing the quality of mental health care within primary care settings was at the heart of the National Service Framework for Mental Health. Standard 2 focused specifically on the treatment of common mental health problems in primary care. Standard 3 focused on 24-hour access to services. Standards 4 and 5 focused on specialist mental health care, but recognised the need for close working between those services and primary care, particularly with regard to enhancing the physical health of people suffering from serious mental illness, and the development of case registers for long-term conditions. Primary care services have a role in the delivery of services for people with the range of mental health difficulties including the most common (anxiety disorders and depression), and the most severe and complex (schizophrenia and bipolar disorder). The point where the majority of people with mental health problems seek assistance and receive care remains general practice (Cape et al 2000).

In addressing these issues the National Service Framework for Mental Health identified the requirement for primary care to be more responsive to mental health need. The NHS National Plan (DH 2000) went further in identifying workforce developments specifically to address these issues in the form of 1,000 Graduate Primary Care Mental Health Workers and 500 Gateway Workers.

There have been major changes to the primary care context since the publication of the National Service Framework for Mental Health. Primary Care Groups were developed to assess and respond to the needs of local populations, and then were transformed into Primary Care Trusts (NHS Executive 1999). Health Authorities transferred their commissioning role to Primary Care Trusts and were then disbanded. Strategic Health Authorities were established, taking on some of the roles of the Regional Health Authorities, which were then disbanded. Latterly Strategic Health Authorities have merged to produce regional bodies, and Primary Care Trusts have merged to produce larger units better suited to the needs of commissioning services (DH 2005). The whole health economy is being re-shaped with an emphasis on multiple providers, choice and competition (DH 2005). General Practice contracts have become more performance-based with the implementation of the General Medical Services contract and the development of the Quality Outcomes Framework (http://www.nhsemployers.org/primary/index.cfm). It is perhaps heartening how much progress has been made within the area in the light of such 'disruptive governance' (Oxman et al 2005, Hunter 2006).

There is a continuing tension within policy regarding the treatment of mental health problems in primary care. One consequence of the re-focusing of community mental health services on the needs of those with serious mental illness has been to reduce access to mental health expertise for staff within primary care. This prioritisation of resources on those with the most serious difficulties has been reiterated in the Chief Nursing Officer's Review of Mental Health Nursing (DH 2006). In contrast, a stream of National Institute for Clinical Excellence guidance continues to highlight the central role of primary care in delivering the majority of mental health interventions. There is little evidence that the production of protocols to manage the referral interface between primary care and specialist mental health services, as recommended within the NSF, has been a viable alternative to the working relationships that were disrupted as a result of this re-focusing (Ricketts et al 2003).

Despite recommendations for a client-centred integrated system of mental health care, with close cooperation between primary care and specialist mental health services within the NSF Workforce Action Team report in 2001, slow progress was reported within the five-year review of the NSF (Appleby 2004). Progress with recruitment of the graduate primary care workers was slower than anticipated, commissioning arrangements were considered to be problematic, and the developments of serious mental illness registers were not reported by the majority of Local Implementation Teams. The inclusion of mental health issues in the Quality Outcomes Framework (Table 15.1) that guides payment within the GMS contract for GPs may represent an opportunity to provide the necessary financial incentives for general practitioners to focus on the needs of a large minority of their populations with mental health problems.

National Institute for Clinical Excellence Guidelines have been produced relating to the mental health problems reported to be most common in primary care – depression and anxiety disorders (CSIP 2006). They reiterate the extent to which the bulk of mental health care is, and should continue to be, provided within the primary care setting, and outline the principles of stepped care as an organising framework within which to manage the high levels of demand for services in a rational and equitable manner.

Stepped care

Stepped care approaches propose the reorganisation of resources such that the most efficient, least intrusive, and least restrictive interventions that have an evidence-base are provided for people with mental health difficulties prior to the consideration of more extensive and intrusive interventions (Davison 2000). The approaches involve the close monitoring of outcomes from the less intensive interventions, so that movement to more intensive approaches can occur appropriately and without disjunction. Stepped care models assume that the majority of the population concerned will respond to lower steps, and that a

Table 15.1

Mental health indicators within the Quality & Outcome Framework (2006)	
Indicator	**Points**
Depression	
Diagnosis and initial management	
DEP 1: The percentage of patients on the diabetes register and/or the CHD register for whom case finding for depression has been undertaken on one occasion during the previous 15 months using two standard screening questions	8
DEP 2: In those patients with a new diagnosis of depression, recorded between the preceding 1 April to 31 March, the percentage of patients who have had an assessment of severity at the outset of treatment using an assessment tool validated for use in primary care	25
Mental health	
Records	
MH 8: The practice can produce a register of people with schizophrenia, bipolar disorder and other psychoses	4
Ongoing management	
MH 9: The percentage of patients with schizophrenia, bipolar affective disorder and other psychoses with a review recorded in the preceding 15 months. In the review there should be evidence that the patient has been offered routine health promotion and prevention advice appropriate to their age, gender and health status	23
MH 4: The percentage of patients on lithium therapy with a record of serum creatinine and TSH in the preceding 15 months	1
MH 5: The percentage of patients on lithium therapy with a record of lithium levels in the therapeutic range within the previous six months	2
MH 6: The percentage of patients on the register who have a comprehensive care plan documented in the records agreed between individuals, their family and/or carers as appropriate	6
MH 7: The percentage of patients with schizophrenia, bipolar affective disorder and other psychoses who do not attend the practice for their annual review who are identified and followed up by the practice team within 14 days of non-attendance	3
Dementia	
Records	
DEM 1: The practice can produce a register of patients diagnosed with dementia	5
Ongoing management	
DEM 2: The percentage of patients diagnosed with dementia whose care has been reviewed in the previous 15 months	15

greater number of individuals as a result will receive some form of appropriate treatment at as early a stage in their care as possible (CSIP 2006).

Stepped care approaches to common mental health problems have proven popular within the UK health system, as evidenced by their inclusion in NICE

Guidelines for Depression; Panic and Generalised Anxiety Disorder; Eating Disorders; Post-Traumatic Stress Disorder; Obsessive-Compulsive Disorder and Body Dysmorphic Disorder (NCCMH 2004, 2005a,b, NICE 2004a,b). Interventions at the lower levels of intensity have developed to the extent that a NICE technology appraisal now recommends the routine availability of Computerised Cognitive Behaviour Therapy (NICE 2006), and there is emerging evidence of the effectiveness of guided self-help approaches based upon cognitive behaviour therapy (Richards et al 2003).

Implications for primary care mental health are that there should be availability of evidence-based psychological and pharmacological interventions for common mental health problems for large numbers of individuals, delivered by suitably trained staff in primary care. This should be combined with simple routine measurement of outcomes, with robust systems to move individuals through the steps rapidly where initial interventions are ineffective (Davison 2000).

Interventions

In this section of the chapter we will outline the interventions currently in development in each 'step' that aim to improve choice and access in primary care settings. As discussed above the first contact for most people who experience mental health problems is with a primary care practitioner. Over the years there have been attempts to add to the skills these clinicians have in relation to the identification and management of mental health issues with equivocal results (Thompson et al 2000). Often it is possible to develop new skills in workers, however the ultimate impact of these upon improving clinical outcomes remains limited. Bower & Sibbald (2000) found that mental health practitioners simply being based in primary care settings resulted in no clinical benefit beyond those patients seen by the practitioners themselves. Gradually it has been recognised that whole systems need to be adapted to promote acceptance that treatment of mental health in primary care is core business and not something to ignore or pass to specialist services.

The development of the Quality Outcomes Framework (QOF) to guide payment for primary care work within the GMS (http://www.nhsemployers.org/primary/index.cfm) has incorporated significant points for managing mental health well within the practice (see Table 15.1). The system allocates 1000 points, which are split into 655 for clinical services, 181 for organisational systems, 108 for patient experience monitoring and 56 for additional services and holistic care issues. The revised QOF allocates points for both the recognition of depression in certain 'at risk' groups and the use of a validated tool to assess the severity of such problems once diagnosed. Three tools are recommended: the Beck Depression Inventory (Beck et al 1961), the Hospital Anxiety and Depression Scale (Zigmund & Snaith 1983) and the Patient Health Questionnaire (PHQ9) (Kronke at al 2001). In addition points are allocated to the physical health checks for those with severe and enduring mental health problems and checks on lithium blood levels. The contract also allows for local enhanced services to be developed that further improve local care (see Fletcher et al 2004).

Associated with this development a new interest has been seen at least in relation to those clinical areas where such points can be earned. Pathways relating to mental health may now be found in many practices and the incorporation of structured screening and symptom measurement tools such as the PHQ9 (Kronke at al 2001) will improve the identification of problems. An implication of increased recognition is that already overburdened services will also have to consider the means by which they respond to anxiety and depression. A move away from the focus on high intensity, low volume approaches to those of high volume and low intensity, with good governance, is required. Below we outline some of the approaches that can be developed to facilitate this.

Step 1 Minimal–mild problems

Watchful waiting is recommended initially at this step (NICE 2004b). Randomised trials have consistently been unable to differentiate outcomes between interventions and placebo at this level of symptoms, possibly due to natural remission. There is more indication that some of the anxiety disorders are less likely to spontaneously remit than mood disorders. When psychological complaints are identified but the clinician and patient agree they are mild, and this assessment is reflected by a tool such as the PHQ9 (scoring <10), agreement can be made that the problem will be reviewed after a set period (2 weeks according to NICE). Patients should be actively followed up at that point. There are some interventions that lend themselves to provision for this step and if available should be offered to the patient.

Community interventions

Large scale educational workshops based upon cognitive behaviour therapy (CBT) models are growing in popularity. These can be used to treat both anxiety and depression in community settings optimising the resource at this level of clinical presentation (White 1998, Brown et al 2000). Courses generally run over a 6–8-week period and are up to 2 hours long. The format is similar to that of adult education environments and teaches participants about the condition (anxiety and depression), methods to understand one's own problems and a simple structure that leads to the development of techniques to gradually overcome the functional and emotional impairment that is being experienced. Groups can be large and no self-disclosure is expected. Such formats lend themselves to family members or friends attending so as to better assist the sufferer with between-class exercises.

Another community intervention is the availability of books on prescription. Such schemes were initially developed in Cardiff but are now available through many libraries in the UK. These schemes allow clinicians to prescribe a book that has been quality-tested and is available in their local library. Ongoing evaluation of such schemes will be informative as unsupported self-help may not be as effective as facilitated self-help (Febbraro et al 1999). To try to offer extra assistance many schemes now have additional drop-in or email support available should they be required. Books are generally based upon CBT models. The aim of such schemes is to help navigate the multitude of self-help literature available in high street bookshops that is often of questionable quality.

In addition to the above, information about accessing web-based information and support can be placed in surgeries or given to patients. Organisations such as No Panic (http://www.nopanic.org.uk), OCD action (http://www.ocdaction. org.uk), triumph over phobia (http://www.triumphoverphobia.com) and depression alliance (http://www.depressionalliance.org) can be recommended.

The aim of all of the above is to inform and empower the person with the problem to start the path to recovery. As can be seen, watchful waiting does not mean simply sitting on the problem; the above resources can create a menu of options for primary care with relatively small resource allocation. It is of importance however to ensure that the watchful aspect of this step is not forgotten; repeated application of validated measures will allow comparison to baseline to assess if additional input is needed.

Step 2 Mild–moderate problems: minimal psychological interventions

The reliance on traditional one-hour sessions for psychological interventions has been under scrutiny for some time now (Lovell & Richards 2000). The situation nationally is one where the number of therapists available does not meet demand (London School of Economics 2006), resulting in unacceptable waiting times for therapy, if therapy is available at all. Guided self-help has emerged as one possible option for managing demand in primary care, with NICE guidelines for both anxiety and depression (NICE 2004a,b) recommending it at this level of problem severity. It appears that such methodologies may lend themselves to primary care settings and achieve positive clinical outcomes (Ekers & Lovell 2003, Lovell et al 2003). The optimum training required to be able to facilitate such technologies is unclear and requires ongoing research (Ekers et al 2006).

Self-help differs from traditional therapy in that roles of the therapist and the literature they use are reversed. In traditional CBT the therapist will use handouts with exercises to support the learning within the session between sessions. In guided self-help the written material is considered the main change agent, with the facilitator supporting this. It follows then that the sessions can be shorter, even down to 15 minutes, as the facilitator role is to deal with problems in the utilisation of the materials. In a similar way to traditional CBT, guided self-help sessions require structure (see Table 15.2 below) and explore the patient's expert knowledge of their own difficulties via exercises in the material. Each material has its own slant (a list of 'web-based' examples is given at the end of this chapter) and a patient can find the approach that best suits them. One of the major advantages of this approach is that it makes significant use of the largest resource the health service has at its fingertips, the patients themselves! Once the material is introduced it can be used at any time of the day or night in the patient's own home. Whilst many staff are now receiving training and such interventions are becoming more common we remain unsure as to how to best make use of these technologies. The ideal placement and structure of guided self-help is yet to be established, although the approach may well be best placed early in a care pathway to provide treatment for patients before their difficulties become entrenched.

Computer delivered treatments

Computer delivered CBT (CCBT) is an alternative way of delivering therapy advocated by NICE (NICE 2006). Whether this approach is seen as self-help or therapist replacement (as sessions are of the same length as traditional therapy and incorporate the same components) it certainly may release therapist time. Both clinical and cost effectiveness of certain packages have been demonstrated when based in primary care settings. The computer packages typically take on the role of the therapist in the explanation of treatment rationale and goal setting tasks. Case examples are given and the patient is encouraged to work through exercises aimed at understanding their own difficulties and setting homework targets to develop new adaptive learning. In addition such approaches lend themselves to a web based format where the GP can prescribe a password so treatment can occur at a time convenient to the patient rather than in a pre-set clinic appointment. Web-based delivery may also be important because of the difficulty in finding suitable venues to place such systems in busy general practice settings.

Step 3 Moderate problems: medication and/or psychological interventions

Antidepressant medication is often seen in primary care as the only option due to limited alternative choices (Ekers & Preston 2006). Indeed the effectiveness of medication for moderate depression is accepted (NICE 2004b) although many problems remain in optimising its effect in routine care. Changes in the way services are delivered can improve the effect of medication with limited additional resource, an issue that is possibly understated in clinical guidelines. Such changes require services to consider depression a chronic and relapsing disorder (Andrews 2001) requiring the same process of pro-active care delivery in primary care as other chronic diseases.

The chronic care model

Six domains require development in the improvement of chronic condition management in primary care (www.improvingchroniccare.org) (Wagner 1998):

- *Community resources*. The integration and development of community resources that complement traditional services. It is important to ensure non-statutory and statutory services do not duplicate what is on offer.
- *Health system development*. Focus on development of health systems in place via clear plans and agreement of roles between all involved. Developments must be linked to incentives (an example of which is the QOF), assertively led and subject to regular audit and subsequent adjustment.
- *Self-management support*. Utilise the resource that is the patient themselves by providing good quality information and self-help. Incorporate clear information regarding treatment and incorporate feedback into subsequent condition management.
- *Delivery system design*. The delivery system provides information to guide interventions that are likely to be effective related to symptom level. This

information provides clarity regarding the suitable level (step) of intervention that is the first offered. Regular reviews are built in to monitor response rate against established benchmarks to ensure treatment is delivered as designed.

- *Decision support.* Decision on care is supported through clear guidance on what is to be offered and when this is to be adjusted. Expected response rates should be linked to interventions on offer so open and frank discussion can take place between clinician and patient regarding choices at any given time.

- *Information systems.* These are available to all involved in care and have the latest up-to-date reviews of progress. Such systems highlight those patients who have not responded to treatment, or have not had contact, and ensure a treatment review is in place. They have access to appointment systems and educational resources. It is also useful to have information systems that allow a review of the system as a whole and the benchmarking of the clinician against best practice.

Case management of depression

Proactive case management has demonstrated marked improvement over usual care (Bower et al 2006). Larger improvement is noted where six or more contacts are scheduled, support is available from specialist mental health services, there is a psychological component and case managers have suitable training. A key factor is the role of a case manager to deliver follow-up and assessment of response to treatment at each session. In doing this we are analysing, in a systematic manner, if the treatment delivered is effective – much in the same way as response to blood pressure treatment is monitored by regular BP checks. The clinical/cost effectiveness of such approaches are clear at 2-year follow-up; the challenge now is the incorporation into routine care (Simon 2006).

Case management of depression commonly combines medication concordance, engagement and education regarding the condition and treatment with a psychological intervention, commonly behavioural activation (Jacobson et al 2001). It is delivered in primary care and notes are included on primary care systems, allowing up-to-date information to all involved in care provision. Generally case management is delivered through phone contacts lasting 10–15 minutes. During these sessions with their case manager patients are able to discuss any problems they may have with the treatment and to instigate problem solving. As treatment progresses the PHQ9 is used to monitor the response to this level of treatment (medication and activation) and at 6–8 weeks change is benchmarked against expected outcomes. If treatment is not working other options are considered with the patient at the earliest possible opportunity. This prevents ongoing administration of insufficient interventions. The typical call structure is outlined in Table 15.2.

Psychological interventions

The above describes a selection of the less intensive but clinically effective approaches suitable to meet patient demand in primary care. It is clear that

Table 15.2

Session structure: depression case management, guided self-help and cognitive behaviour therapy		
DCM structure (10–15min)	**GSH session structure (15–30min)**	**CBT session structure (50min–1 hour)**
• Introduction • General review in relation to last week's call • PHQ9 and discussion of score • Medication discussion • Activity scheduling discussion/planning • Problem solving • Wrap up	• Introduction and agenda • Recap on material used and exercises developed from this • Review progress • Problem solve any issues • Summarise ongoing work • Arrange next review	• Negotiation of agenda • Review last session • Review homework exercises • Discussion of issues pertaining to the above • In session exercises • Review and link to homework plan • Feedback on session • Arrange next appointment

not all patients will respond to such limited interventions and this is where the importance of systematic monitoring of outcomes is critical. Those not achieving the expected responses can be 'stepped up' to more intensive psychological or pharmacological intervention.

Currently the psychological treatment of choice for anxiety disorders and depression is cognitive behaviour therapy (NICE 2004a,b, NCCMH 2005a,b). Typically this takes the form of a short-term problem-focussed intervention that explores the cognitive and behavioural maintaining factors of a problem. Sessions are generally 1 hour and treatment can last between 8 and 20 sessions. Patients are encouraged to undertake between-session tasks that allow them to recognise thinking and behaviour patterns and modify these in experiments. This allows for the development of new and adaptive behaviours and cognitions. The longer sessions allow more detailed exploration of underlying factors that may be contributing to the problem and thus are most suited to those with complex problems or problems that are not responding to interventions lower in the stepped care system. A typical CBT treatment session is outlined in Table 15.2. There are many approaches to CBT from the more behavioural (Jacobson et al 2001) to more cognitive (Beck 1976) and combinations of the two (Hawton et al 1989). Therapists are required to be trained to an acceptable standard via established courses (see: www.babcp.org.uk).

Interpersonal therapy (IPT) is also recommended by NICE in the treatment of depression (NICE 2004b). In IPT the main problem areas focussed upon are grief, interpersonal deficits, role dispute and role transition (Klerman et al 1984). The therapist uses the therapeutic relationship as the 'workshop' within which understanding and changes of response can be developed, much in common with brief psychodynamic psychotherapy. IPT is time-limited, generally being delivered over 20 sessions or fewer. There are indications that IPT may be particularly useful for older adults, an important consideration given the incidence of depression amongst that group (Clarkin & Levy 2004).

Counselling is an intervention commonly found in primary care, with between one-third and one-half of general practices having on-site counselling services provided by a range of mental health professionals. Although the term counselling is used to describe a range of brief approaches to emotional distress, in general it is viewed as concerned with a skilled, facilitative relationship in which the counsellor enables the patient to explore problems in a non-directive, person-centred manner (DH 2001). Generally counselling in primary care is time-limited to 6–8 sessions. It is most effective for short-term psychological distress associated with life events (DH 2001). Counselling in primary care is significantly more effective than treatment as usual in the short term, but not at long-term follow-up (Bower & Rowland 2006). Patients are generally satisfied with the receipt of counselling.

Primary care and serious mental illness

The role of primary care in the treatment of patients with severe and enduring mental illness has again been highlighted within the GMS contract. Many patients with such complaints remain treated within primary care alone or if not solely treated use primary care for their physical health needs. It is clear that the physical health of this population is generally poor with increased rates of heart disease, diabetes, obesity, cancer, hypertension and respiratory problems. This population has a greater mortality rate in relation to such problems, does not receive adequate testing and follow-up and has difficulty in accessing general practice (Disability Rights Commission 2006).

The GMS has sought to ensure that the problem of 'passing the buck' in relation to these issues is stopped and all patients in a practice are included on a register, and are offered both physical and mental health checks yearly to highlight and resolve any issues found. In addition those on lithium have bloods monitored to ensure the safety of this medication is maintained in relation to the increased risk of hypothyroidism and hypocalcaemia and to maintain therapeutic levels in the bloodstream. It is to be hoped that by the inclusion of such quality indicators the health inequalities experienced by this population can be reduced.

Remaining challenges

Whilst a great deal of progress has been made in enhancing primary care mental health services since 1999 there remain significant challenges. Primary care mental health services have not adequately addressed the call within the National Service Framework for all people with a common mental health problem to be able to access effective interventions 24 hours a day (Appleby 2004). The availability of evidence-based psychological therapies remains limited (London School of Economics 2006). The effectiveness of stepped care systems in widening access is largely unproven, although there is increasing evidence for the impact of component parts of such systems.

There have been recent calls for psychological therapists in primary care (largely CBT) to address the impact of chronic ill-health on the employment prospects of parts of society. The Layard proposals (London School of Economics 2006) have resulted in pilot sites in Newham and Doncaster that will not produce evidence of effectiveness for some years. Whether the primary care health system is suitably placed to expand massively the national availability of cognitive behavioural therapy remains uncertain.

A continuing concern amongst those developing approaches in this field is that the approaches developed and applied to primary care mental health are congruent with the culture of general practice, and recognise the factors that motivate clinicians in that setting. Initiatives derived from a specialist mental health perspective are unlikely to flourish in the context of primary care (Bower & Sibbald 2000).

Successful implementation of the primary care proposals contained within the National Service Framework for Mental Health will have the greatest impact on the largest body of the population suffering from mental ill-health. The recent priority that this part of the mental health system has been receiving is both welcome and long overdue.

References

Andrews G 2001 Should depression be managed as a chronic disease? British Medical Journal 322:419–421

Appleby L 2004 The National Service Framework for Mental Health – Five Years On. DH, London

Beck A T 1976 Cognitive therapy and the emotional disorders. International Universities Press, New York

Beck A, Ward C, Mendelson M, Mock J, Erdbaugh, J 1961 An inventory for measuring depression. Archives of General Psychiatry 4:561–571

Bower P, Gilbody S, Richards D, Fletcher J, Sutton A 2006 Collaborative care for depression in primary care. Making sense of a complex intervention: Systematic review and meta-regression. British Journal of Psychiatry 189:484–493

Bower P, Sibbald B 2000 Systematic review of the effect of on-site mental health professionals on the clinical behaviour of general practitioners. British Medical Journal 320:614–617

Bower P, Rowland N 2006 Effectiveness and cost effectiveness of counselling in primary care (review). The Cochrane Collaboration

Brown J, Cochrane R, Hancox T 2000 Large scale health promotion stress workshops for the general public: a controlled evaluation. Behavioural And Cognitive Psychotherapy 28:139–151

Cape J, Barker C, Buszewicz M, Pistrang N 2000 General practitioner psychological management of common emotional problems (I): definitions and literature review. British Journal of General Practice 50:313–318

Care Services Improvement Partnership 2006 Improving primary care mental health services. DH, London

Clarkin J F, Levy K N 2004 The influence of client variables on psychotherapy. In: Lambert M J (ed) Bergin and Garfield's Handbook of psychotherapy and behavior change, 5th edn. Wiley, New York, p194–226

Davison G C 2000 Stepped care: Doing more with less? Journal of Consulting and Clinical Psychology 68:580–585.

Department of Health 2000 The NHS plan: A plan for investment, a plan for reform. HMSO, London

Department of Health 2001 Treatment Choice in Psychological Therapies and Counselling: Evidence Based Clinical Practice Guideline. DH, London

Department of Health 2005 Health reform in England: update and next steps. DH, London

Department of Health 2006 From values to action: The Chief Nursing Officer's review of mental health nursing. DH, London

Disability Rights Commission 2006 Equal treatment: closing the gap. Interim report of a formal investigation into health inequalities. Disability Rights Commission, London (http://www.drc-gb.org)

Ekers D, Preston J 2006 Depression case management in a stepped care system. Progress in Neurology and Psychiatry 10(7):31–36

Ekers D, Lovell K 2003 Self -help for anxiety and depression in primary care: an audit of a pilot clinic. Clinical Effectiveness in Nursing 6:129–133

Ekers D, Lovell K, Playle J F 2006 The use of CBT based, brief, facilitated self-help interventions in primary care mental health service provision: evaluation of a 10-day training programme. Clinical Effectiveness in Nursing 9(Suppl 1):e88–e96

Febbraro G A R, Clum G A, Roodman A A, Wright J H 1999 The limits of bibliotherapy: A study of the differential effectiveness of self-administered interventions in individuals with panic attacks. Behavior Therapy 30:209–222

Fletcher J, Bower P, Richards D, Saunders T 2004 enhanced services specification for depression under the new GP Contract. National Institute for Mental Health in England, London

Hawton K, Salkovskis P, Kirk J, Clark D 1989 Cognitive behaviour therapy for psychiatric disorders. Oxford University Press, Oxford

Hunter D J 2006 The tsunami of reform: The rise and fall of the NHS. British Journal of Healthcare Management 12(1):18–23

Jacobson N, Martell C, Dimijan S W 2001 Behavioural activation treatment for depression: returning to contextual roots. Clinical Psychology: Science & Practice 8(3):255–270

Klerman G, Weissman M, Rounsaville B, Chevron E 1984 Interpersonal psychotherapy of depression. Basic Books, New York, NY

Kronke K. Spitzer R, Williams J 2001 PHQ9 validity of a brief depression measure. Journal of General Internal Medicine 16:606–613

London School of Economics 2006 The depression report: a new deal for depression and anxiety disorders. The Centre for Economic Performance's Mental Health Policy Group. London School of Economics, London

Lovell K, Richards D A 2000 Multiple Access Points and Levels of Entry (MAPLE): Ensuring choice, accessibility and equity for CBT services. Behavioural and Cognitive Psychotherapy 28:379–391

Lovell K, Richards D, Bower P 2003 Improving access to primary care mental health, uncontrolled evaluation of a pilot self-help clinic. British Journal of General Practice 53:133–135

National Collaborating Centre for Mental Health 2004 Eating Disorders: Core interventions in the treatment and management of anorexia nervosa, bulimia nervosa, and related eating disorders. British Psychological Society, Leicester

National Collaborating Centre for Mental Health 2005a Post-traumatic stress disorder: The management of PTSD in adults and children in primary and secondary care. Royal College of Psychiatrists, London

National Collaborating Centre for Mental Health 2005b Obsessive-compulsive disorder: core interventions in the treatment of obsessive-compulsive disorder and body dysmorphic disorder. Royal College of Psychiatrists, London.

National Institute for Clinical Excellence 2004a Anxiety: Management of anxiety (panic disorder with or without agoraphobia, and generalised anxiety disorder) in adults in primary, secondary and community care. NICE, London

National Institute for Clinical Excellence 2004b Depression: Management of depression in primary and secondary care. NICE, London

National Institute for Health and Clinical Excellence 2006 Technology Appraisal 97: Computerised cognitive behaviour therapy for depression and anxiety. NICE, London

NHS Executive 1999 Establishing Better Services. NHS Executive, Leeds

Oxman A D, Sackett D L, Chalmers I, Prescott T E 2005 A surrealistic mega-analysis of redisorganization theories. Journal of the Royal Society of Medicine 98:563–568

Richards A, Barkham M, Cahill J, Richards D, Williams C, Heywood P 2003 PHASE: a randomised, controlled trial of supervised self-help cognitive behaviour therapy in primary care. British Journal of General Practice 53:764–770

Ricketts T, Saul C, Newton P, Brooker C 2003 Evaluating the development, implementation and impact of protocols between primary care and specialist mental health services. Journal of Mental Health 12(4):363–377

Simon G 2006 Collaborative care for depression. British Medical Journal 332:249–250

Thompson C, Kinmonth A, Stevens L et al 2000 Effects of a clinical-practice guideline and practice-based education on detection and outcome of depression in primary care: Hampshire Depression Project randomised controlled trial. The Lancet 355(9199):185–191

Wagner E H 1998 Chronic Disease Management: What will it take to improve care for chronic illness? Effective Clinical Practice 1(1):2–4

White J 1998 'Stress control' large group therapy for generalized anxiety disorder: two year follow-up. Behavioural and Cognitive Psychotherapy 26:237–245

Zigmund A, Snaith R 1983 The Hospital Anxiety and Depression Scale. Acta Psychiatrica Scandinavica 67:361–370

16

A national survey of Crisis Resolution Teams:
an evaluation of implementation in England

S. Onyett • K. Linde

Introduction

Crisis Resolution Teams (CRTs) were introduced in the UK in the late 1980s, during a wave of government funded demonstration projects. Their design was particularly influenced by pioneering work in Australia (Hoult 1986), where in order to provide an alternative to hospital admissions, teams delivered a 24-hour service to users at home, with the maximum opportunity to resolve crises in the contexts where they occurred. Their implementation in England was prompted by the National Service Framework for Mental Health (NSF) (DH 1999). NSF Standard 4 was explicit: people should be able to access services 24 hours a day, 365 days a year; while Standard 5 stated that people should be able to access care in the least restrictive environment and as close to home as possible.

The NHS Plan (DH 2000) set the national target of 335 CRTs serving 100,000 users by December 2004. These requirements were performance managed through a new Local Delivery Plan process (DH 2002), which included the Public Sector Agreement (PSA) targets. Crisis services were referred to generically as part of the PSA aim of: '...transforming the health and social care system so that it produces faster, fairer services that deliver better health and tackle health inequalities'.

The NHS was required to set in place arrangements for 24-hour crisis resolution to all eligible patients by 2005, based on the national target of 335 functioning CRTs set in 2004. The Mental Health Policy Implementation Guide (MHPIG; DH 2001a) specifies the principles of care in such teams:

- A 24-hour, 7-day a week service
- Rapid response following referral
- Intensive intervention and support in the early stages of the crisis

- Active involvement of the service user, family and carers
- An assertive approach to engagement
- Time-limited interventions, with sufficient flexibility to respond to differing service user needs
- An emphasis on learning from the crisis, with the involvement of the whole social support network.

CRTs represent a major new investment area. Spending on access and crisis services rose from £152 million in 2001/02 to £229 million in 2003/04 – a real terms increase of 51%. In 2004, £17 million was made available to Mental Health Trusts to improve access to services for people in crisis (Appleby 2004). Trusts were expected to use this sum to improve the coordination of crisis services, for example mental health teams providing liaison to emergency departments, through CRTs and gateway staff.

Do CRTs work?

Crisis resolution is a comparatively new model internationally and the evidence base for effectiveness is still developing. A systematic review of crisis intervention (Joy et al 2001, updated 2006) reported only a limited effect on admissions, but found home care to be as cost-effective as hospital care with respect to loss of people to local services, deaths and mental distress.

Recent studies of CRT report significant impact on admissions. Johnson et al (2005a) in a before and after study found significant differences in bed use (20% lower for CRT group) and admissions (77% of pre and 49% of post introduction of CRT were admitted). A randomised control trial (Johnson et al 2005b) found CRT users were less likely to be admitted to hospital in the 8 weeks after the crisis and there was a reduction in admissions (59% to 22%). Glover et al (2006) employed NHS admission statistics to consider evidence of impact on admissions following the programmatic implementation of teams. A 10% overall reduction was shown for all CRTs, but where the team operated over 24 hours seven days per week (24/7) this was more marked, reaching 20%.

Clinical and social CRT outcomes have generally been judged to be similar to in-patient treatment, though the focus to date has been on clients diagnosed with a functional psychosis (Smyth et al 2000). CRTs were also judged to have reduced the burden on families, and were preferred by both users and families (Dean et al 1993, Joy et al 2001).

Joy et al's 2006 review found that positive results from CRT depended on effective implementation. In particular, routing all referrals for in-patient care through the CRT appeared to be critical to success in fully offering a realistic alternative to admission. Such teams are therefore likely to be highly dependent on support from those practitioners who can circumvent the system, by making direct admissions to in-patient care. Ford & Kwakwa (1996) also observed that poorly delivered crisis services can have a detrimental effect on clients and increase hospital admissions. To date there has been limited in-depth description of day-to-day CRT policies and practices and their relative potency in achieving outcomes.

This chapter will explore some of those policies and practices, informed by a recent national survey of CRTs (Onyett et al 2006). This national survey aimed to provide a team level description of services, adapting a schedule from a study of community mental health teams (CMHTs; Onyett et al 1994). Entry criteria for the survey was permissive and included any local arrangements that had been designed to achieve the outcomes required of a CRT locally. Most of the data collection occurred between October 2005 and January 2006, with a response rate of 73%. The majority of respondents defined their role in managerial terms (deputy, project manager) and most were CRT managers (90% of the total sample).

How have CRT services developed in England?

In March 2004, the national reported number of CRTs had risen to 168 from only 35 in 2000. These teams mostly met the MHPIG criteria, although 64 of the 168 did not operate 24/7 (Appleby 2004). In 2005, the national survey (drawing on intelligence from crisis leads in regional development centres) found 243 CRTs and a detailed profile was derived from the 177 teams included in the study – 55% of respondents described their locality as urban, 9.6% of the respondents as rural and 36% as mixed/suburban.[1] Teams were relatively young, with 63% taking referrals for less than two years. The mean age of teams was 30 months, with distribution heavily skewed towards younger teams. Half were 20 months old or less. Urban teams were the oldest and rural the youngest.

Is there sufficient CRT capacity?

National targets for the number of teams needed to be underpinned by local need assessment as the main determinant of staffing capacity to see a given number of clients. The MHPIG refers to a norm of 14 designated named workers covering populations of approximately 150,000 who should carry a caseload of 20–30 users at any one time. Clearly this will vary according to the mental health needs of populations and demographics, so that inner city teams may cover populations of 40,000–60,000, while in less deprived areas this could rise to 200,000.

The national survey found that staffing capacity fell below expected levels and varied related to region. Using a simple projection to estimate the deviation of actual size from projected team size based on MHPIG recommendations (14 staff per 150,000, excluding admin), the East and West Midlands were the most adequately staffed. Teams were least staffed in the South East and South West. For England overall, the figures suggest that CRTs have achieved 88% of their recommended staffing.

---

[1]Using survey definitions adapted from Perlman et al (1984) – urban: worked within a city or town with a population of at least 50,000; rural: worked in localities defined as having no town of 10,000 or more, less than half the population live in towns/villages of 2500 of more.

Staff shortfalls were mirrored in levels of caseload activity. The survey found that the current caseload mean was 20 and current caseloads were positively correlated with both team size and age. Teams aged two years or more were in the lower range of the MHPIG recommendations (20–30). Teams between 1–2 years were close to the minimum recommended caseloads (20), but teams less than a year old fell well below (16). Younger teams had experienced significant changes in staff and rapid expansion over a short period. In addition to capacity, the stability of teams (level of staff turnover) and their maturity were important variables in meeting caseload expectations.

Compared with MHPIG guidance, teams in the South East and South West were seeing the lowest numbers, while the West and East Midlands saw the most clients. Overall, CRTs were estimated to see 59% of the numbers of clients recommended by MHPIG; caseload size mirrored staff capacity by region.

Team composition

CRT working requires a focus on the interaction of health and social factors in crisis and thus the input of staff with differing perspectives, disciplines and life histories is vital to bringing this kind of understanding to bear on team practices. Intensity of provision is not sufficient. For example, Muijen et al (1994) found comparatively poor outcomes from a uni-disciplinary community mental health nurse (CMHN) team, even when they were providing intensive support.

The MHPIG specified an appropriate skill mix to deliver interventions with a range of professions and support workers designated. Given their initial training in acute care it is perhaps therefore not surprising that the survey found that CMHNs were the main professional group (and the main nursing category) in teams (Table 16.1). The largest proportion of teams (48%) employed 7–9 nurses while only 13% had five or less. Levels of part-time working were low.

Recruitment strategies had made good use of opportunities for expanding the skill base for unqualified workers in this new area. Community support workers were making a significant contribution (e.g. compared with only 0.69 FTE in CMHTs in 1994) with likely benefits to a user focus in teams and more accessible and continuous relationships with staff. In other settings, when compared with professional staff, community support workers have been found to be more likely to be active in those areas of provision that users most rated as important (Murray et al 1997).

In a review of the future for social work in mental health (CSIP/NIMHE 2006), the new teams have been expected to add scope by developing the social work role in social inclusion. Social work input was a mean of 0.80 input and 1.1 for approved social workers, and levels of part-time working were low. However, there was considerable variation in the nature of coverage and 27% of teams did not have input from any social workers.

The input of other professions was more fragmented in form and less evident. While 30% of teams reported input from occupational therapists, the majority had just one post (24% of all responders) and 18% were part-time.

Among those employing a psychologist (13 teams or 8%), only 6 teams had full-time posts and 54% of posts overall were part-time, representing very small

Table 16.1

Profile of disciplines within teams				
	Mean number of people	Percentage of teams with input	Mean FTE per team	Percentage part-time
Community mental health nurses	9.9	98	9.7	6
Nurses (other than CMHNs)	0.3	12	0.3	4
Approved social workers	1.1	49	1.1	10
Other social workers	0.8	45	0.8	7
Occupational therapists	0.4	30	0.3	18
Consultant psychiatrists	0.5	44	0.4	44
Staff grade medical staff	0.3	27	0.3	39
Junior medical staff	0.1	11	0.1	25
Social time recovery workers	0.8	24	0.7	7
Support workers, other generic mental health workers	2.6	70	2.5	8
Clinical psychologists	0.1	8	0.1	54
Other specialist therapists	0.0	2	0.0	25
Administrative staff (including receptionists)	0.9	50	0.8	26
Others	0.4	19	0.4	21
All disciplines	18.3		17.6	10
All except administrative, others	17.0		16.4	9

amounts of input into teams. Specialist therapists (e.g. family therapists) were rare – only 2% (3 teams) reported a post.

Only 44% of teams reported any medical input at all – and even in those cases, the actual amount of input from psychiatrists was small at a mean 0.4 FTE (e.g. when compared to the mean 0.75 equivalent input in CMHTs in 1994; Onyett et al 1994). Twenty-four percent (or 39 teams) had one full-time consultant post; 16% had part-time posts ranging from 0.2 to 0.8. Only 4% of teams had more than one full-time equivalent.

The scope for involving service users as employees or advisors in CRTs was underdeveloped in services. Only 24% of teams had support time and recovery worker posts which had been explicitly designed to be open to service users as employees. A small number of teams had dedicated posts for service users and carers. Only 18 teams (10%) reported having a post filled by a service user and seven teams (4%) had a post filled by someone specifically to support work with carers. However, the majority of these posts were dedicated to developing practice with service users, rather than a wider service development role.

What do CRTs provide?

The key role of CRTs is to provide intensive support for the duration of an acute mental health crisis, while fully utilising the community, social and family context in resolution and prevention of future relapse.

Teams are resourced to enable an extended assessment process in the home, facilitating greater familiarity with the realities of service users' lives and neglected factors such as social support or housing, which may have led to recurrent hospital admission. Practical support has been found to be a core component of such work (Minghella et al 1998).

Access to emotional support and recognition of the impact of crisis on wider family and friends figure highly in what service users want from such services (Bristol Mind 2004). The MHPIG specifies provision of a range of therapies (problem solving, brief supportive counselling and social interventions) to support engagement, assessment and educative roles. However, there has been no high quality research of how therapies are provided, their sequencing, structure or efficacy in this setting – or the continuity of such work with other teams, working over the longer term.

The survey asked teams about the interventions they made. Those most usually and intensively provided were: risk assessment; monitoring of mental state; help with self-help strategies; delivering psychosocial interventions and administering medication. Small numbers of teams were providing and delivering medication less than weekly (17% and 13% respectively) and this was associated with lack of dedicated medical cover. The majority of teams provided 'early warning signs' training for family members or supports, forty per cent of teams did this daily or more often. However, one-third of teams reported never using advance directives. The majority of teams provided either weekly or daily therapeutic work with families and supports. Practical help formed a core activity. Over half of teams provided this on a daily or more frequent basis to service users, while 62% of teams also provided this on a daily or weekly basis to families and supports.

Wider 'whole life' issues – such as attending to issues of housing, finance and employment – were provided much less frequently. The majority of teams provided help with maximising income and housing needs weekly or less often. Reports of direct involvement in employment (i.e. more than signposting) suggest that this is undertaken less often than housing or income management. Figure 16.1 shows the scope of team interventions.

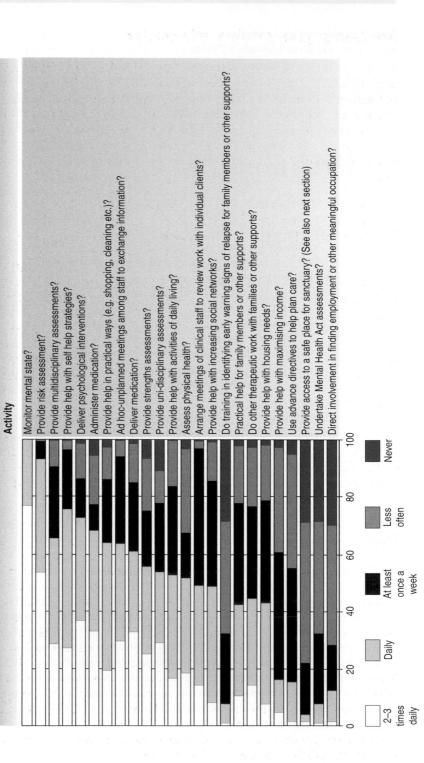

Figure 16.1 • Team interventions

Are teams gate-keeping effectively?

As we saw above, how well placed CRTs are to gate-keep within the wider system will impact strongly on their capacity to reduce admissions and to achieve and sustain a focus on their core client group. Recent guidance (DH 2006) defines 'full' gate-keeping and the breadth of team involvement required. This needs to encompass all requests for admission, including pending MHA assessments and assertive outreach. This also requires a consistent process, through which all service users at risk of admission can access assessment for home treatment as a potential option in care.

The requirement to involve a reflexive multidisciplinary team process (in the form of CRT involvement) has invoked some resistance and controversy, not least because it challenges medical autonomy and authority. The national survey found that although almost all teams aimed to provide an alternative to admission, only 68% (115) teams agreed that they acted as a gate-keeper to the acute in-patient beds, indicating a difference between aspiration and practice. Only 14% of teams claimed to be involved in all assessments for admission. Similar levels have been reported in a survey of acute in-patient care (SCMH 2004) where ward managers estimated only 12% of CRTs fully gate-kept beds.

Failure to gate-keep may be associated with a poor focus on the core client group, particularly given that the survey revealed there were high levels of demand on teams to do assessments. Levels of targeting varied, with a mean of 65% of case loads comprising people diagnosed with serious mental illness. Over a fifth of referrals were not even deemed appropriate for assessment, and even when assessed, only two-fifths of referrals were taken on for ongoing work.

The influences on gate-keeping are many, relating to team capacity, the supportiveness of other teams and stakeholders, and the clarity of local protocols and pathways to care. Positive outcomes for effective gate-keeping are apparent in the extant literature with respect to the presence of 24/7 access and dedicated medical cover. The relative availability of these nationally is discussed here in more detail.

Medical input and gate-keeping

Hoult (1986) advocated the contribution of a dedicated psychiatrist to gate-keeping, as this enhances the clinical authority of teams and enables a collegial approach to dealing with the attitudes of other doctors. Working in a dedicated way involves redefinition of psychiatrists' traditional generic role and there has been national direction and support for such transitions (DH 2005) The national survey found that dedicated cover was not well established in teams. Around half of teams had a dedicated consultant and other medical staff (46%), with a small number of teams accessing a dedicated consultant only (9%). The other main arrangement in teams was for support to come from a CMHT consultant (29%). Dedicated medical input had an impact on a number of variables relating to team fidelity. It was strongly associated ($p<0.01$) with whether a senior consultant can undertake home visits through an on-call rota and with the provision of a home-visiting service.

Of most importance in relation to gate-keeping, dedicated input was associated with whether teams considered they were able to override decisions to admit from others such as junior doctors (51% of teams reporting that the team was able to override others' decisions overall).

The impact of a senior medic within the team seemed therefore to be associated with the authority and confidence of the team and its ability to respond effectively out of hours.

How available is CRT support out of hours?

The national survey found that full provision was proving slow to develop, particularly in rural areas, and a widely varying national profile was apparent. Only 112 teams (67% of respondents) reported being available (on call or on duty) between 10pm and 8am. Availability was highest in urban teams (74%) and a similar proportion of suburban and rural teams offered this cover (58% and 60% respectively).

Only 53% (91) of respondents operated a 24/7 home visiting service, and these were mostly urban teams (64% compared with 39% of suburban teams and only six rural teams). Sixty-three percent of respondents reported providing a 24-hour telephone support service and again this was most prevalent among urban teams (77% compared to 59% of suburban teams and 44% of rural teams).

Where full 24/7 arrangements were not in place the mean length of cover of services was only 12 hours (for both telephone support and home visiting). The reasons for such variability of provision are not well established. In the case of rural teams, differing arrangements for the delivery of such services may be required. Although 41% of teams reported there were plans to change the hours of the service (and all teams described plans to extend their out-of-hours function), the extent to which this target included 24-hour provision varied considerably. The financial position of funding bodies, competing priorities and recruitment difficulties were cited as local barriers.

What was the extent of team fidelity?

The national survey data enabled rudimentary appraisal of the fidelity of teams, using a simple six point scale from the range of variables studied:

1. The team aims to provide an alternative to hospital admission for those experiencing acute mental health difficulties.
2. The team provides a 7-day per week, 24-hour home-visiting assessment service.
3. The team provides 7-day per week, 24-hour telephone support service.
4. The team is available (on call or on duty) between 10pm and 8am.
5. The team stays intensively involved as long as necessary for the immediate crisis to be resolved.
6. The team acts as the gate-keeper to the acute in-patient beds by assessing people referred for hospital admission.

All six questions were answered by 150 teams. Nearly all (98%) indicated that they aimed to be an alternative to hospital admission and that they would stay involved with a case until the crisis was resolved (97%). Seventy-two percent reported gate-keeping hospital admission; 67% as being on-call between 10pm and 8am, and 55% and 63% respectively as providing 24/7 home visiting and telephone based support. Using cleaned data which excluded teams giving incompatible answers (39 of the 150), teams reported meeting a mean of 4.9 of the criteria.

Teams were also asked to state whether they would describe themselves as 'fully set up' to meet the MPIG guidelines as 70 teams (40%) said they were. Those rating themselves as fully set up also had significantly higher fidelity scale ratings (mean 5.3 vs 3.9, $p<0.0001$). The lowest proportion of teams that were reporting themselves as fully set up were suburban (25%), followed by rural (38%) and urban (50%) teams. Fully set up teams were also older (34 vs 25 months) and fidelity and team age were weakly but significantly correlated ($p<0.01$). Differences with respect to fidelity were most evident on whether the team provided a 24-hour home visiting assessment service.

Workforce and training issues for the future

The National Plan (DH 2000) outlined the sheer scale of workforce expansion involved in recruiting rapidly to a range of new teams (early intervention, assertive outreach and CRT) and a number tensions are evident in the development of educational and workforce strategies over the longer term.

How can services secure the flow of appropriate numbers and range of staff while avoiding undermining development in other parts of the local service? Recruitment to CRTs appears to have been relatively easy and 48% of teams described their team as being easy to recruit to, when compared with other parts of the mental health service. Nursing was the discipline reported as easiest to recruit.

Staff groups with low representation in teams were also seen as difficult to recruit and reflect national trends in staffing shortages. Social work was identified as the most difficult to recruit, followed by psychology and occupational therapists (45%, 28% and 12% respectively).

When teams described recruitment strategies the local service was described as a main source of new workers, particularly from wards and CMHTs. Such success may have been at the cost of other parts of the acute care pathway – underlining the importance of ensuring parity of reward structures with community teams to ensure improvement across the whole system occurs (Sainsbury Centre for Mental Health 2004).

Initiatives such as use of rotational contracts, joint and link posts have the potential to develop practice across settings and were underdeveloped in services. Integrated workforce plans (Workforce Action Team; DH 2001b) form a key mechanism to ensure local services take into account the dynamics of new service models, consider the way skill mix is deployed between teams and use the widest range of recruitment strategies to mitigate uneven development of staff capacity.

These have proved difficult to implement, particularly with respect to the effective involvement of all stakeholders (Readhead & Brooker 2003) but will form a vital support for a longer term strategic approach to workforce development.

How can full CRT staffing be achieved and reflect a broader disciplinary mix in the future? Teams viewed themselves as still in development. Only 40% of teams could describe themselves as fully set up, primarily because of lack of staff and particularly to support out-of-hours working. Resourcing of CRTs appears to have been insufficient in some areas and it is possible that a sustainable critical mass of CRT activity has yet to be established nationally. Recruitment strategies will need to address the multifactorial barriers to employment of a wider disciplinary mix, such as the unpopularity of out-of-hours working, disparities in reward for out-of-hours work between health and social care, and the lack of joint investment and ownership of CRT across health and social care. Services were taking various initiatives to improve the acceptability of out-of-hours working such as the organisation of shift patterns to enable extended time out (e.g. 12-hour shifts and three days off), but there is a lack of guidance on effective recruitment strategies.

The skills in a crisis that staff within CRTs and across the whole mental health work force should have is specified within a national framework for a modern skill base of capabilities in mental health (SCMH 2000). However, the implementation of CRTs indicates a number of difficulties in the availability and access to appropriate training programmes, for what forms a relatively small new constituency of CRT staff.

The survey found many teams had been established with limited skill development to support the transition to new working practices. Only 52% of respondents had received some formal training on the establishment or running of crisis resolution services. Only one national training programme dedicated to crisis team has been developed and training was almost wholly accessed from this independent provider (Sainsbury Centre for Mental Health), with a minimal role for universities.

Aspects of training need for CRT may be difficult to respond to within mainstream programme development. Team working requires an innovative approach to learning that is site-based, tailored to the objectives sought and which can embrace the wider local service system in an iterative process of review.

Such an approach has been developed by NIMHE in partnership with other organisations (such as the Creating Capable Teams Approach, www.newwaysofworking.org.uk; and the Effective Teamworking and Leadership Programme, www.icn.org.uk/leadership) but capacity to deliver it is limited. Such sustained and sophisticated team support programmes pose a challenge for universities, but would fit well with their recent focus on knowledge transfer. Practice-based expertise on site-based, action learning orientated team and leadership development work is scarce in the UK and will involve careful consideration of its organisation in the face of consistent national demand.

Embedding CRTs in a whole system of care

The importance of a whole system approach to care is explicit in the NSF and multi-agency Local Implementation Teams were charged with coordinating local processes. However, the introduction of a range of specific interventions and team models has also been viewed as lacking coherence (Perri & Peck 2004), increasing the number of care interfaces and potentially contributing to fragmentation in service systems (Hall & Newbiggin 2004). Thus, the implementation task is complex and it is important that CRTs are considered as a central part of a new local service configuration.

Rummler & Brache (1995) identify a number of features of organisations when considered as whole systems: they have the potential to go wrong; they are multi-faceted; have multiple parts and processes and interdependencies; they have a sense of interconnectivity that is often undisclosed or ill considered and when adapted or developed in one part, it has a knock on effect in another. When CRTs were asked about local barriers to implementation, problems in relationships across the whole service system figured strongly and were interwoven with issues of inadequate resourcing. Ninety-three percent of respondents reported delays in referring on to the local CMHT when the crisis had resolved. CMHTs were seen as poorly resourced, often burnt out and evasive of contact. Poor joint working was reported at practice levels and other teams appearing to be jealous or threatened by CRTs. Medical culture, practices or attitudes were manifest in vocal opposition to CRTs or more covert obstructiveness such as not using CRTs, unless beds were full. At the level of the wider organisation senior managers were target driven and seen as lacking understanding of CRT operational and sustainability issues. Poor whole system ownership (or understanding of the home treatment philosophy of care) was illustrated in a lack of consensus around risk taking. Competition between different parts of the service arose, where for example, the threshold for admission was reportedly lowered as CRTs made an impact on the numbers of people presenting.

In a review of experiences of supporting CRTs, McGlynn (2007) also indicates that service strategies have been insufficient and may have mirrored divisions within systems. The following sources of conflict were identified:

- Teams becoming highly identified with their own ethos – MHPIG guidance for differing teams has not been consistent or related to a whole system.
- Teams lacking understanding of their role and having unrealistic expectations of other teams with gaps or duplication of functions.
- Rigid exclusion criteria and lack of flexibility creating conflict and confusion among service users and referrers accessing the system.

More sophisticated local whole system approaches that link service capacity to demand need to be achieved. Tribal, the Sainsbury Centre for Mental Health, and Research and Development in Mental Health have produced a briefing document on 'Capacity Planning'[2] which provides a dynamic planning tool for modelling demand and capacity within local service systems based on an iterative process of analysing local data (e.g. on in-patient bed use), agreeing assumptions (e.g. on the functions of parts of the local service system), producing a model and reviewing future activity against the model. A Capacity Management Framework for teams has also been developed by Training and Development for Health

---

[2] Download at www.tribalgroup.co.uk/?id=348&ob=2&rid=223

(www.td4h.co.uk). Development also needs to be informed by evidence on how to provide effective care in the least restrictive setting. This will require dedicated service improvement support and strong local leadership to enable teams to see beyond their own part of the service. There is also potential for the care programme approach, when effectively implemented, to contain tensions around interfaces introduced by new teams (Kingdom & Shabbir 2005). Teams themselves emphasised the importance of structural interventions to improve the integration of services, such as a whole system management of admission requests (based on a clear provider-wide clinical risk assessment and management strategy), strategic management of all emergency services, and one consultant wards to promote effective gate-keeping.

Conclusion

Subsequent to the introduction of the National Service Framework, the growth of crisis resolution services across the UK has been extensive and rapid, mobilising considerable local energy and investment. The majority of CRTs are urban, where they operate with greatest fidelity to the MHPIG. The reasons why rural teams find it difficult to achieve fidelity merits closer examination (e.g. proposed levels of out-of-hours cover might not be deemed necessary by local stakeholders). Different approaches to implementation may be warranted, informed by the more sophisticated and whole systems technologies described above.

The survey scoped the development needs of teams. Over half of the CRTs are newly established, experiencing high levels of internal staff change. Many have had no formal training in CRT development. Integrated, locality-based working was a challenge, particularly with respect to acceptance and understanding of the gate-keeping role; the supportiveness of medics as a key stakeholder; the ease of transfer back to CMHTs and opportunities for working on early discharge with in-patient staff.

The centrality and boundary spanning nature of CRT work make them an ideal focus for further inquiry. The national survey revealed very patchy and incomplete implementation alongside evidence that when properly implemented the impact on the rest of the service system is both radical and positive (Glover et al 2006).

The challenge now regarding CRTs, their commissioners, managers and development support is to learn what works – and then do more of it, taking into account the wider local service context within which CRTs form such an important part.

References

Appleby L 2004 The National Service Framework for Mental Health – Five Years On. Department of Health, London

Bristol Mind 2004 Crisis? What crisis? The experience of being in crisis in Bristol. Mind, Bristol

Care Services Improvement Partnership NIMHE 2006 The Social Work Contribution to Mental Health Services: The Future Direction. NIMHE, London

Dean C, Phillips J, Gadd E, Joseph M, England S 1993 Comparison of a community based service with a hospital-based service for people with acute, severe psychiatric illness. British Medical Journal 307:473–476

Department of Health 1999 National Service Framework for Mental Health: Modern Standards & Service Models. DH, London

Department of Health 2000 The NHS Plan. DH, London

Department of Health 2001a Mental Health Policy Implementation Guide. DH, London

Department of Health 2001b The National Workforce Action Team: Final Report. DH, London

Department of Health 2002 Improvement, expansion and reform: The next 3 years. Priorities and planning framework 2003–2006. DH, London

Department of Health 2005 New ways of working for psychiatrists: Enhancing effective, person centred-centred services through new ways of working in multidisciplinary and multiagency contexts. DH, London

Department of Health 2006 Crisis Resolution and Home treatment Guidance Statement. DH, London

Ford, R, Kwakwa J 1996 Rapid reaction, speedy recovery. Health Service Journal 18 April: 30–31

Glover G, Gerda A, Babu K 2006 Crisis resolution home treatment teams and psychiatric admission rates in England. British Journal of Psychiatry 189:441–445

Hall J, Newbiggin K 2004 Developing Mental Health Services in Northumberland. HASCAS, London

Hoult J 1986 Community care of the acutely mentally ill. British Journal of Psychiatry 149: 137–144

Johnson S, Nolan F, Hoult J et al 2005a Outcomes of crisis before and after introduction of a crisis resolution team. British Journal of Psychiatry 187:68–75

Johnson S, Nolan F, Pilling S et al 2005b Randomised controlled trial of acute mental health care by a crisis resolution team; the North Islington crisis study. British Medical Journal 331: 599

Joy C B, Adams C E, Rice K 2001 Crisis Intervention for those with a severe mental illness. The Cochrane Library, Issue 4, Oxford

Joy C B, Adams C E, Rice K 2006 Crisis intervention for people with severe mental illnesses. Cochrane Database of Systematic Reviews, Issue 4, Oxford

Kingdom D, Shabbir A 2005 Care programme approach: relapsing or recovering? Advances in Psychiatric Treatment 11:325–329

McGlynn P 2007 Crisis Resolution and home-treatment teams; a practical guide. The Sainsbury Centre for Mental Health, London

Minghella E, Ford R, Freeman T et al 1998 Open all hours. The Sainsbury Centre for Mental Health, London

Muijen M, Cooney M, Strathdee G, Bell R, Hudson A, 1994 Community psychiatric nurse teams. Intensive support versus generic care. British Journal of Psychiatry 176:116–120

Murray A, Shepherd G, Muijen M 1997 More than a friend: The role of Support Workers in Community Mental Health Services. The Sainsbury Centre for Mental Health, London

Onyett S R, Heppleston T, Bushnell D 1994 A national survey of community mental health teams. Journal of Mental Health 3:175–194.

Onyett S R, Linde K, Glover G, Floyd S, Bradley S, Middleton H 2006 A national survey of crisis resolution teams in England. (http://www.nepho.org.uk/view_file.php?c=1788) North East Public Health Observatory, Stockton-on-Tees

Perlman et al 1984 A study of mental health administrators and systems utising a four-part urban/rural taxonomy. Community Mental Health Journal, 203:202–211

Perri 6 P, Peck E 2004 New Labour's Modernisation in the Public Sector: A neo-Durkheimian Approach and the case of mental health services. Public Administration 82(1):83–108

Readhead E, Brooker C 2003 Developing the Workforce: Review of local implementation teams in the northern and Yorkshire Region. Northern Centre for Mental Health, Leeds

Rummler G, Brache A 1995 Improving Performance: how to manage the white space on the organisation chart. Jossey-Bass, San Francisco

Sainsbury Centre for Mental Health 2000 The Capable Practitioner: A framework and list of the practitioner capabilities required to implement the National Service Framework for Mental Health. The Sainsbury Centre for Mental Health, London

Sainsbury Centre for Mental Health 2004 Acute Care Survey. The Sainsbury Centre for Mental Health, London.

Smyth M, Hoult J, Jackson G 2000 The Home-treatment Enigma. British Medical Journal 320:305–309

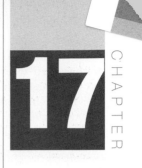

Research and development

M. Clark • C. Chilvers

Introduction

Research has been a key, but not sole, part of the knowledge base for the National Service Framework (NSF) for Mental Health. Research answers specific questions vital in implementing the highly complex NSF. The NSF drew on the best evidence available when written, yet this was patchy, given the long-term, highly developmental nature of the NSF. Hence, many of the recommendations in the framework were based on informed experience from service users, carers and professionals, with weaker research evidence. A challenge, then, in implementing the NSF was to develop the evidence base to assess how these recommendations worked following national implementation.

In this chapter we examine the research base for the NSF when first written and the research recommendations made within it. We then discuss what is to be learnt from the literature to improve the interactions between research, policy and practice. We conclude with a brief look to the future.

The NSF and other evidence based documents since 1999

It ought to be noted at the outset that the NSF was the first of several significant documents drawing on research evidence to make prescriptions for mental health services. The NHS Plan (DH 2000) and the Mental Health Policy Implementation Guides (MHPIGs) were other notable documents here.

The NHS Plan, for example, set targets for the development of mental health services, such as a number of new community services, based on research evidence and expert opinions, including those of service users and carers.

The MHPIGs translated knowledge into detailed standards and models to guide local service improvements outlined in the NSF and NHS Plan. Services addressed in these documents included established ones, such as Community Mental Health Teams and Psychiatric Intensive Care Units. They also attended to new developments, including Crisis Resolution and Home Treatment,

Assertive Outreach Teams, and Early Intervention in Psychosis Services. Most of these had weaker research bases than was desired. At such times, policy has leapfrogged the research evidence, but always with a commitment to further research to assess policy and its implementation.

During the life of the NSF, other documents were published codifying the best evidence available into guidance for practice. Examples include policy statements on personality disorder and women's mental health services. Further, the National Institute for Health and Clinical Excellence (NICE) (www. nice.org.uk) developed evidence based guidelines detailing best practice in such topics as schizophrenia, depression and obsessive–compulsive disorder.

When examining the interaction between research and the NSF, then, we need to bear in mind a whole range of other documents too. For clarity and brevity, though, we will confine the rest of this chapter to discussion of the NSF as the overarching policy document.

Research and the development of the NSF

The NSF had an assurance that recommendations for improving mental health care are based on the best available research evidence. The External Reference Group, which included academics, service users, carers and care professionals, distilled a range of knowledge, including research, into the NSF.

There were, though, significant gaps in the evidence base for the NSF. Further, the NSF noted that during its 10-year implementation period, new knowledge would emerge and, hence, implementation should remain flexible to take account of this. As such, systematic means to improve the evidence base and its links to policy and practice were seen as priority challenges. Hence, commitments to research and development were made, summarised in the intention that: 'Department of Health investment in mental health R&D will focus on the knowledge base required to implement the National Service Framework' (p116).

A number of priorities were listed for research, including:

- Evaluating the individual and collective performance of the component parts of the NSF
- Investigating variations in the use of in-patient beds, and their implications
- The management of comorbidity, and the interfaces between primary care, specialist mental health services and substance misuse services
- Investigating ways to enhance staff morale, retention, recruitment and performance, and thereby improve service user engagement and outcomes
- Evaluating the effectiveness and cost-effectiveness under usual service conditions of psychological and psychosocial interventions
- Comparing the outcomes for self-harm between different types of services
- Assessing relative cost-effectiveness, service user satisfaction and concordance rates of:
  - atypical antipsychotic drugs
  - newer antidepressants
  - complementary therapies compared to standard management

— evaluating the better management of antisocial attitudes/behaviours that attract the label of severe personality disorder.

Service user satisfaction is an important outcome measure in these priorities, manifest in various ways, including:

* Developing and evaluating a range of occupational activities to maximise social participation, enhance self-esteem and improve clinical outcomes
* Developing research tools with service users to assess their view on how services can best meet their needs.

Service user involvement in research cuts across all priorities.

The NSF, then, set a challenging agenda for mental health research, with an action plan for mental health R&D being promised.

Research developments in support of the early implementation of the NSF

The Mental Health Research and Development Portfolio

To advance R&D in priority policy areas (initially cancer, coronary heart disease and mental health), the Research and Development Directorate in the Department of Health appointed portfolio directors for them. The portfolio director was to work with national service directors, policy makers, research funders and the research community to identify research priorities, seek funding, and deliver findings to be disseminated for implementation into policy and practice. In the mental health portfolio, two pieces of work were needed: a stock-take of the state of mental health research and its relevance to the national service framework, and the determination of immediate priorities for funding.

The Strategic Review of Mental Health Research

The Strategic Review of Research and Development – Mental Health (DH 2002) aimed to assess the state of mental health research in the UK. It was overseen by a steering group, chaired by the Mental Health R&D Portfolio Director, that reviewed multiple sources of data covering recent and ongoing mental health research. In summary, the review found that:

* although there were more than 30 externally funded research units, centres and programme grants, there were relatively few large-scale, multi-centre projects in progress
* randomised controlled trials were few
* many projects were small with no external funding
* there was a lack of systematic reviews of research evidence
* there was a lack of expertise in many NHS organisations carrying out mental health research
* there was little research carried out within social services

- there was a lack of funding sources for mental health research; in particular, unlike most other major disease areas there is no dedicated research charity covering mental illness
- there were significant gaps in research relating to NSF standards, notably mental health promotion, access to care and services to support carers
- many members of NHS staff were involved in research, yet relatively few were working at PhD or post-doctoral level
- there was a need to involve mental health service users and carers at all stages of the research process.

Setting research priorities and the action plan for mental health research

Two early pieces of work to determine research priorities for the NSF were a thematic review of NHS R&D funded mental health research commissioned in 2000, and a synthesis of researchable questions to support mental health policy (Thornicroft et al 2002).

The importance of the user voice in determining research priorities was acknowledged and a Service User Panel was convened, chaired by Professor Peter Beresford. The findings of the panel are in Box 17.1. It is noteworthy that many of the priorities identified by the Service User Panel have become more accepted ways of viewing the world. For example, many research funders require service users to be fully involved in the development of research proposals, as does the Mental Health Research Network before adopting projects.

In addition, there is now a programme of work on mental health and race equality (Box 17.2), and the Social Exclusion Unit's (SEU) Report on Social

---

Box 17.1

Priorities from the Strategic Review of Mental Health Research in the NHS Service User Panel

- Service users should be involved in an ongoing way in developing research priorities
- Research to address issues about race equality in mental health service provision
- Research for social inclusion
- Development of user-defined outcomes
- Full user involvement at all stages in the research process
- Research into broader public policy and how it impacts on mental health service users
- Research that addresses positive risk management and a more holistic approach to service-users' lives
- Research on user-controlled services including the strengths and weaknesses of complementary forms of support
- Research focusing on the abuse of mental health service users
- Research to explore and challenge the conflation of violence with madness and distress
- Research into positive initiatives to support other groups of service users that might be applied in the context of people with mental illness.
- Exploring user involvement in policy and practice

Box 17.2

Research projects commissioned in support of the improving mental health services to Black and ethnic minority individuals and communities

- Evaluation of community engagement in BME mental health
- A review of BME mental health research on the National Research Register
- A systematic review of BME suicide and interventions to prevent suicide
- An evaluation of the Focused Implementation Sites
- Experiences of Acute Mental Health Services among BME groups
- Ethnic Pathways Improvement Centres (EPIC) project

Inclusion and Mental Health (SEU 2004) highlighted areas for research which are being taken forward. Independently, the Prince of Wales Foundation for Integrated Healthcare is carrying out a review of research into complementary therapies and mental well-being.

Research commissioned over the first 5 years of the NSF

The 5-year review of the National Service Framework (DH 2004) describes in the chapter on research and development how the national research plan promised in the Framework was developed (Table 17.1). By the end of 2004, 69 projects costing over £9million had been commissioned (Table 17.2). These

Table 17.1

Literature reviews and scoping exercises supporting the Mental Health National Service Framework

NSF standard	Title	Start date of award	Amount of award (£000)
1	Occupational outcomes of mental health interventions	2001	34.8
1 + 2	Self-help interventions for mental health problems	2001	29.7
2 + 3	Primary care mental health workers	2001	10.9
2 + 3	Effectiveness of post-qualification mental health training in primary and secondary care	2001	29.9
4 + 5	Assertive outreach: workshop on research priorities	2001	20.0
4 + 5	Dual diagnosis: workshop on design of randomised control trial	2001	(1)
4 + 5	Early intervention and management of first episode psychosis	2001	41.4
4 + 5	Treatment of sex offenders: workshop	2001	0.2

(Continued)

Table 17.1

(Continued)			
NSF standard	**Title**	**Start date of award**	**Amount of award (£000)**
4 + 5	Clinical effectiveness and cost consequences of SSRIs in the treatment of sex offenders	2001	90.0
4 + 5	Psychological treatment for sex offenders	2002	34.0
4 + 5	Psychological treatment for juvenile sex offenders	2004	25.5
4 + 5	Prevention strategies for the population at risk of engaging in violent behaviour	2002	66.0
4 + 5	Effectiveness of pharmacological and psychological strategies for the management of people with personality disorder	2002	63.0
4 + 5	In-patient care for mental health problems: a review of research and identification of researchable questions	2001	5.0
4 + 5	A literature review of staff morale on in-patient units	2003	59.5
4 + 5 + 6	Rehabilitation of people with severe personality disorder	2001	7.0
6	Services to support carers of people with mental health problems	2001	76.8
6	Measuring outcomes for carers of people with mental health problems	2003	64.0
6	Respite services for carers of people with dementia	2003	75.5
7	Suicide prevention: workshop	2001	3.0
7	Scoping review of services for people bereaved by suicide	2004	29.9
All	Thematic review of NHS R&D-funded mental health research in relation to the NSF for mental health	2000	27.0
All	Scoping review of the effectiveness of mental health services	2000	40.0
All	Researchable questions to support mental health policy	2000	(2)
All	Women-only and women-sensitive mental health services: an expert review	2001	35.0
All	Development of prison mental health services	2002	75.0
Total funding			943.1
(1) Funded by Medical Research Council (2) Information not available			

Table 17.2

Projects supporting the Mental Health National Service Framework			
NSF standard	**Title**	**Start**	**Total cost (£000)**
1	Occupational outcomes of mental health interventions	2001	34.8
1 + 2	Self-help interventions for mental health problems	2001	29.7
2 + 3	Primary care mental health workers	2001	10.9
2 + 3	Effectiveness of post-qualification mental health training in primary and secondary care	2001	29.9
2 + 3	Primary care mental health workers: best practice to facilitate managed care pathways in primary care settings	2004	(1)
2 + 3	Graduate primary care mental health workers	2003	53.0
2 to 5	Comparing needs and satisfaction with services between psychiatric patients in prison and forensic mental health teams	2001	104.5
2 to 5 + 7	Development of prison mental health services	2003	75.0
2 to 5 + 7	Development and evaluation of a new telepsychiatry service for prisoners	2001	110.0
4 + 5	Assertive outreach: workshop on research priorities	2001	20.0
4 + 5	Dual diagnosis: workshop on design of randomised control trial	2001	(2)
4 + 5	Early intervention and management of first episode psychosis	2001	41.4
4 + 5	Treatment of sex offenders: workshop	2001	0.2
4 + 5	Clinical effectiveness and cost consequences of SSRIs in the treatment of sex offenders	2001	90.0
4 + 5	Psychological treatment for sex offenders	2002	34.0
4 + 5	Psychological treatment for juvenile sex offenders	2004	25.5
4 + 5	Development of a scale to measure sadism in sex offenders	2001	81.0
4 + 5	Feasibility study for randomised control trial of treatments for sex offenders	2002	17.2
4 + 5	Use of polygraph in the monitoring of high-risk behaviour on community supervision	2001	59.0
4 + 5	Processes of disengagement and engagement with assertive outreach for African-Caribbean and white British men	2002	24.0
4 + 5	In-patient care for mental health problems: a review of research and identification of researchable questions	2001	5.0

(Continued)

Table 17.2

(Continued)			
NSF standard	**Title**	**Start**	**Total cost (£000)**
4 + 5	A literature review of staff morale on mental health in-patient units	2003	59.5
4 + 5	Large-scale change in multi-professional organisations: the impact of leadership factors in implementing change in complex health and social care environments – NHS Plan clinical priority for mental health crisis resolution teams	2003	295.6
4 + 5	A national study of the association between observation practice and adverse events on acute psychiatric wards	2003	298.5
4 + 5	Social and cognitive correlates of anti-social and violent personality disturbance	2002	108.0
4 + 5	Differential access to services for individuals with severe personality disorder	2001	186.0
4 + 5	Prevention strategies for the population at risk of engaging in violent behaviour	2002	66.0
4 + 5	Interpersonal processes and their importance in the treatment of personality disorder	2002	112.1
4 + 5	Black and minority ethnic groups' pathways into forensic mental health services	2002	135.0
4 + 5	Intensive multi-modal cognitive behaviour therapy programme for adolescent offenders in secure care	2003	143.2
4 + 5	Clinical, genetic and environmental risk factors for juvenile ASPD in a high-risk group	2003	146.0
4 + 5	Aetiology and developmental pathways related to the emergence of psychopathic tendencies in children	2003	144.0
4 + 5	Pilot study of a new intervention for hard-to-treat children with conduct disorder	2003	43.0
4 + 5	Services for older people moving out of high secure hospitals	2002	158.0
4 + 5	Assertive outreach in England: a national survey of service organisation	2004	133.0
4 + 5	Operational and individual predictors of outcome of assertive outreach throughout England	2005	233.0
4 + 5	The City 128 Study observation and outcomes on acute psychiatric wards	2003	298.5
4 + 5	In-patient alternatives to traditional in-patient care	2004	301.9
4 + 5	Psychological intervention for clients with schizophrenia and co-morbid substance abuse (MIDAS)	2004	1,871.9

Table 17.2

(Continued)			
NSF standard	**Title**	**Start**	**Total cost (£000)**
4 + 5	Development of prison mental health services	2003	75.0
4 + 5 + 6	Structured community-based treatment for people with personality disorders	2001	183.0
4 + 5	Evaluation of pilot training packages on personality disorder for NHS staff	2004	200.0
4 + 5	Outcomes of involuntary hospital admission in England	2003	329.0
4 + 5	Survey of Black and minority ethnic service user views of cultural competency of in-patient services	2004	200.0
4 + 5	Effectiveness of pharmacological and psychological strategies for the management of people with personality disorders	2002	63.0
4 + 5	A meta-regression study to explain the heterogeneity in assertive outreach study outcomes	2002	66.0
4 + 5	A randomised controlled trial of assertive outreach services in North London	2002	112.0
4 + 5 + 6	Structured community-based treatment for people with personality disorders	2001	183.0
4 + 5 + 6	Rehabilitation of people with severe personality disorders	2001	7.0
6	Services to support carers of people with mental health problems	2001	76.8
6	Measuring outcomes for carers of people with mental health problems	2003	64.0
6	Respite services for carers of people with dementia	2003	75.5
6	Enabling partnerships in carer assessments: the way forward	2003	299.1
6	Professionals sharing information with carers: examples of good practice in mental health	2003	80.0
7	Suicide prevention: workshop	2001	3.0
7	Suicide prevention: research training fellowship	2002	109.0
1 + 7	Evaluation of a health promotion intervention for suicide prevention in young men	2004	50.0
7	Investigation of methods of suicide using coroners' records	2004	122.0
7	Scoping review of services for people bereaved by suicide	2004	29.9
7	Multi-centre monitoring of deliberate self-harm	2004	(3)
All	Thematic review of NHS R&D-funded mental health research in relation to the NSF for mental health	2000	9.6

(Continued)

Table 17.2

(Continued)			
NSF standard	Title	Start	Total cost (£000)
All	Scoping review of the effectiveness of mental health services	2001	40.0
All	Researchable questions to support mental health policy	2001	(3)
All	Women-only and women-sensitive mental health services: an expert review	2001	30.0
CC	Psychiatric morbidity survey	2001	492.2
CC	Outcome measurement in mental health – evaluation of pilots	2001	229.0
All	Development of prison mental health services	2002	51.0
All	Prison academic network	2004	598.9
All	Psychiatric morbidity and mental health treatment needs among women in prison mother and baby units	2003	36.5
Total			9,392.8
(1) Included in National Primary Care R&D Centre Programme (2) Funded by Medical Research Council (3) Information not available			

projects covered primary, secondary and social care, and particular groups of service users such as those from Black and minority ethnic groups, prisoner-patients, and patients in secure hospitals. This was in addition to existing research, such as that ongoing in Trusts.

The National Institute for Mental Health in England and the Mental Health Research Network

The establishment of the National Institute for Mental Health in England (NIMHE) gave a focus to the implementation of the NSF, as described elsewhere in this volume. Including research in the work programmes of NIMHE put research into context in its role of supporting the transformation of mental health services. To give two examples: the Black and Minority Ethnic Groups Programme Board of NIMHE has, as we have seen, commissioned a number of research projects in support of its work (see Box 17.2) and the National Suicide Prevention Advisory Group has a Research Forum advising on and undertaking research priorities (Box 17.3).

The small number of randomised controlled trials in Mental Health R&D indicated the need for an infrastructure to support mental health research. Research funders also revealed that mental health research was regarded as high risk because of the lack of a solid infrastructure to ensure successful completion of projects. To develop capacity in this area, NIMHE commissioned a mental health research network.

The Department of Health commissioned cancer research network, based on the clinical cancer networks, already covered the whole country. In this model local research networks coterminous with clinical networks were progressively funded, leading to a marked increase in recruitment into cancer trials. Although an impressive model, mental health services are not organised in the same way as cancer services and, hence, required a different approach.

The Mental Health Research Network (MHRN) aimed to:

- deliver large-scale research projects to inform policy and practice
- broaden the scope of research and gain full involvement from service users and carers
- identify research priorities
- develop research capacity.

The network is organised around a managing partnership, comprising the Institute of Psychiatry and the University of Manchester, and eight research hubs across England (Fig. 17.1). At the time of writing, the network includes 20 universities and 38 NHS Trusts, covering more than 60% of the population of England. It includes a diverse range of expertise and supports the involvement of service users and carers in mental health research.

In March 2004, new funding for science was announced by the UK Government. This included a substantial increase in funding for research networks, including the MHRN. The success of the network has yet to be established in terms of speed of recruitment into large scale research projects. The network supports an impressive number of projects and early indications of delivering successful projects are encouraging.

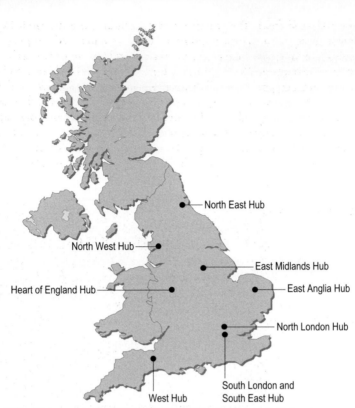

Figure 17.1 • The organisation of the UK Mental Health Research Network

The network also funds Research Topic Groups to identify research priorities and write applications to research funders. The biggest barrier to increasing mental health research is not the capacity of the network but lack of funding for mental health research.

Funding for mental health research

The Mental Health Research Funders' Group brought together the main funders of mental health research in the UK from the statutory sector and charities. In 2005 the Group published a strategic review of its combined research funding to create a national picture of mental health research funding in the UK to:

- provide a broad thematic overview of research for strategic analysis and planning of future metal health research
- develop a shared understanding of what each organisation contributes to the wider profile of research activity
- create a basis for greater cooperation and collaboration in setting and improving research priorities.

Data were collected from 20 research funders, including the Research Councils, Government sources and charities, and found that the annualised spend on mental health and related neuroscience research was £74 million. Internationally mental health receives proportionally less funding than cardiovascular disease and cancer compared to total economic cost of disease (Kingdon 2006, Sobocki et al 2006).

The report of the strategic analysis highlighted the considerable diversity and strengths of current research funding and activity, but also notable gaps. For example, there is a relatively low level of funding for research on anxiety and stress related and somatoform disorders, and into suicide and self-harm. Figure 17.2 shows the spend across different disorders. Only 2% of research

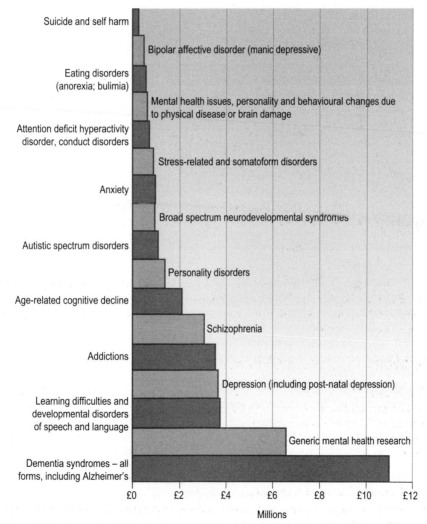

Figure 17.2 • Annualised spend on research for the mental health relevance categories (Source: Mental Health Research Funders' Group (2005) Strategic Analysis of Mental Health Research Funding, p15)

spend was on prevention of mental ill-health and promotion of well-being. Other gaps were in clinical trials (21 trials were identified by the analysis) and in secondary analysis (literature reviews and meta-analysis).

Funding streams

The main sources of funding for research into mental ill-health are the Medical Research Council (MRC), Department of Health Research programmes and the Wellcome Trust. Whilst notable charities support research, there is no large, dedicated mental health research charity, in sharp contrast to most major groups of diseases.

Recently the MRC funded a large programme of work on Brain Science, including pilot studies for clinical trials (Trial Platforms), which should increase the number of clinical trials in the future. Of the main Department of Health Research Programmes, i.e. the Health Technology Assessment (HTA) Programme (www. hta.ac.uk) and the Service Delivery Organisation (SDO) Programme (www.sdo. lshtm.ac.uk), the former has not historically funded much research into technologies for the treatment of mental disorders, with some notable exceptions such as counselling for depression. In contrast, the SDO Programme has funded a substantial body of very informative research, for example on alternatives to mental health in-patient care for both adults and children.

The Forensic Mental Health Research Programme (www.nfmhp.org.uk), although small in size (less than £2 million per annum spend), was a specialist Department of Health programme to build capacity in this demanding area. It has funded primary and secondary research and fellowships at PhD and post-doctoral levels into the health of people with mental illness who are offenders or at risk of offending and includes research into the mental health of prisoners, as well as those in secure psychiatric hospitals. The programme concluded in 2007.

Notable gaps in funding from the Department are in public mental health and in epidemiology. Another is the lack of a coordinated approach to funding recommendations for research from guidelines and technology appraisals from NICE to develop evidence in areas close to policy. Recent welcome developments include fast-tracking a small number of these recommendations by the HTA Programme, and a pilot of dissemination of NICE Guidelines alongside mental health policy.

Changes in the organisation of research and development in the NHS following publication of 'Best Research for Best Health' (DH 2006a) will present a challenge to future mental health research. How effectively mental health researchers can compete with other health areas for funding remains to be seen. Closure of the Forensic Mental Health Research Programme is a blow to researchers in that particularly difficult area. Establishing post Cooksey report (Cooksey 2006, DH 2006b) a single research fund combining Research Council and Department of Health funding streams may or may not be beneficial: the benefit may be protecting research funding previously at risk of being diverted into patient care; a danger may be to the balance between basic and applied/ health services research and investigator-led and nationally commissioned research.

Balancing established research approaches with new paradigms emerging from user-led research is another challenge. Mental health service users are well-organised and rightly vocal in their demand to be heard. Many funding organisations expect service users will be included in the research process. A consultation with mental health service users and carers of people with mental ill-health on their research priorities for user and carer-centred services further illuminates this issue (Naylor et al 2006).

Summary

In summary then, the above amounts to a significant national effort to close gaps in the knowledge base for the NSF. A key feature of this effort, though, is that none of it is done in isolation. Infrastructure development is not for its own ends. No single project is expected to deliver all answers. The work is integrated to provide a comprehensive approach to improving the knowledge base.

Relationships between research, policy and practice

As well as providing a strategic framework for mental health policy and service development, the Mental Health NSF provided a similar function for research to support policy and practice. It is, then, timely to reflect on the relevant literature and the evidence on improving research-policy-practice interactions.

Relationships between research and policy

The concept of *evidence-based policy making* is often used akin to that of evidence-based medicine, defined as 'the integration of best research evidence with clinical expertise and patient values' (Sackett et al 2000). Evidence-based policy has become commonplace rhetoric in the UK. Yet it is not always clear what this means, nor how possible or desirable it is. However, 'it is widely agreed that health policies do not reflect research evidence to the extent that in theory they could' (Hanney et al 2003). There is an additional general problem across British public services of significant evidence gaps for policy making (Nutley 2003).

The NSF marked a systematic effort to break away from this pattern in mental health. Yet, it was a classic case of that situation noted by others (Knott & Wildavsky 1980, p549) in which policy makers usually have better evidence for old policies than new, just at a time when this evidence is really desired. Evidence was used where it existed, and, as noted above, work was put in place on a deliberate approach to address evidence gaps.

Organising a better interaction between research and policy requires a better understanding of the 'integration' of knowledge referred to by Sackett et al in their definition quoted above. Some prescriptions of evidence-based policy suggest a model in which research evidence is the sole knowledge that should be leading policy development. The model is of a simple, linear link from research findings directing policy making and them implementation.

Studies of policy making, though, show it to be more complex than this model [for examples see Weiss (1977, 1979), and Hanney et al (2003) for an overview of issues]. Research evidence is but one contributing factor amongst several in policy making (Ham 2005). Indeed, some find policy making so political and contingent that they caution against notions of evidence-based policy (Clarence 2002, Parsons 2002). Others argue for evidence-*informed* policy making (Davies & Nutley 2002, Nutley 2003), accepting that policy making is open to diverse influences, such that we are unlikely to see a situation where research routinely leads the process. Rather, the expectation is for research findings to have the best possible level of impact in policy making alongside other forms of knowledge. Simplistic models of *evidence-based* are seen as unrealistic and unhelpful (Nutley 2003), particularly on the scale of policy and practice development and implementation in the Mental Health NSF.

It is helpful, then, to reflect on the meanings attached to research 'impact' and 'utilisation'. The ways in which knowledge can be utilised, or have an impact, have been delineated (Huberman 1992, Weiss 1998, Nutley et al 2002, Nutley 2003):

- *Instrumental* – research leads policy making.
- *Conceptual* – rather than directly informing the content of the policy, research influences the thinking of people and how they see situations.
- *Mobilisation of support* – research used for persuasion to garner support and legitimacy.
- *Wider influence* – research contributes to a broader development in knowledge, being synthesised for influence in areas beyond the original context.
- *Tactical use* – commissioning research to assuage immediate public concern and pressure for action.

We can see how research can play such roles in relation to the NSF. For research to play any of these roles it is important to specifically translate the findings to suit the role and the given context (Knott & Wildavsky 1980, p552). For example, research on ethnic minority inequalities in mental health care needs to be translated into a meaningful form to improve services.

A further challenge in building bridges between research and policy making is managing expectations of what research can deliver (Nutley 2003). The generally long-term nature of research and its focus on particular questions mean it may not deliver what policy makers are expecting, when they want it. For supporting the NSF it has been important to sustain an interaction across research and policy to manage such issues. In undertaking this we have to recognise that (Nutley 2003):

'The relationship between research, knowledge, policy and practice are always likely to remain loose, shifting and contingent. Initiatives to improve the linkages between policy and research need to be designed with this in mind.'

Various means of building better understanding between policy makers and researchers have been employed in other contexts (Nutley 2003). Whilst the evidence bases for them are not strong, it is likely that several work some of the time, but none all of the time. We echo Ham's (2005) 'welcome refrain' of 'the need for researchers and decision makers to work together closely at all stages' on shared work. We need 'sustained interactivity' (Huberman

1987) between researchers and users of research. The NSF provided a foundation (the permission and incentive) and structure (the shared language and framework) for enacting this. It has been augmented by 'communicative action' (Habermas 1984) in which 'the actions of the agents involved are coordinated not through egocentric calculations of success but through acts of reaching understanding'. The shared values in the NSF supported this.

As we have seen in the preceding parts of this chapter, this mode of communication included a broad range of people and knowledge to inform and implement the NSF. For example, diverse expert knowledge shaped the NSF, including public[1] opinion.

The reality of the interaction between research and policy making in the context of the NSF, then, has been far from the naive, linear model of evidence-based. Indeed, it has moved some way towards 'democratising' (Parsons 2002) policy making. The 'policy network' underpinning the NSF and its implementation continues to reach beyond government departments to other, diverse relationships to influence policy. In this research has developed a strengthened link to policy making.

Travelling this far in linking research and policy, we see the requirements for stronger research–policy interaction, namely (Davies & Nutley 2002):

1. Agreement as to the nature of evidence.
2. A strategic approach to the creation of evidence, together with the development of a cumulative knowledge base.
3. Effective dissemination of knowledge; together with development of effective means of access to knowledge.
4. Initiatives to increase the uptake of evidence in both policy and practice.

The NSF established a terrain for debate for point 2, with a view to facilitating greater understanding and communicative action. There is always potential for debate with regard to point 1, but pragmatic working agreements can be achieved, particularly if given a cohesive framework such as the NSF.

The intention of this development has been to facilitate debate and initiatives, not to close them down. The NSF facilitated focused debate and developing initiatives (including more research) within a common understanding. Flexibility and responsiveness have been maintained.

For the third and fourth points, the existence of the Mental Health R&D Portfolio, interaction with the National Director for Mental Health, and links to NIMHE, now part of the Care Services Improvement Partnership (CSIP), have all helped. They are themes we will turn to next with regard to improving links between research and practice.

Relationships between research and practice

For effective change, the long run requires a two-way relationship between research and practice, with each informing the other's agendas. In this section, though, we can only cover one direction of this relationship, namely research informing practice to successfully implement the NSF.

---

[1]In this we include patients, service users, families, carers and community and voluntary sector organisations.

Getting research findings into practice is generally a known, persistent challenge. An improving evidence base on tackling this does help (e.g. Haines & Donald 1998, Bero et al 1998, Haynes & Haines 1998, Greenhalgh et al 2004). Applying it remains a challenge though.

Many of the points made in the previous section on policy–research links apply here. Some of the structures discussed there, such as NIMHE and Portfolio Directors, may also help with dissemination into practice. Dissemination for implementation is often enacted on the basis of a 'push' model, i.e. processes to push information out to those who need it in their practice. In many ways it is a sensible model, and strong institutions have been established to support its operation, such as the Cochrane Collaboration and the mental health specialist library in the National Library for Health. They are, though, not sufficient in themselves to address dissemination/implementation across all complex services. As in the previous section, simplistic, linear models can be limited in understanding and enacting the desired changes. Rather, as Davies & Nutley (2002) wrote:

'One crucial lesson is the need to move to more holistic models that bring research producers, research funders and commissioners, policy makers, and practitioners into much closer and more sustained collaborations. It is through open partnerships that span the creation, validation and incorporation of research evidence that we are likely to see more effective use of such evidence for the betterment of public services.'

Such partnerships enable the ongoing discussion required for knowledge transfer, including translating findings into helpful information for practitioners and others. Arenas such as NIMHE and CSIP work programmes can be helpful in this undertaking. Helpful communication arenas become akin to a jazz improvisation ensemble. The participants in it work within a shared understanding of the boundaries of their working together, including an accepted background of values and sense of direction. As each musical piece develops, the acceptance of each other's abilities and authority allows ensemble members to come to the foreground for solo displays of skill, against a collaborative backcloth. The overall piece develops to a conclusion based on the best mixture of individuality and collective input.

The evolving nature of the evidence base and of practice requires ongoing attention to the research–practice interface, and innovation in means of supporting dissemination/implementation. New means of understanding the challenge, then, will be helpful.

Beyond current achievements

There are still many important gaps in the evidence for implementing the NSF. For example, research for promotion of mental well-being and preventing mental ill health, for better primary mental health care, to support better services for particular groups, such as ethnic minorities and carers, and research for employment and social inclusion for people with mental health problems all remain topics for more systematic research. Work to identify the specific research questions continues with policy and practitioner colleagues. The dialogue with research funders to then commission the required projects also continues, although within an environment of generally increased demand on health research budgets, and the challenges of new research funding arrangements discussed earlier.

Linking research to policy and practice will stay as challenges, requiring new work for particular contexts. The notion of developing a sustained interaction between research, policy and practice remains a helpful way of conceptualising the challenge. It has led to successful work tackling some of the challenges, such as processes for developing national guidance documents. Infrastructure developments such as NIMHE were, and continue to be, helpful to engage a wide range of stakeholders in meeting dissemination/implementation challenges.

Such involvement may move us beyond only the 'push' analogy for dissemination. Rather than relying on pushing out research findings, the opposite approach is to support people to demand the evidence, or pull it to them as they need it. This could include the public as well as practitioners and managers in mental health.

In this context, approaches such as social movements offer potential for increased impact of research. Social movements, like the civil rights movement in the USA, develop when networks of people, motivated by a cause, drive societal change. How they draw down evidence and other knowledge to support this is a topic worth further investigating for supporting dissemination/implementation. Such 'pull' approaches to addressing implementation of research findings are tantalising concepts with promise to be explored.

More and better involvement of the public in mental health research is a continuing priority. Work continues on this through NIMHE, the Department of Health and the MHRN. Exciting new developments are taking it further, such as:

- The James Lind Alliance (www.lindalliance.org) argue that the public should be more involved, with clinicians and others, in establishing research priorities across all health care. Linked early work to identify the research questions, or uncertainties, for treatments has started with schizophrenia.
- Better information to the public about mental health clinical trials is important for recruitment and general support for such research. A web site (www.trime.org.uk) has been developed specifically aimed at this challenge.

Conclusion

The NSF was a significant landmark, not only in terms of directly reorganising mental health care, but also for providing a broad framework to guiding a systematic national effort to improve the evidence base for that care. In many ways there has been a helpful sustained interaction between research, policy and practice.

Whilst it is difficult (and probably ultimately not helpful) to directly manage knowledge and its production, it is possible to better organise the environment for healthier production and sharing of useful knowledge (Collinson & Parcell

2004). The work discussed in this chapter has adopted this approach. Many challenges remain with regard to R&D, the NSF for mental health, and life beyond its original 10-year plan, but it clear that at the time of writing there is a better foundation on which to tackle these.

References

Bero L A, Grilli R, Grimshaw J M, Harvey E, Oxman A D, Thomson M A 1998 Closing the gap between research and practice: an overview of systematic reviews of interventions to promote the implementation of research findings. British Medical Journal 317:72–75

Clarence E 2002 Technocracy reinvented: the new evidence based policy movement. Public Policy and Administration 17(3):1–11

Collinson C, Parcell G 2004 Learning to fly – practical knowledge management. Capstone Books, London

Cooksey D 2006 A review of UK health research; report for HM Treasury. HMSO, London

Davies H, Nutley S 2002 Discussion Paper 2. Evidence-based policy and practice: moving from rhetoric to reality. Research Unit for Research Utilization, St Andrews University, St Andrews

Department of Health 2000 The NHS Plan: a plan for investment, a plan for reform. DH, London

Department of Health 2002 Strategic Review of Research and Development – Mental Health. DH, London

Department of Health 2004 The National Service Framework for Mental Health – Five Years On. DH, London

Department of Health 2006a Best Research for Best Practice – a new national health research strategy. DH, London

Department of Health 2006b Sir David Cooksey's review of UK Health Research. DH, London

Greenhalgh T, Robert G, MacFarlane F, Bate P, Kyriakidou O 2004 Diffusion of knowledge in service organisations: systematic review and recommendations. The Milbank Quarterly 82(4): 581–629

Habermas J 1984 The theory of communicative action. Vol. 1, Reason and the rationalization of society. Beacon Press, Boston

Haines A, Donald A 1998 Making better use of research findings. British Medical Journal 317:465–468

Ham C 2005 Don't throw the baby out with the bathwater. Journal of Health Services Research and Policy 10(Suppl 1):S51–S52

Hanney S R, Gonzalez-Block M, Buxton M J, Kogan M 2003 The utilisation of health research in policy-making: concepts, examples and methods of assessment. Health Research Policy and Systems 1:2 (accessed August 2006: www.health-policy-systems.com/content/1/1/2)

Haynes B, Haines A 1998 Barriers and bridges to evidence based clinical practice. British Medical Journal 317:273–276

Huberman M 1987 Steps toward an integrated model of research utilization. Knowledge: Creation, Diffusion, Utilization 8(4):586–611

Huberman M 1992 Linking the practioner and researcher communities for school improvement. Address to the International Congress for School Effectiveness and Improvement, Victoria, B.C.

Kingdon D 2006 Letter: Health research funding. Mental health research continues to be underfunded. British Medical Journal 332:1510

Knott J, Wildavsky A 1980 If dissemination is the solution, what is the problem? Knowledge: Creation, Diffusion, Utilization 1(4):537–578

Naylor C, Wallcraft J, Samele C, Greatley A 2006 Research priorities for service user and carer-centred mental health services. Consultation report. SDO Research Programme, London

Nutley S, Walter I, Davies H 2002 Discussion Paper 1. From knowing to doing: A framework for understanding the evidence-into-practice agenda. Research Unit for Research Utilization, St Andrews University, St Andrews

Nutley S 2003 Bridging the policy/research divide: reflections and lessons from the UK. Paper presented at 'Facing the Future: Engaging stakeholders and Citizens in Developing Public Policy'. National Institute of Governance Conference, Canberra, Australia

Parsons W 2002 From muddling through to muddling up – evidence based policy making and the modernisation of British Government. Public Policy and Administration 17(3):43–60

Sackett D L, Straus S E, Richardson W S, Rosenberg W, Haynes R B 2000 Evidence-based medicine: how to practice and teach EBM, 2nd edn. Churchill Livingstone, Edinburgh

Sobocki P, Lekander I, Berwick S, Olesen J, Jonsson B 2006 Resource allocation to brain research in Europe. European Journal of Neuroscience 24(10):1–24

Social Exclusion Unit 2004 Mental Health and Social Exclusion. Office of the Deputy Prime Minister, London

Thornicroft G, Bindman J, Goldberg D, Gournay K, Huxley P 2002 Researchable questions to support evidence-based mental health policy concerning adult mental illness. Psychiatric Bulletin 26:364–367

Weiss C 1977 Introduction. In: Weiss C (ed) Using social research in public policy making. Lexington Books, Lexington

Weiss C 1979 The many meanings of research utilization. Public Administration Review 39:426–431

Weiss C 1998 Have we learned anything new about the use of evaluation? American Journal of Evaluation 19(1):21–33

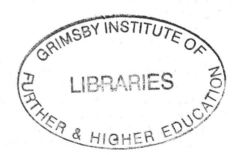

NICE guidelines

K. Gournay

Introduction

This chapter will provide an account of the work of NICE and look specifically at how such work impacts on mental health policy and implementation. NICE (or more correctly the National Institute for Health and Clinical Excellence) is an independent organisation responsible for providing national guidance on the promotion of good health and the prevention of ill health. NICE was originally set up as the National Institute for Clinical Excellence. The functions of another NHS organisation, the Health and Development Agency, were transferred to NICE on 1 April 2005. NICE's role is described in the 2004 White Paper, 'Choosing Health: Making healthier choices easier'. In this, the government set out key principles for helping people make healthier and more informed choices about their health. The government sees NICE as a way of bringing together knowledge and guidance on ways of promoting good health. NICE has guidance in three areas of health:

- Public Health – guidance on the promotion of good health and the prevention of ill health for those working in the NHS, local authorities and the wider public and voluntary sector
- Health Technologies – guidance on the use of new and existing medicines, treatment and procedures within the NHS
- Clinical Practice – guidance on the appropriate treatment and care of people with specific diseases and conditions within the NHS.

The topics that NICE issue guidance upon are chosen by three main groups of people:

- Health professionals, patients, carers and the general public
- The National Horizon Scanning Centre, which suggests which technologies might need to be assessed by NICE
- The Department of Health's National Clinical Directors and Policy teams. In the case of mental health, the National Clinical Director is currently Professor Louis Appleby.

NICE guidance on public health

NICE produces public health interventions and programme guidance. It provides recommendations on various types of interventions provided by local organisations with public health responsibility. These interventions set out to promote or maintain a healthy lifestyle, or reduce the risk of developing a disease or condition; for example, giving patients advice at home, in GP practices or in clinics to encourage them to take more exercise. Public health programme guidance deals with the broader activities for the promotion of good health and the prevention of ill health. This guidance may focus on a topic, such as strategies to help people give up smoking, or in a particular population such as young people or pregnant women, or in a particular setting such as the workplace. Little work published by NICE on public health has any implications for mental health care. However, there are several public health programmes of NICE that do have relevance, which are currently in progress and which will be published in the future. These will be referred to in more detail below.

Health technologies

Health technology appraisals are recommendations on the use of new and existing medicines and treatments within the NHS and centre on:

- medicines
- medical devices – e.g. hearing aids or inhalers
- diagnostic techniques – i.e. tests used to identify diseases
- surgical procedures
- health promotion activities – e.g. ways of helping people with diabetes to manage their condition.

As will be demonstrated below, there have been a number of health technology appraisals that are relevant to mental health. Health technology appraisals are based upon reviews of the clinical and economic evidence, particularly taking account of how well a specific treatment works, how much it costs the NHS and whether it represents value for money.

Health technology appraisals provide recommendations that are prepared by an independent committee. Members of these committees include professionals working in the NHS and people who are familiar with the issues affecting patients and carers. The Committee seeks the views of organisations representing health professionals, patients, carers, manufacturers and government and its advice is independent of any invested interests.

Clinical guidelines

Clinical guidelines are recommendations by NICE on the appropriate care and treatment of people with specific diseases and conditions within the NHS.

They are based upon the best available evidence. Guidelines help health professionals in their work, but they do not replace their knowledge and skills. Clinical guidelines often take two to three years to develop. Guidelines development is generally based in one of NICE's National Collaborating Centres, where teams with a wide range of expertise are based.

At the beginning of the process, a Guidelines Development Group (GDG) is set up. This is usually chaired by a leading expert in the particular area where the guideline is developed. A GDG is appointed with representation of all the main stakeholders. Thus, for example, for Mental Health guidelines there would generally be representatives from psychiatry, psychology, nursing, social work and occupational therapy. In addition, there will be at least one (and usually two) service users and various experts from other relevant fields – for example pharmacology and law. GDGs usually include a health economist, who provides the group with expertise in the costing of recommendations. The work of the health economist is usually supported by the work of other health economists who are employed or contracted by the National Collaborating Centre. The GDG meets regularly and usually works systematically through a range of topics relating to the area. Thus the GDG will look at areas such as assessment, effective psychological interventions, effective medications, the needs of particular groups (e.g. women, various ethnic groups) and so on. The GDG begins guideline development by conducting systematic Cochrane-style reviews of the literature and identifying the relevant literature in each of the areas to set out for the GDG the most effective approaches. The GDG then considers the literature and develops recommendations that allow the most effective approaches and interventions to be implemented. In order to ensure that the recommendation is realistic and acceptable to the patient/service user, the GDG also considers information obtained from surveys and focus groups of the relevant individuals.

The National Collaborating Centre is able to access expertise from various centres of expertise – for example, Cochrane Centres, centres for statistics, clinical effectiveness, and so on. At various stages during the development of a guideline, the GDG is able to access expertise from particular subject specialists and may invite these specialists along to meetings of the GDG in order to provide members with particular advice. At the end of the process, the GDG, with the assistance of the National Collaborating Centre, will have produced draft guidelines, which will contain recommendations and good practice points. The Guideline is then subject to review. NICE has established a number of Guideline Review Panels, which are linked to the National Collaborating Centres. After this review and any subsequent modifications, the guideline will then be widely circulated among stakeholders and one, or sometimes two, public consultations with stakeholders and a wider audience take place. One of the essential features of a guideline is that it is a document that is agreed by all members of the GDG. In order for recommendations and good practice points to be included, each and every recommendation and good practice point has to be the subject of a vote by the GDG. If there is any significant dissent, a recommendation or a good practice point will not be included.

NICE and mental health

At the time of writing, NICE has carried out work in all three areas – public health, technology appraisals and clinical guidelines. What follows is a description of the outputs of NICE on these three topic areas. However, the reader should be informed that this information is correct at the time of writing (February 2007) and, by the time that this textbook is published, it will be necessary for the reader to refer to the NICE website (www.nice.org.uk) to obtain a completely up-to-date picture of NICE and Mental Health topics. However, the description that follows may assist the reader in appreciating how NICE has contributed to the respective areas.

Prior to providing specific detail of the work of NICE on specific mental health topics, it is worth making some general comment about the evidence in Mental Health and the strength of the evidence. One major difficulty for NICE in the area of mental health care is the relative paucity of evidence. While, in disorders such as hypertension and cancer, there are thousands of very well designed clinical trials, many areas in mental health are, by comparison, greatly deficient. Whilst the evidence for the efficacy of medication in various mental health conditions is quite extensive, the ability to delineate the particular effects of pharmacological interventions is, by comparison with other areas of medicine, somewhat problematic. For example, if one is conducting a randomised controlled trial on the effectiveness of a new drug for schizophrenia, one needs to be aware that other variables, such as social and psychological factors, may influence clinical outcomes in particular individuals. It is therefore very difficult to tease out the respective effects of drugs and other variables.

There is also a problem with drug treatments in respect of the diagnosis of mental health problems. The making of a diagnosis in many mental health conditions is much less a science than, for example, in cancer or heart disease, where very accurate diagnostic techniques are available and the models of illness are quite different. In many interventions in mental health care, the number of randomised controlled trials may number a dozen or less. Thus, for example, while cognitive behaviour therapy is known to be a much favoured treatment for schizophrenia, there are, at the time of writing, only five or six well-designed studies of cognitive behavioural therapy (CBT) with schizophrenia and it has to be said that these studies were conducted on relatively small numbers of people, with relatively short post-treatment follow up – usually no more than a few months. Thus, overall, whilst NICE's work is based on evidence, one needs to consider each piece of NICE guidance on a mental health topic separately and to ask questions about the volume and quality of the evidence that underpins the particular guidance.

One final point needs to be made about evidence. While there is widespread acceptance that the randomised controlled trial presents the gold standard in research, it is becoming increasingly obvious that there is a need to consider qualitative evidence, particularly regarding the experience of service users/patients during treatment and their overall views regarding acceptability.

Turning now to the specific work carried out by NICE under the three areas of its work, what follows is a description of NICE's completed work and some information concerning work in progress, which will be completed during 2007 and 2008. The reader will appreciate that what follows is not a comprehensive account and that the reader should go directly to the NICE website (www.nice.org.uk) in order to obtain precise and detailed information. At the website, the reader will find a range of publications on the topic. The website contains detail of how the guidance was commissioned, with relevant timelines. It will also provide a complete text of the full review. In some cases, this may run to over 400 pages. However, the website also breaks down the full guideline into chapters that can be downloaded separately. The site also contains details of the publications that underpin the guideline, so that the reader can source material with confidence. The website also contains a Quick Reference Guide (QRG) for each guideline; these QRGs are intended to provide an executive summary and can be used by clinicians as a ready source of guidance and information in the course of their clinical work. The QRG is constructed to provide the most important and clinically relevant aspects of the guidance. In the case of medication, the QRG often includes well-designed charts or algorithms for use by busy clinicians.

All NICE guidance is also published in a form for the general (lay) public, patients and carers. NICE also provide a newsletter, which is free. All one needs to do to obtain the newsletter is visit the NICE website, register and this will be sent by email or post. The NICE website also contains details of guidelines under development.

One a NICE Guideline has been published, it becomes subject to another review after five years. The Guideline is revisited and, as necessary, amended and/or re-written.

Implementing NICE guidance

The public health guidance issued by NICE has to be implemented within the context of wider economic, organisational and political changes. Obviously, interventions on areas such as smoking need to be supported by legislative approaches and be part of more general, strategic health policy.

With regard to the implementation of clinical guidance, NICE admits that implementation happens more quickly in some places than in others. In 2004 the Department of Health published 'Standards for Better Health', which set out how NHS organisations should respond to NICE guidance. Technology appraisals and interventional procedures guidance are 'core' standards (the minimum level of service that patients can expect); the clinical guidelines are 'developmental' standards (frameworks for planning improvements in services). The distinction between 'core' and 'developmental' standards is very important. For example, a core standard such as provision of a specific medication usually means that the patient has a right to receive that medication and could, if necessary, argue this right in court. On the other hand a developmental standard, for example a particular psychological intervention as recommended by a clinical guideline, is aspirational and although the patient should expect that this intervention will probably be available, they have no 'rights' which could be pursued in a court of law.

The Health Care Commission is responsible for monitoring progress on the implementation of NICE guidance and more information on this topic can be found at the Health Commission's website (www.healthcarecommission.org. uk). Finally, NICE has set up an implementation support programme and provides reports and active assistance to organisations in implementation. NICE has set out to actively engage with NHS Trusts, has provided a wide range of publications; taken active steps to engage those responsible for providing undergraduate training programmes, established links with the Health Care Commission and Audit Commission for monitoring and inspection and attempts to show items of good practice and disseminate these over the country.

NICE and public health

As noted above, there has been very little work on public health that has direct implications for mental health. However, at the time of writing, there are at least five NICE groups working on various topics and their work will be published over the next couple of years. Brief details of this work follow.

Mental health and older people

This work, which is expected to be completed in March 2008, concerns the development of guidance for primary care and residential care institutions in the promotion of good mental health in older people. This work has been prompted by the National Service Framework for Older People (DH 2001) and will particularly focus upon increasing the feelings of well-being in later life and also identifying common mental health problems in older people, so that interventions may be delivered.

Workplace mental health

This Public Health Guidance is expected to be published in August 2008 and will assist employers and occupational health departments in the promotion of good mental health in employees.

Mental well-being of children in primary education

This Public Health Guidance is expected to be published in February 2008 and the published work on this topic, thus far, outlines a wide range of interventions that will be aimed at teachers, school support staff and school governors and all those responsible for primary school education.

Alcohol and schools intervention

This Public Health Guidance was published in November 2007 and concerns all aspects of alcohol education and intervention. Obviously this preventative approach is to be welcomed as most initiatives still centre on long established alcohol problems and could be seen as too little too late.

Substance misuse interventions

This Public Health Guidance focuses on community based interventions to reduce substance misuse among the most vulnerable and disadvantaged groups of young people.

Public health briefing

NICE has produced a very helpful briefing, entitled 'Public Health Interventions to Promote Positive Mental Health and Prevent Mental Health Disorders Among Adults'. This was published in January 2007. It identifies all relevant systematic reviews and review papers on non-drug treatments, which promote positive mental health and prevent mental disorders in adults aged over 16 years. It is designed to be accessed by a variety of readers, including those who simply want to look for headline findings, as well as those who might want to search.

Technology appraisals

The majority of technology appraisals conducted by NICE concern drug treatments and NICE has published very helpful guidelines on a number of conditions where drug interventions are used. However, the technology appraisals for mental health have extended their remit from drug treatments to computerised cognitive behaviour therapy, ECT and the new technique for treating severe depression, transcranial magnetic stimulation. In addition, technology appraisals also cover education and training programmes and this is particularly so for the treatment of conduct disorders in children. The list below sets out the technology appraisals which have either been published or are soon to be published:

- Conduct Disorder in Children – Parent Training/Education Programmes
- Depression and Anxiety – computerised cognitive behaviour therapy (CCBT)
- Attention Deficit Hyperactivity Disorder (ADHD) – Methylphenidate, Atomoxetine, Dexamphetamine
- Bipolar Disorder – new drugs
- Electro Convulsive Therapy (ECT)
- Schizophrenia – atypical antipsychotics
- Insomnia – new hypnotic drugs
- Drug misuse – Naltrexone
- Drug misuse – Methadone, Buprenorphine
- Dementia (non-Alzheimer) – new pharmaceutical treatments
- Transcranial Magnetic Stimulation for severe depression.

To access any one of these topics simply go to the NICE website and type in the details as set out above.

Clinical guidelines

As the list below shows, there are now a very wide range of clinical guidelines available in mental health. These are:

- bipolar disorder
- antenatal and postnatal mental health

- obsessive compulsive disorder
- depression
- schizophrenia
- self-harm
- depression in children and young people
- post-traumatic stress disorder
- anxiety
- violence
- eating disorders
- substance misuse interventions.

Example of a guideline – obsessive compulsive disorder

It might be helpful to examine a particular guideline to see how an individual disorder, in this case obsessive compulsive disorder (OCD), is treated, how effective interventions are set out and how the guideline describes how it should be implemented within the NHS, taking into account the real world problems of cost and staff shortages. For a fuller discussion of the condition and NICE Guideline, the reader is referred to Gournay et al (2006).

The Guideline sets out what is known about OCD and describes, in full, the features of the condition, based upon a review of the relevant literature and the current systems of classification. The Guideline then describes the background literature on epidemiology and causation, emphasising the probability that the condition is caused by a mixture of biological and psychological factors. The literature review on treatment effectiveness identifies the effectiveness of psychological treatments, based upon a cognitive behavioural model, and pharmacological interventions. The psychological treatments known to be most effective for OCD are clearly the behavioural intervention, exposure and response prevention and cognitive therapy, which has been adapted for specific use with OCD. Of the pharmacological interventions, the Guideline is clear in stating that tricyclic antidepressants, apart from Clomipramine, monoamine oxidase inhibitors and anxiolytics are not recommended. However, the Guideline makes clear that patients benefit from Selective Serotonin Reuptake Inhibitors, SSRIs), usually in a dose which is much higher than that used to treat depression. The Guideline also notes that pharmacological interventions are characterised by a much longer period before there is an onset of therapeutic effect, i.e. up to 12 weeks or more.

NICE sets out five core principles of care for people with OCD. These are:

- The promotion of public understanding of OCD and the provision of information and explanation
- The provision of continuity of care, so that treatment can be delivered in a seamless and effective way
- Ensuring that due respect is given to differences that may exist between religious or cultural practice and obsessive compulsive symptoms
- Ensuring that information and support are provided and that the individual patient's needs and preferences are taken into account when offering

treatment. The role of self help and support groups is also emphasised for people with OCD and their families and/or carers

- Providing an emphasis on giving families and carers appropriate information about assessment and treatment. In addition, the Guidance emphasises a need to conduct a needs assessment for the family and/or carer when the patient's condition is moderate, severe or chronic.

The Guideline recognises that, whilst the evidence for the effectiveness of both psychological and pharmacological treatments (or a combination of both) is clear, the modern NHS has considerable problems ensuring that people with OCD are provided with adequate treatment. First, there are simply not enough professionals trained to deliver treatments and only a small minority of sufferers can expect to receive a reasonable course of psychological therapy. With regard to pharmacological treatment, a barrier to the implementation of the Guideline is the relatively poor state of knowledge among general practitioners, such that most GPs will not be familiar with the specific issues in prescribing medication, in particular the higher dose required and the long period of onset of action.

The NICE Guideline sets out a 'Stepped Care' model to ensure that scarce resources are used to greatest effect. For a more detailed account of Stepped Care in psychological therapies, the reader is referred to an excellent review article by Bower & Gilbody (2005). Essentially, Stepped Care has two central features. First, the recommended treatment within a stepped care model should be the least restrictive of those currently available, but still likely to produce significant health gains and, second, the Stepped Care model is self correcting. Therefore, in the treatment of people with OCD, the NICE Guideline recommends six steps:

- Step 1 involves the general public and the NHS in general and focuses on awareness and recognition of the condition. The aim of this step is to provide, seek and share information about OCD and its impact on the general public, sufferers of the condition and families and/or carers.
- Step 2 involves general practitioners and primary care staff who may come across the condition and should be able to recognise and make an initial assessment. The aim of this step is to increase detection and education and to consider treatment options, which might include referral to more specialist services.
- Step 3 involves a wider range of primary care workers and child and adolescent mental health services. The focus of this step is on the management and initial treatment of OCD and the treatments involved in this step include brief Cognitive Behaviour Therapy (CBT) with self help materials, drug treatments or a combination of both.
- Step 4 involves a greater level of care, probably involving some mental health professionals. This is aimed at OCD complicated with the presence of another mental health problem and/or where the simple approaches used in step 3 have failed to work.
- Step 5 involves care and treatment by the multidisciplinary mental health team and includes professionals who have expertise in treatment and management. The focus of this step is on patients with OCD who have

severely impaired function and have not responded to steps 3 and 4. Treatment usually involves drug therapy and/or CBT, but may also include care coordination, admission and social care. In the case of children and young people, consideration should be given to a referral to specialist services outside of the general services available.

- Step 6 involves in-patient care or intensive home treatment programmes and focuses on those patients at the very severe end of the spectrum. There may be risk to life, to severe self neglect and severe distress or disability.

Thus Stepped Care provides a systematic approach to delivering interventions, leaving the specialist services the task of focussing on the most difficult to treat patients, whilst patients with less severe conditions are managed with simpler, but effective interventions.

Conclusion

NICE has now become a central feature of health care delivery in England and Wales and the outputs of the organisation are widely used not only in other parts of the United Kingdom, but also in many parts of the English-speaking world, including the USA. The main contribution of the body is the systematic and rigorous collection and analysis of evidence for treatments, procedures and technology in health care, with an over-arching emphasis on an approach to various conditions by wider public health initiatives. All health professionals can now readily access very detailed information about the various problems from which their patients suffer and, in mental health care, guidance on topics such as management of violence, the use of education and training materials and the management of self harm provide invaluable assistance. At the technical level, NICE's work is detailed and precise. However, one of its main assets is the stream of work that converts specialist and, often complex, technical knowledge into everyday language, thus facilitating the education of patients, families, carers and the general public at large. It is clear that NICE is still undergoing developments that will improve outputs. The writer of this chapter was privileged to chair a Guideline Development Group over a period of three years and was able to observe that NICE is for ever refining its procedures and examining its functions. Anyone with access to the internet can respond to any one of the hundreds of outputs of the organisation and take part in the feedback process, which shapes our approach to various problems.

Although the above has demonstrated that NICE has a very significant mental health portfolio, there are clearly many aspects of mental health care which deserve further attention. In a sense, NICE's job will never be complete, because guidelines need to be refined at regular intervals in view of emerging evidence.

References

Bower P, Gilbody S 2005 Stepped care in psychological therapies: access, effectiveness and efficiency. British Journal of Psychiatry 186:11–17

Gournay K, Curran J, Rogers P 2006 Assessment and management of obsessive compulsive disorder. Nursing Standard 20(33):59–65

19

Developments in education and training:
towards a whole system reform

D. Rushforth • I. Baguley

Introduction

This chapter examines the challenges facing education and training providers to deliver a modern mental health service in the wake of a fundamental programme of reform outlined in Modernising Mental Health Services (DH 1998) and the National Service Framework (NSF) for Mental Health (DH 1999a) which sets standards for mental health care across both health and social care.

Particular attention is given to emerging policy and workforce initiatives, which, guided by the NSF standards, aim to influence mental health education programme development and review. Further consideration is given to strategies to promote service users' involvement in education and training – from initial commissioning through to the delivery and evaluation of programmes of learning. To achieve this requires a radical rethink of core values which embraces the whole system of care, questions traditional clinical practice, workforce skills mix and in particular recognises the role of the service user in redesigning education and training provision which is responsive to user need, evidence based and fit for purpose.

Promoting social inclusion, extending choice and access to psychological treatments in order to improve standards of care are the touchstones of the NSF for mental health. Recent evidence indicates that education and training providers do not fully reflect these key standards in current curricula (Brooker et al 2002). Initiatives to improve dialogue between stakeholders are considered and illustrations of new ways of working to deliver balanced user and carer focussed training are highlighted.

The aims of policy change

We are witnessing a redesign of service provision, away from traditional services to more diverse service models based on person centred care, skills mix, core values and evidence based practice (Chadwick et al 2006, Rushforth et al

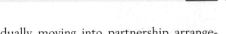
2007). Mental health provision is gradually moving into partnership arrangements across health and social care. In addition, a number of mental health trusts have applied for foundation status leading to more local control and less government direction.

The importance of modernising education and training is to ensure that the workforce is properly equipped to deliver the new mental health agenda in an ever changing landscape. The 'Pulling Together' report (SCMH 1997) highlighted the need to ensure that the skills, knowledge and attitudes of both existing and future mental health staff are appropriate to the demands of this changed environment and that they are properly prepared to function in continually evolving services.

Research evidence indicates that many staff are inadequately prepared for present day services, with particular shortfalls being identified in severe mental illness (Holmshaw 1999), for roles in primary care (DH 2001a) and for acute care (DH 1999a). Current courses have been found to be inappropriate and not relevant to support the implementation of NSF standards (DH 1998, Brooker et al 2002).

In addition, there is a raft of new workers in mental health whose role is directed by the needs of service users: Community Development Workers for the Black and Minority Ethnic Community (CDW) (DH, 2005a), Graduate Workers for Primary Care Mental Health (GWPCMH) (DH 2003a, NIMHE 2004b), Support, Time and Recovery Workers (STR) (DH 2003b).

To support new workers and new ways of working guidance has been issued about the roles and education needs of the existing workforce – Breaking the Cycle of Rejection: the personality disorder capabilities framework (NIMHE 2003), Women's Mental Health (DH 2003d) Developing Positive Practice to Support the Safe and Therapeutic Management of Aggression and Violence (NIMHE 2004a), Acute Inpatient Mental Health Care (DH 2002a, Clarke 2004), Dual Diagnosis (DH 2002b) and Community Mental Health Teams (DH 2002c).

Concerns have been expressed about the competency of the current mental health lecturer workforce to deliver these radical new approaches, and recommend an urgent need to update their knowledge and skills (SCMH 1997, Ferguson et al 2003). Practice staff consider that lecturers lack robust recent clinical experience, are not regarded as clinically credible, have little experience in the skills and interventions they are required to teach, and have unmet training needs of their own (DH 2001a, Lindley & Lemmer 2001, Brooker et al 2002).

The current and ambitious changes to modernise health and social care services have necessitated a far reaching rethink regarding the education and training of the future workforce. Reviews (SCMH 1997, Holmshaw 1999, DH 1999a, 2001a) and mapping exercises (DH 1999b, 2001b) have highlighted the gaps in educational provision for the mental health workforce. They have also questioned the ability of Higher Education Institutions to prepare practitioners with the skills, knowledge and attitudes to implement the NSF for mental health (Ferguson et al 2003).

In summary, the standards set out in the NSF set challenging goals to improve mental health practice, which, in turn, has generated considerable debate on the capacity of traditional education and learning provision to deliver on these standards. A series of reports have highlighted key issues and recognises that revising education and training programmes requires a whole system strategy which fully addresses workforce planning, recruitment, new ways of working across professional boundaries and the creation of new roles.

Recruitment and retention

The recruitment and retention of good quality staff, who reflect the profile of the community they serve, is central to the growth and development of the mental health workforce. Three key documents have been published recently on recruitment and retention issues within higher education, nursing and psychiatry (Ferguson et al 2003, McDonald et al 2004, DH 2005b).

Work is currently taking place as part of the Chief Nursing Officers (CNO) response to the Review of Mental Health Nursing (DH 2005c) to produce good practice guidance on recruitment and retention, recommend action that might be taken and describe resources that exist currently to help achieve such action.

Currently, mental health is not seen as an attractive place to work. This needs to be addressed by demonstrating that mental health provides an interesting, stimulating and challenging environment, good career opportunities, a fair rate of pay and a family friendly working environment. In addition, there is an urgent need to recruit from a different pool of people to expand the mental health workforce (Box 19.1). This means targeting people who do not have the required academic qualifications and those who may be graduates in health or social science related degrees. Many of these people do not necessarily want to enter traditional professions, but with the bespoke training could carry out important roles supporting other people.

Building workforce capacity and developing new roles

Two new workforce initiatives are exemplars of new investment to build capacity in order to meet National Service Framework standards to reduce social inclusion and improve access to psychological treatments.

Box 19.1

Recruitment of Asian people into mental health nursing

> A recruitment initiative led by Northern Birmingham Mental Health Trust has launched a major campaign to recruit Asian people into mental health nursing as part of their ongoing work to reduce stigma associated with mental health issues within Asian communities. The campaign includes a photography show, briefing pack and a 15-minute video featuring contributions from Asian nurses already working in mental health and from leaders of Birmingham's Asian communities.

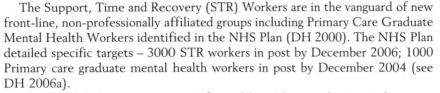
The Support, Time and Recovery (STR) Workers are in the vanguard of new front-line, non-professionally affiliated groups including Primary Care Graduate Mental Health Workers identified in the NHS Plan (DH 2000). The NHS Plan detailed specific targets – 3000 STR workers in post by December 2006; 1000 Primary care graduate mental health workers in post by December 2004 (see DH 2006a).

The STR Worker concept was informed by wide consultation with service users and carers as to what they regarded as the most valuable type of support (Russell 2000). It was acknowledged that many staff currently working in support worker roles are unfamiliar with recovery models, with little or no consistency in their training and supervision. These people are from diverse backgrounds, including existing and former service users and carers, and had the potential to become STR Workers (Box 19.2).

Front line professionally qualified staff were burdened by increasing workloads. Many reported that they were struggling to achieve a balance between spending time with service users and fulfilling other work requirements (Russell 2000).

Early in 2003, six small pilot sites were set up across England, facilitated by the then NHS Modernisation Agency's Changing Workforce Programme (CWP). These sites began to work through such issues as terms and conditions of employment; education and training; and joint working across health and social care organisations.

From late 2003, the Changing Workforce Programme in partnership with the National Institute for Mental Health in England (NIMHE) supported a much wider implementation initiative, through an Accelerated Development Programme (ADP), in order to achieve the DH target of 3000 STR Workers. Two national Programme Leads from the CWP Mental Health Team were assigned to facilitate and support the ADP, which was formally launched in November 2003 and will end in December 2006. There are 1275 STR Workers in post and 166 being actively recruited across health, social and voluntary

---

Box 19.2

Key features of the STR Worker role

- STR Workers work with people who are experiencing enduring mental health problems, particularly the elderly, spending negotiated time with them to provide appropriate support, so aiding their recovery.
- They have a specified education and training pathway.
- They work in a variety of statutory or non-statutory mental health service settings, and work across traditional service boundaries. They work as part of a team, under supervision, and contribute to the provision of individualised, flexible and holistic care.
- Their work focuses on providing practical help; promoting service users' independence and integration into the community; supporting service users in self-management of their health, and access to employment, community support and resources. In short, STR Workers empower service users to live ordinary lives.

settings. Funding for a further 549 workers has been identified with a projection of 1990 STR workers in post by the summer of 2006.

To recap, the Support, Time and Recovery (STR) Worker role was developed at the request of service users and carers. The STR Worker who would spend time with them, providing support and time, mainly people over 65 years, to achieve recovery to live an ordinary life. Carers and people with experience of using mental health services form 20% of the workforce in the majority of sites. The implementation of the role has been through an Accelerated Development Planning process, instigated and led by the Changing Workforce Programme (now within the NIMHE National Workforce Programme) in collaboration with NIMHE/CSIP regional development centres.

The readiness of primary care workers to address common mental health problems

Whilst many common mental health problems are minor and transitory, primary health care professionals face considerable difficulty in detecting commonly presenting health problems, such as depression. Fewer than 35% of general practitioners have undertaken any staff development education relevant to primary mental health (Kerwick et al 1997).

There is some evidence that other primary care workers may not always deliver high standards of care for people with mental health problems. Practice nurses encounter particular difficulties and miss up to 77% of people presenting with depression (Plummer 1997). Less than 2% of practice nurses have undertaken appropriate training to manage depression (Crossland & Kai 1998). The Department of Health recognises that the current demands on front line primary care are such that a new workforce capacity was needed to provide support to people with mild to moderate mental health problems (DH 2001c).

Investment in primary mental health care

The capacity of secondary mental health to address the huge demand from service users with anxiety and depression is limited by both financial and long-standing recruitment difficulties. The Department of Health is now actively encouraging primary care trusts to take a lead role in commissioning and delivering redesigned primary care services, which builds new workforce capacity, and review existing skills mix within general practice (DH 2006a).

The NHS Plan for England signalled investment in the primary care workforce to support the wider 10-year plan for mental health and social care. The Graduate Workers in Primary Care Mental Health are in the forefront of a diverse group of new workers appointed to complement and expand existing mental health workforce provision as advised by the Workforce Action Team (DH 2001d).

The Priorities and Planning Framework set out a target to appoint 1000 new graduate primary care workers by December 2004 supported by a national mental health delivery plan to monitor performance and review progress managed by the Strategic Health Authorities in England (DH 2006b).

Additional revenue to fund the appointment of new graduate primary care workers and their training fees were delivered with the uplift in general allocation, on the basis of weighted capitation, to Primary Care Trusts (PCTs) (DH 2003b;c). Local implementation teams (LITs) were required to submit progress reports on mental health targets to the service mapping database at the Centre for Public Mental Health at the University of Durham.

Expansion of the new primary care mental health workforce has not been uniform across England with significant local differences emerging (Rushforth 2004). A number of PCTs failed to meet the local target numbers (Centre for Public Mental Health 2002), citing competing spending priorities in other target areas. Significantly, where Strategic Health Authorities sent a clear message, that primary care mental health worker recruitment is an important performance indicator, workforce targets were achieved. The majority of PCTs have delivered on target numbers and a small, but growing number are investing strategically in primary care mental health workers above these targets to build workforce capacity to meet local delivery plans. An audit of higher education programmes offering the Post-Graduate Certificate programme identified 735 entering training between January 2004 and August 2006 (Baguley et al 2006).

Whilst these new workers are a tangible product of a commitment to invest in new workforce capacity, there are wider issues of service redesign and professional working practices to be addressed in order to integrate new workers into multidisciplinary teams and respond imaginatively to user dissatisfaction with current service provision

New ways of working

The burgeoning demand for redesigned services articulated by user, carer and voluntary sector groups contrasts sharply with long-standing difficulties in recruiting professionally qualified staff.

Implementing New Ways of Working presents a number of challenges; first, professional bodies can be protective of current practice and professional boundaries; second, staff may be worried about the long-term implications of change for them and their professional role; third, there may be insufficient change management processes in place to support and drive forward the modernisation agenda.

Significant progress has been made at a national level with the professions but if modernisation is to be meaningful at a local level then NHS trusts will need support from CSIP regional development centres. New Ways of Working for Psychiatrists (DH 2005b,d) clarified medical responsibility in a multidisciplinary setting and issued revised guidance on the employment of consultant psychiatrists.

A new role for clinical pharmacists is currently under development as part of a mental health pilot for the Changing Workforce Programme (Newcastle, North Tyneside and Northumbria Mental Health Trust 2005). Patients can now access advice and support and information from a clinical pharmacist who participates in patient reviews and takes medication histories with the aim to provide early interventions that improve safety and reduce risk. The patient potentially benefits from the nursing staff having more time, freed of routine tasks such as drug checks. The integration of clinical pharmacists into the multidisciplinary team is intended to provide additional advice and support to staff on medication issues.

Work is underway across other professional disciplines and a 'Creating Capable Teams' toolkit is under development to assist teams to examine their function, capabilities and skill mix.

The wider implications for education and training

Although the numbers of people employed to provide a service are important, numbers alone are insufficient. An educated and capable workforce that is well supported and supervised is key to delivering effective services. In addition to providing services that will support changes and improvements in patient care, access to education and training will allow people to take advantage of wider career opportunities and realise their potential.

There are a number of challenges for agencies concerned with education and training for mental health services including:

- establishing learning needs across sectors, professional groups, and agencies, including non-professionally affiliated staff groups
- ensuring that appropriate and relevant training and education is both commissioned and provided at all levels including training for entry into a professional group and continuing education
- incorporating learning for new and changing roles in mental health services, and new and changing services
- ensuring that the principles and values which underpin mental health services today inform personal and professional development
- developing local capacity for training and education programme development and delivery
- commissioning and quality assuring training and education.

Whilst the development of National Occupational Standards (NOS) for mental health and the Knowledge and Skills Framework (KSF) are an important central plank in aligning future education and training strategies within and across all staff groupings, neither the NOS nor the KSF apply to all staff in all settings.

The Ten Essential Shared Capabilities (ESC) for mental health practice were developed following consultation with service users and carers and describe the core values that should drive service activity across all sectors and settings (DH 2004). The development of the ESC was, in part, informed by the outcome of the Mapping of Mental Health Education & Training in England.

This exercise revealed significant omissions in both the pre and post qualifying training of all professional groups, with notable gaps within existing curricula which undermine progress towards meeting the NSF standards. The most significant omissions included:

- *Standard 1 Mental health promotion*
  - — User involvement
  - — Working with diversity
  - — Values
- *Standard 4 Effective service delivery*
  - — Evidence based practice
  - — Multidisciplinary working
- *Standard 6 Caring about carers*
  - — Carer involvement
  - — Working with families.

The Ten Essential Shared Capabilities apply to all staff groups, whether qualified or unqualified, and across all settings – health, social care and the non-statutory sector (Box 19.3). The ESC framework should be viewed as a fundamental building block to support the development of education programmes and as complementary to the CPF and NOS frameworks (SCMH 2001, Skills for Health 2002).

Whilst the primary aim of the ESC is to influence education and training provision, implementation of this framework will require a whole range of activities within mental health education to be addressed. Future developments to support implementation anticipates working with a range of key influencers to refine frameworks for personal development plans for individual practitioners, training needs analysis and joint education plans which influence both the commissioning process and subsequent purchasing decisions.

Investment in training and service delivery

The Centre for Clinical Academic Workforce Innovation at the University of Lincoln invested heavily in resources to assist graduate workers in primary care mental health to enhance their practice skills and demonstrate their potential

---

Box 19.3

The Ten Essential Shared Capabilities

1. Working in Partnership
2. Respecting Diversity
3. Practising Ethically
4. Challenging Inequality
5. Promoting Recovery
6. Identifying Peoples Needs and Strengths
7. Providing Service User Centred Care
8. Making a Difference
9. Promoting Safety and Positive Risk Taking
10. Personal Development and Learning

value to primary care teams. The main focus of this investment was the production of the interactive CD-Rom toolkit launched in January 2006. 'Primary Care Mental Health' is a flexible learning programme which offers a comprehensive teaching resource both to complement existing course programme delivery within the higher education institutions and also provides the teaching materials to support the development of reconfigured blended learning programmes (CCAWI 2006).

During the development of this toolkit, wider issues informed the structure and content of the final product. First, the skills based training needed to be congruent with emerging service development models which was not only responsive to user need but grounded in evidence-based cognitive behavioural assessments and treatments which improve outcomes for people presenting with common mental health problems (Lovell et al 2003, Mead et al 2005).

Core to preparatory training are skills based units which develop: client centred interviewing skills, risk management, and specific brief low intensity interventions based on tried and tested cognitive behavioural therapies, for example in behavioural motivation and problem solving. It is anticipated that Graduate Workers for Primary Care Mental Health will spend an average of 3–4 days each week in clinical contact when fully trained. It is therefore vital that education and training programmes build in the financial resource and timetabled sessions to fully brief practice areas and support both clinical supervisors and line managers within the employing PCTs.

Second, the interactive learning toolkit has to be a readily available resource to both learners and learning support teams at the end point of use. The 'Creative Commons Licence' allows permission for use on internal learning intranet platforms with freedom to replicate the CD-Roms for remote use on work-based platforms and personal computers, subject to conditions.

The gradual easing of professional boundaries which has fostered wider access to skills training and the resources to support accurate and efficient assessment and treatment are pivotal to the expansion of a competent workforce trained to meet the needs of service users.

The development of interactive learning tools in CD-Rom format for common mental health problems and managing psychosis (Myles 2004) are in the forefront of new ways of accessing learning that challenges traditional commissioning arrangements. The potential to build and expand upon conventional university based training deploying remote PC platforms, intranet and web-learning to integrate academic learning with practice based resources is high on the agenda of an increasing numbers of higher education institutions. They are strategically developing resource centres to realign academic staff training, technological infrastructure and establish dialogue with stakeholders to identify training needs; the support mechanisms required for safe practice; ethical probity and quality standards.

In tandem, we are witnessing the development of commercially available web based learning resources aimed at specific service users, for example, Fear Fighter for the treatment of phobic conditions (Kenwright et al 2001). However, the Primary Care Mental Health toolkit is uniquely identified as a product to support staff training. It is currently under further development, in partnership with a commercial publisher to provide a web-based learning resource to support low intensity cognitive behavioural therapy training for the treatment of mild to moderate anxiety and depression.

A second funding stream was directly invested in pilot book prescription schemes. These initiatives are developing rapidly with approved interactive treatment guides (Norcross & Santrock 2003) and self-help manuals increasingly available through local public libraries in England and Wales (Frude 2004). Borrowing arrangements vary slightly, but most libraries issue these books subject to normal borrowing conditions. They aim to promote self-help, widen access to psychological treatments, reduce stigma and foster user empowerment (Hicks 2003). Book prescription schemes have also alerted primary care teams to specific ways in which graduate workers in primary care mental health and other staff can facilitate guided self help.

User involvement in education and training

To date, service user involvement in mental health provision has mainly focused on specialist mental health services, rather than health and social care training provision; for example, service user and voluntary sector representatives sit on Local Implementation Teams (LITs). Local LITs are charged with delivering change at a local level and this has provided an opportunity to influence the Local Implementation Plans for mental health guided by the NSF standards.

This obligation to consult service users has been formalised by statute through a system of Patient and Public Involvement Forums (PPIFs), Patient Advice and Liaison services (PALs) and individual redress through the Independent Complaints Advocacy Service (ICAS).

No such level of scrutiny and accountability has been focused on training providers to date. However, the regulation of personal counselling services has focused attention on training standards and in particular the competencies required for practice on completion of training (BABCP 2006).

Meaningful revision of education programmes and in service training priorities requires user involvement. A report commissioned by Trent Workforce Confederation sought to identify good practice in higher education institutions (Gell 2004). Nottingham Advocacy was commissioned to undertake interviews with academic leads providing mental health training in higher education and report back on the findings. The report recommended engaging service users in the active planning of curricula, their involvement in the delivery and evaluation of course programmes. It further identified good practice for employment of service users in higher education and an activity check list for service user involvement in all aspects of mental health training.

Further consultation with a range of service user and user involvement networks by Trent Workforce Confederation, NIMHE West Midlands, and Mental Health in Higher Education (MHHE) led to the development of a framework for involving service users which aims to facilitate a consistent approach across England (NIMHE 2004b) (Box 19.4).

The MHHE report (Tew et al 2004) recommends that higher education institutions and mental health stakeholders undertake regular structured reviews of programme delivery using the National Continuous Quality

Box 19.4

Framework for involving service users in education and training

- *Open events* Local sites should establish promotional events inviting service users, to raise awareness of new workers
- *User reference group* At promotion events information should be given as to how users can be involved in training people recruited to a reference group for training programmes. The reference group can be involved in many aspects of training including design and delivery decisions. Consideration should be given to payment for involvement and adequate support
- *Developing the curriculum* Service users should be part of the group that plans the curriculum and can be involved in designing materials
- *Training and preparation* Service users will need adequate preparation to be trainers and good support. They should be involved in the process of and training in research skills, such as interviewing and focus groups
- *Ongoing monitoring of programmes* Service users who are reference group members should be involved in ongoing monitoring of the course programme
- *Evaluation* Service users should be involved in evaluating training as part of a reference group or training planning group
- *Assessor* Training collaborations including higher education institutions need to identify how service users can be involved in assessing learners

Improvement Tool for Mental Health Education (Brooker et al 2003). This tool serves a dual purpose: to assist workforce planning in the commissioning of mental health education programmes and as an audit tool to assist local stakeholder groups to assess carer and user involvement in their educational programmes.

Summary

Although mental health education and training will continue to face challenges over the next few years, it is important to note the achievements that have been made so far towards improving access and widening choice of treatments.

Investment in workforce capacity has supported the development of new roles and the increasing number of new mental health workers is tangible; with over 1900 STR workers in post and 735 Graduate Workers in Primary Care Mental Health entering training and they have been very well received by service users and carers.

Pilot training programmes are now underway to develop further roles, for example, psychology associates, graduate workers in child and adolescent mental health services and in prison health settings.

Whilst financial pressures present immediate challenges, over the long term they also provide opportunities to develop further new roles and service models that may meet the needs of people who use services and their families and carers. Further research examining the cost-benefit of graduate workers in primary care mental health teams is underway and due to report in 2007. The outcomes of this research may influence commissioning decisions by PCTs on future investment in additional mental health workforce capacity in primary care settings.

References

Baguley C, Rushforth D, Whyte M et al 2006 The graduate primary care mental health worker programme: a view from higher education training providers. Higher Education Academy Psychology Network, University of York, York

British Association of Psychological Therapies 2006 BABCP training newsletter. February. BABCP, Accrington

Brooker C, James A, Readhead E 2003 National continuous quality improvement tool for mental health education. Northern Centre for Mental Health, York

Brooker C, Gournay K, O'Halloran P, Saul C 2002 Mapping training to support the implementation of the National Service Framework for mental health. Journal of Mental Health 11:103–116

Centre for Clinical & Academic Workforce Innovation 2006 Primary care mental health: an interactive toolkit for professionals working with common mental health problems. CCAWI, Lincoln

Centre for Public Mental Health 2002 Mental Health Service Mapping Strategy. Centre for Public Mental Health, Durham

Chadwick S, James A, Rushforth D 2006 Implementing a new national role in mental health; the Support, Time and Recovery worker. Journal of Mental Health Workforce Development 1:30–36

Clarke S 2004 Acute inpatient mental health care: education, training and continuing professional development for all. NIMHE & SCMH, London

Crosland A, Kai J 1998 They think they can talk to nurses: practice nurses views of caring for mental health problems. British Journal of General Practice 48:1383–1386

Department of Health 1998 Modernising mental health services: safe, sound & supportive. HMSO, London

Department of Health 1999a National Service Framework for mental health: Modern standards and service models. HMSO, London

Department of Health 1999b Report by the Standing Nursing & Midwifery Advisory Committee (SNMAC). Mental health nursing: addressing acute concerns. HMSO, London

Department of Health 2000 The NHS Plan: a plan for investment, a plan for reform. DH, London

Department of Health 2001a Primary care key group report in the final report by the workforce action team – mental health national service framework, workforce planning, education and training. DH, London

Department of Health 2001b Workforce action team – key area H: mapping of education and training. DH, London

Department of Health 2001c Shifting the balance of power in the NHS: securing delivery. DH, London

Department of Health 2001d Mental health national service framework and the NHS Plan: workforce planning, education and training. An underpinning programme for adult mental health services: Workforce Action Team final report. (www.doh.gov.uk/mentalhealth/wat. htm) DH, London

Department of Health 2002a Mental health policy implementation guide: adult acute inpatient care provision. DH, London

Department of Health 2002b Mental health policy implementation guide: dual diagnosis good practice guide. DH, London

Department of Health 2002c Mental health policy implementation guide: community mental health teams. DH, London

Department of Health 2003a Fast-forwarding primary care mental health: graduate primary care mental health workers: best practice guide. DH, London

Department of Health 2003b Mental health policy implementation guide: support, time and recovery workers. DH, London

Department of Health 2003c Primary care trust revenue resource limits 2003–06. DH, London

Department of Health 2003d Mainstreaming Gender and Women's Mental Health. DH, London

Department of Health 2004 The ten essential shared capabilities: a framework for the whole of the mental health workforce. DH, London

Department of Health 2005a Mental health policy implementation guide: community development workers for black and ethnic minority communities: interim guidance. DH, London

Department of Health 2005b Joint guidance on the employment of consultant psychiatrists. (http://www.dh.gov.uk/PublicationsAndStatistics/Publications/PublicationsPolicyAnd Guidance/PublicationsPolicyAndGuidanceArticle/fs/en?CONTENT_ID=4122352& chk=CWEIUX) DH, London

Department of Health 2005c From values to action: the chief nursing officer's review of mental health nursing. DH, London

Department of Health 2005d New ways of working for psychiatrists: enhancing effective, person-centred services through new ways of working in multi-disciplinary and multi-agency contexts. DH, London

Department of Health 2006a The competence and curriculum framework for the physician assistant. DH, London

Department of Health 2006b The priorities and planning framework 2002–03. DH, London

Ferguson K, Owen S, Baguley I 2003 The clinical activity of mental health lecturers in higher education institutions. Report for the mental health care group workforce team. (http://www.lincoln.ac.uk/ccawi/RsrchPublications.htm) Trent WDC, Nottingham

Frude N 2004 A book prescription scheme in primary care. Clinical Psychology 39:11–14

Gell C 2004 Guidance for user involvement in mental health training in higher education. (http//:www.mhhe.heacademy.ac.uk/docs/projects/gudelines.doc) Trent WDC, Nottingham

Hicks D 2003 Reading and health mapping research project. The Reading Agency, Huddersfield

Holmshaw J 1999 Fitness to practice in community mental health. Nursing Times 34:52–53

Kenwright M, Liness S, Marks I 2001 Fear Fighter, reducing demands on clinicians by offering computer-aided self-help for phobia & panic: a feasibility study. British Journal of Psychiatry 179:456–459

Kerwick S, Jones R, Mann A, Goldberg D 1997 Mental health care training priorities in general practice. British Journal of General Practice 47:1383–1386

Lindley P, Lemmer B 2001 Clinical effectiveness training: a role development programme for lecturers in mental health. Sainsbury Centre for Mental Health, London

Lovell K, Richards D, Bower P 2003 Improving access to primary mental health care: an uncontrolled evaluation of a pilot self-help clinic. British Journal of General Practice 53:133–135

McDonald R, McQuade C, Patel K 2004 Mental health workforce recruitment and retention research project: final report. (http://www.uclan.ac.uk/facs/health/ethnicity/reports/documents/MHRetentionrecruitmentresearchprojectfullreport.pdf) UCLAN, Preston

Mead N, MacDonald W, Bower P, Lovell K, Richards D, Bucknell A 2005 The clinical effectiveness of guided self help versus waiting-list control in the management of anxiety and depression: a randomised controlled trial. Psychological Medicine 35: 1–11

Myles P 2004 Praxis: a cognitive behaviour therapy training package. North Tyneside and Northumberland Mental Health NHS Trust, Newcastle

National Institute for Mental Health in England 2003 Breaking the cycle of rejection: the personality disorder capabilities framework. NIMHE, Leeds

National Institute for Mental Health in England 2004a Developing positive practice to support the safe and therapeutic management of aggression and violence in mental health inpatient settings: mental health policy implementation. NIMHE, Leeds

National Institute for Mental Health in England 2004b Primary care graduate mental health workers: a practical guide. NIMHE North West Development Centre, Hyde

Newcastle, North Tyneside and Northumberland Mental Health NHS Trust 2005 Mental Health Services Directory. NNNMH NHS Trust, Morpeth

Norcross J, Santrock J 2003 Authoritative guide to self help resources in mental health, 2nd edn. Guilford Press, New York

Plummer S 1997 A controlled comparison of the ability of practice nurses to detect psychological distress in patients who attend their clinics. Journal of Psychiatric and Mental Health Nursing 4:221–223.

Rushforth D 2004 The graduate primary care mental heath worker – a progress report. Trent WDC, Nottingham

Rushforth D, Patel J, James A, Chadwick S 2007 Developing the mental health workforce capacity in primary care: implementing the role of graduate primary care mental health workers in England. Journal of Mental Health Workforce Development 2(1):42–49

Russell T 2000 A Primary Responder, the missing link: an unpublished report. Breakthrough, London

Sainsbury Centre for Mental Health 1997 Pulling together: the future roles and training of mental health staff. Sainsbury Centre for Mental Health, London

Sainsbury Centre for Mental Health 2001 The capable practitioner framework: a framework and list of practitioner capabilities required to implement the national service framework for mental health. Sainsbury Centre for Mental Health, London

Skills for Health 2002 National Occupational Standards for Mental Health. (http://www.skillsforhealth.org.uk/)

Tew G, Gell C, Foster S 2004 Learning from experience: involving service users and carers in mental health education and training. MHHE, Nottingham

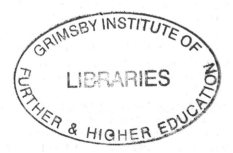

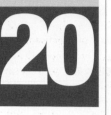

20

The National Service Framework for mental health:
costs of implementation

M. Parsonage

Introduction

The main aims of this chapter are: first, to set out some broad estimates of the costs of implementing the National Service Framework (NSF) for mental health in England; and second, to set these estimates in the context of past and prospective trends in total expenditure on mental health services for adults of working age. As will be explained below, little official information has been made publicly available on the resource requirements of the NSF, so use is also made here of the results of an independent costing study (Boardman & Parsonage 2007). Drawing on this work, the main conclusion of the analysis is that, while substantial extra resources have been provided for mental health services since publication of the NSF in late 1999, these are unlikely to be sufficient to deliver the NSF in full by 2010/11, i.e. within the approximate 10-year time-scale that was originally envisaged. Seen in an expenditure context, good progress has been made in implementing the NSF, but there is still likely to be some shortfall in the overall availability of resources at the end of the planning period. One obvious question that arises in the light of this prospective funding gap concerns the choice of key priority areas on which resources should be targeted over the next few years.

Official estimates of cost

The National Service Framework for Mental Health (DH 1999) was published in September 1999 and set out for the first time a set of officially sanctioned minimum standards which mental health services were expected to achieve. A chapter in the NHS Plan (DH 2000) published the following year contained further details on some of the services needed to be provided in support of the NSF, and the Framework was also amplified in the Mental Health Policy Implementation Guide (DH 2001a) and a number of subsequent guides. Notwithstanding the extensive nature of NSF-related policy statements and guidance, these documents say relatively little on the financial or resource requirements of the Framework, particularly at the aggregate level. For example, the NHS Plan included an announcement that extra investment of over £300 million a year by 2003/04 was being provided to fast-forward the NSF, but said nothing about the overall scale of expenditure needed to deliver the Framework that would have put the extra £300 million in context.

In passing, it is worth noting a rather different approach that has been pursued in New Zealand, where a 10-year national mental health strategy was launched in 1994 with the publication of 'Looking Forward' (New Zealand Ministry of Health 1994) and developed further in a 1997 report 'Moving Forward' (New Zealand Ministry of Health 1997). In 1996 the New Zealand government set up an official watchdog, the Mental Health Commission, whose main role has been to promote and monitor implementation of the national strategy. In 1998 the Commission produced a 'Blueprint for Mental Health Services in New Zealand' (New Zealand Mental Health Commission 1998), setting out a detailed description of the service developments needed to implement the national strategy and the associated requirements for extra resources. Subsequent annual reports produced by the Commission give a detailed account of the progress being made towards the delivery of these service and spending objectives, including an explicit quantitative statement of the overall distance travelled in resource terms. For example, the Commission's 2005 report notes that between 1993/94 and 2003/04 total funding for mental health services increased by 141.7% after allowing for general inflation and that at 30 June 2004 'funded clinical capability was at 74% of 'Blueprint' while the funded non-clinical capacity was at 83%' (New Zealand Mental Health Commission 2005, p3).

In England, monitoring the implementation of the NSF has mainly been based on a new system of service and financial mapping carried out annually by Local Implementation Teams (LITs) across the country. Service mapping is managed and coordinated by the Centre for Public Mental Health at Durham University, while the same functions in relation to financial mapping are undertaken by the Manchester-based consultancy, Mental Health Strategies. Regular reports are produced by these two organisations which provide valuable information on the development of mental health services and on trends in spending on these services by the NHS and local authorities (Centre for Public Mental Health 2006, Mental Health Strategies 2006). Particularly in the case of finance, the mapping returns have led to a step change in the quantity and quality of information that is now regularly available on mental health provision in England – an important and welcome development. On the other hand, a limitation of the exercises is that there is no equivalent in this country of the New Zealand 'Blueprint', giving a comprehensive statement of NSF-related service and spending objectives against which progress can be monitored on an annual basis. In the absence of such a statement, it is not straightforwardly possible to say, as it is in New Zealand, whether the funded provision of mental health care in England is currently near the overall target level implied by the NSF or a long way short and, if so, by how much.

As far as is known, the only official published estimate of the cost of implementing the NSF for mental health is given in the Treasury-sponsored Wanless review of long-term health spending, the final report of which was published in April 2002 (Wanless 2002). This includes a table giving cost estimates, attributed to the DH, of implementing all five disease-based NSFs that had been prepared up to that time (coronary heart disease, cancer, renal disease, mental health and diabetes). The figures for mental health indicate that, to deliver the NSF in this area, spending on services for adults of working age would need to increase in real terms (i.e. over and above general inflation) from £3.3 billion in 2002/03 to £6.4 billion in 2010/11, equivalent to an average real increase of 8.8% a year (assuming general inflation of 2.5% a year, this corresponds to an average increase in cash or money terms of around 11.5% a year). No information is provided on how this estimate was prepared, nor is any breakdown given of the target figure of £6.4 billion, for example by type of service (in-patient care, day care, community teams etc) or between the various NSF standards.

Information from the financial mapping returns indicates that between 2002/03 and 2005/06 total spending on mental health services for working age adults increased in cash terms by 32.2% (Mental Health Strategies 2006). Allowing for general inflation (as measured by the GDP deflator), this translates into an increase in real terms of 22.4%, or an average increase of 7.0% a year. This is a substantial annual rise but still less than the required increase of 8.8% a year noted above, implying that if the target figure for spending in 2010/11 is to be achieved, expenditure must now rise at an even faster rate over the remainder of the period. Thus it can be estimated that, after allowing for the actual growth in spending up to 2005/06, expenditure over the remainder of the period to 2010/11 needs to increase in total by 58.4% in real terms to deliver the NSF as costed in the Wanless review, equivalent to an average real increase of 9.6% a year (or 12.3% a year in cash or money terms, assuming general inflation of 2.5% a year).

An independent estimate of costs

As noted in the Introduction, an independent assessment of the costs of implementing the NSF has been undertaken by the Sainsbury Centre for Mental Health. Full details of this project are available elsewhere (Boardman & Parsonage 2007), so what follows is a short summary, with a particular focus on findings rather than methodology.

The cost estimates were built up in stages, as follows. The first and most time-consuming was to prepare a detailed specification of the full range of services needed to deliver the seven standards set out in the NSF. Wherever possible, use was made of the Policy Implementation Guides published in support of the NSF as the basis for these service descriptions. However, despite their extensive nature, the Guides are not always very explicit or prescriptive about service structures and models and, where this was the case, use was made of alternative approaches to service specification, including reference to NICE guidelines, current examples of good practice or a consensus of professional opinion.

The second stage was to relate these service specifications to needs for mental health care, as represented by the underlying epidemiological base. As far as possible, population-based figures of existing rates of mental health conditions based on population surveys were used. In some cases this was not possible and usage figures or official projections were employed instead. For example, in the case of hospital in-patient services, use was made of the estimated numbers of mental illness beds required in 2010/11 as given by the National Beds Inquiry (DH 2001b).

Third, the volumes of service provision generated by the first two stages of analysis were translated into matching workforce requirements disaggregated by type of staff (psychiatrists, psychologists, nurses, social workers etc). Other inputs are also needed for the supply of services, but staff are by far the most important, accounting for about 75% of total costs (Audit Commission 2006). For the purposes of analysis it was assumed that there is a broadly fixed or constant relationship between staff and non-staff inputs, so no separate calculations were undertaken for the non-staff element.

Finally, the estimated workforce requirements, which – like all the projections made in the study – relate to the assumed target or end year for the NSF of 2010/11, were converted into expenditure terms using appropriate pay rates, including an allowance for assumed annual real increases in pay between 2005/06 and 2010/11 in line with historical trends, and also grossed up to allow for non-pay inputs so as to give an estimate of total required expenditure in 2010/11, covering all forms of mental health provision for adults of working age.

A simple schematic representation of these various stages of analysis is shown in Figure 20.1.

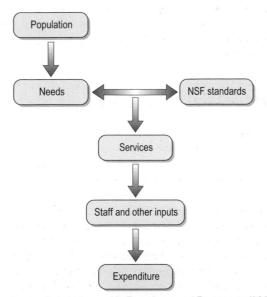

Figure 20.1 • The stages of analysis used in Boardman and Parsonage (2007) to calculate the service, staffing and expenditure implications of implementing the NSF

In effect, the end-product of the analysis is a quantitative model of the mental health system, one important feature of which is that it can readily be recalibrated to incorporate different assumptions or data (for example, local rather than national population figures) and to quantify the resource implications of such changes. This capacity to model the effects of different assumptions is particularly useful having in mind the point made earlier, that the NSF and its associated implementation guides are not always very explicit about the service structures needed to deliver the seven standards. The service specifications in the Sainsbury Centre study are as far as possible evidence-based, but they represent only one possible version of a mental health service that might deliver the objectives of the NSF, hence the value of being able to assess the workforce and cost implications of alternative patterns or methods of service provision.

To illustrate the results, the most straightforward calculations were those relating to the new specialist mental health teams proposed in the NSF (assertive outreach, crisis resolution and early intervention). This is because the 2001 Policy Implementation Guide gives fairly detailed recommendations on workload and staffing for these teams. For example, in the case of assertive outreach, the Guide suggests that each team should cover a total population of 250,000 and have a workload of 90 service users at any one time, with an ideal 10:1 ratio of users to care coordinators. The team should be made up of CPNs, ASWs, OTs, a clinical psychologist, a consultant psychiatrist and other medical staff.

The Sainsbury Centre study notes that according to epidemiological evidence there are, on average, 177 people with severe and enduring mental illness who are difficult to engage and thus suitable for assertive outreach in a total population of 250,000. Following the 10:1 ratio recommended in the Policy Implementation Guide, this implies a need for 17.7 care coordinator staff. Allowing for some additional workers, such as employment specialists and dual diagnosis workers, and grossing up to the national level, it is estimated that by 2010/11 assertive outreach teams will have a total caseload of nearly 37,000 people and an associated requirement for care staff of just over 4900. The latest available data from the Durham service mapping returns indicate that the total number of care staff currently working in assertive outreach teams is about half this number (Centre for Public Mental Health 2006). This and similar calculations for crisis resolution teams and early intervention teams are summarised in Table 20.1.

Taking all specialist teams together, overall numbers of care staff are currently just over half the total required in 2010/11, but there is clearly very substantial variation by type of team, with progress towards target being much greater for crisis resolution teams than for those providing early intervention services.

At the other end of spectrum, mental health care in primary care provides an example of service provision where the NSF and its associated guides provide relatively little by way of clear guidance on appropriate levels and methods of service delivery. In the absence of an agreed model for delivering mental health interventions in this setting, it was decided to adopt an approach which identified the main evidence-based types of treatment for common mental disorders

Table 20.1

Comparison of required and actual numbers of care staff in specialist teams				
	AOTs	**CRTs**	**EITs**	**Combined**
Care staff required in 2010/11	4906	5382	4264	14,552
Numbers working in 2005/06	2551	4322	932	7805
Actual as % of required	52.0	80.3	21.9	53.6

Sources: required numbers of staff given in Boardman & Parsonage 2007 and actual numbers of staff in Centre for Public Mental Health 2006.

and to cost these. The two major forms of treatment delivered in primary care are medication and psychological therapies. As summarised in NICE guidelines, there is a good evidence base for drug treatments in anxiety and depression and for a range of psychological therapies, particularly cognitive behavioural therapy (CBT) (NICE 2004a,b).

In assessing the appropriate level of provision for these services, use was made of a recent survey of people consulting in general practice which not only gives rates of consultation for mental disorders seen in general practice but also provides information on the actual needs for treatment as measured in the same individuals as surveyed (Boardman et al 2004). For example, in the case of depression, the survey found a consultation rate of about 150 per 1000 people consulting their GP, of whom 65% had developed depression during the previous 12 months (i.e. they had new onsets of depression during that year, with many having experienced previous episodes). The study judged antidepressant medication to be suitable for 70% of these consulters and CBT to be suitable for 55%. The further assumption was made in line with NICE guidelines that CBT should be given only to those who do not adequately recover after being given antidepressants. Approximately 60% of people recover after antidepressants, so 40% will require CBT.

On the basis of these and other assumptions, it was estimated that in a typical catchment population of 250,000 people (all ages), there will be around 13,200 new onsets of depression and anxiety among working-age adults in any one year. If treatment is given to all those for whom antidepressant medication or CBT are judged suitable and all these cases are detected by GPs, a total of 8975 people should receive antidepressants and 4400 should receive a course of CBT (of 12 sessions on average). The provision of CBT on this scale would require about 55 therapists per 250,000 population, corresponding to a national requirement in 2010/11 of 11,400 therapists.

The estimates for required levels of medication are broadly in line with current levels of provision, but those for CBT are far higher. Grossed up to national totals, the above figures suggest that around 2.75 million people will consult their GP with new onsets of depression or anxiety each year and 33% of these (0.9 million) should receive CBT. Current figures are that, among people treated by their GP for mental health problems, only about 1% receive CBT, 3% receive some other form of psychotherapy and a further 4% receive counselling (GPs employ about 5000 counsellors) (Layard et al 2006).

Table 20.2

Comparison of current and required staff numbers (all adult mental health services)		
	Actual numbers 2005/06	Required numbers 2010/11
Consultant psychiatrists	2229	4075
Other medical staff	3686	6844
Qualified nurses	42,529	70,790
Social workers	5077	10,211
Clinical psychologists, psychotherapists, counsellors	11,294	16,320

Sources: actual numbers are given in NHS Information Centre 2006, except for social workers (where the number is given in Centre for Public Health 2006) and counsellors (where use is made of the estimate of 5,000 cited in Layard et al 2006), while the required numbers are taken from Boardman & Parsonage 2007.

Service specifications as required to deliver the NSF standards and associated workforce requirements were assessed on these lines across the full range of mental health services for adults of working age. Pulling together the findings, Table 20.2 shows estimates for 2010/11 of required numbers of staff in the key clinical groups and compares these with the numbers currently working in the NHS and social service departments.

These estimates indicate that, in crude unweighted terms, overall numbers of staff in the groups shown need to increase by 67.0% from the 2005/06 base in order to deliver the NSF by 2010/11. A number of adjustments are needed to convert this figure into a corresponding estimate of the requirement for total additional public spending on mental health services.

First, the figures in Table 20.2 need to be weighted to allow for differences in relative pay between the various groups. It costs more to employ an additional consultant psychiatrist than an additional nurse and, as can be seen in the table, the required numbers in these two groups grow at different rates. The effect of weighting according to relative pay is to increase slightly the aggregate growth requirement between 2005/06 and 2010/11, from 67.0% to 68.5%.

Second, allowance needs to be made for staff groups other than those shown in Table 20.2 and also for non-pay inputs. As noted earlier, it has been assumed in the case of non-pay inputs that these bear a fixed or constant relationship to staff inputs and no separate calculations have been made. Partly because of a lack of data on numbers currently employed, a similar assumption has been made with respect to staff groups not shown in Table 20.2, including staff in management, administrative and clerical grades and other support workers. In other words, it has been assumed that, to deliver services effectively, staff numbers in these groups need to increase proportionately in line with numbers in the key clinical groups.

Third, an adjustment is needed to allow for the fact that the figures for 2005/06 in Table 20.2 relate to staff directly employed by the NHS and local authorities, whereas those for 2010/11 give an overall staff requirement for the provision of publicly funded mental health services, whether supplied by the NHS and social services or by the independent and voluntary sectors on a contractual basis. Thus the figures for 2005/06 need to be increased to allow for staff numbers in the non-statutory sector providing publicly funded care. According to the financial mapping returns, purchases of services from the non-statutory sector accounted for 17.1% of all public expenditure on adult mental health care in 2005/06 (Mental Health Strategies 2006) and in the absence of further information it has been assumed that the same ratio applies to staff numbers. Because staff numbers in the base year are increased while those in the end year are unchanged, the net effect of this adjustment is obviously to reduce the estimated growth requirement, from 68.5% to 39.7%.

Finally, an allowance needs to be made for real increases in pay between 2005/06 and 2010/11 and for this purpose it has been assumed that pay in health and social services will increase over and above general inflation in line with historical trends. This is the same as the assumption made in the Wanless review of long-term health spending, where it was noted that the relevant increase was 2.4% a year. Given that pay accounts for three-quarters of total mental health service costs and assuming that prices for non-pay inputs rise at the same rate as general inflation, the effect of this adjustment is to increase the estimated requirement for total expenditure by 1.8% a year, leading to a final estimate that, for full implementation of the NSF, spending on adult mental health services needs to increase between 2005/06 and 2010/11 by 52.7% in real terms. This is equivalent to an average increase of 8.8% a year in real terms, or 11.5% a year in cash or money terms, assuming general inflation of 2.5% a year.

Discussion

As noted earlier, the cost estimate for implementing the NSF given in the Wanless report implies that spending on adult mental health services needs to increase by 9.6% a year in real terms between 2005/06 and 2010/11 if the standards specified in the Framework are to be delivered in full. The corresponding figure of 8.8% a year independently produced by the Sainsbury Centre study is broadly similar. While a detailed comparison of the two estimates is ruled out by a lack of published information on the calculations quoted in Wanless, it does seem that generally comparable conclusions have been reached on the key requirements of NSF implementation, particularly concerning numbers of additional staff. Given a degree of consensus on expenditure implications, an obvious question for discussion is whether additional resources are likely to become available on the scale required, having regard to past and prospective trends in spending on mental health care.

Dealing first with the historical record, the financial mapping returns are the most comprehensive source of information on expenditure related to services for adults of working age but are available only from 2001/02 onwards. For earlier years use has to be made of data published by the DH which covers public spending on mental health for all age groups combined (DH 2004). Assuming that the share of working-age adults in total spending remained broadly constant over time, a series combining the two sources can be constructed as shown in Table 20.3. All figures are at 2005/06 prices, taking into account general inflation as measured by the GDP deflator.

Table 20.3

Year	£ million
Expenditure on mental health services for working age adults	
1999/00	3333
2000/01	3573
2001/02	3623
2002/03	4006
2003/04	4136
2004/05	4615
2005/06	4904
Sources: based on figures given in DH 2004 and Mental Health Strategies 2006.	

These figures show that over the period from 1999/2000 (the year in which the NSF was published) to 2005/06, expenditure on adult mental health services increased in total by 47.1% in real terms, equivalent to an average growth rate of 6.7% a year. By any standards this was a rapid rate of increase in spending and undoubtedly allowed good progress to be made in improving mental health services along the lines envisaged in the NSF.

Suppose that spending continues to increase at 6.7% a year in real terms between 2005/06 and 2010/11. Will this be sufficient to deliver the NSF in full? Perhaps illustrating the very ambitious nature of the policy, the short answer is no, whether use is made of the Wanless estimate of expenditure requirements or that produced by the Sainsbury Centre. The percentage increases in these studies quoted earlier imply that spending in 2010/11 needs to reach £7768 million (Wanless) or £7488 million at 2005/06 prices (Sainsbury Centre) if the NSF is to be implemented in full. A growth rate in expenditure of 6.7% a year from 2005/06 onwards would take spending to £6781 million by 2010/11, a shortfall of 12.7 % relative to Wanless and 9.4% relative to the Sainsbury Centre.

The spending increases for mental health shown in Table 20.3 were achieved at a time when overall expenditure on the NHS and social services was growing at an unprecedentedly rapid rate. For example, in the six years between 1999/2000 and 2005/06 total health spending increased by 57.3% in real terms, which compares with an increase over all of the previous 12 years of just 50.9% (HM Treasury 2006a, Table 3.3); in other words, the expenditure growth rate more than doubled. In the years after publication of the NSF, the general climate for spending on mental health was therefore very favourable, although it is noteworthy that – despite its supposed priority status – expenditure in this area grew less rapidly than spending on health generally (47.1% compared with 57.3% over the period 1999/2000 to 2005/06). Consideration now needs to be given to the question of whether, looking ahead, the generous annual increases of the recent past can realistically be expected to continue.

Departmental spending plans to 2007/08 were set in the Government's 2004 Spending Review (HM Treasury 2004, Chapter 8) and these indicate that in 2006/07 and 2007/08 overall spending on the NHS will increase by an average of 7.1% a year in real terms. This is very much in line with the rapid growth rates of the recent past. On the other hand, spending on local authority personal social services – representing about 20% of all public expenditure on adult mental health care – is planned to increase much less rapidly, at only 1.3% a year in real terms. On the possibly favourable assumption that spending on mental health will grow at the same rate as spending on health and social services generally, it can be calculated that combined NHS and local authority expenditure on mental health will increase by 5.9% a year in real terms over the two years in question. This is less than the average growth rate of 6.7% a year achieved over the six years to 2005/06, but not by much.

Looking further ahead, it is far less plausible to assume that annual increases on this scale will be maintained in the last three years of the NSF planning period, i.e. 2008/09–2010/11. This is mainly because aggregate public spending will be growing at a significantly slower rate than in the recent past and even priority programmes such as the NHS seem certain to be affected by the slowdown. Expenditure plans for individual programmes will not be announced until completion of the Comprehensive Spending Review reporting in 2007, but at the aggregate level the public finance projections published with the 2006 Budget indicate that total public spending will grow at only 1.8% a year in real terms during the three years in question (HM Treasury 2006b, Chapter C). This is well under half the growth rate of 4.4% a year achieved on average between 1999/2000 and 2005/06.

In the light of these considerations a possible set of assumptions is that in the three years beginning in 2008/09 total spending on the NHS will grow at half the annual rate that is planned for 2006/07 and 2007/08, total spending on social services will grow at the same rate and mental health will maintain a constant share of spending in both these programmes. The combined effect of these assumptions is a projection that expenditure on mental health services will increase by 3.1% a year in real terms in the last three years of the NSF planning period. As with public spending generally, this is less than half the annual growth rate achieved over the period 1999/00 to 2005/06.

Bringing together the planned increases for 2006/07 and 2007/08 and the projected increases for the following three years, the overall scenario suggested here as a plausible central case is that, over the five-year period to 2010/11, spending on mental health will increase by 22.0% in real terms. From a base level of expenditure of £4904 million in 2005/06, this implies total spending in 2010/11 of £6027 million, a shortfall of 22.4% relative to the NSF expenditure requirement implied by the Wanless review and 19.5% relative to the requirement suggested by the Sainsbury Centre study. Rounding these figures and expressing them in the language used by the New Zealand Mental Health Commission, funded capacity for adult mental health care in 2010/11 is likely to be at around 80% of the NSF target level.

As noted in the Introduction, an important question that arises in the light of this likely funding shortfall concerns the choice of priority areas within mental health on which additional resources should be focused over the remaining years of the planning period. Detailed consideration of this issue is beyond the scope of this chapter, but as factual background to the debate it may be

Table 20.4

Changes in the pattern of spending on adult mental health services 2001/02 to 2005/06			
	Share of spending 2001/02 (%)	Change in spending 2001/02 to 2005/06 (%)	Share of increase in total spending (%)
CRTs, AOTs, EITs	5.9	+127.5	23.6
Secure care	11.4	+109.9	39.2
Services n.e.s.	7.0	+50.0	10.4
Hostels, care homes etc	10.4	+26.0	7.2
CMHTs	16.6	+19.1	7.8
Psychological therapies	4.3	+18.8	2.0
Rehab/continuing care	12.0	+15.3	4.1
Acute hospital services	26.3	+15.0	8.8
Day services	6.1	−11.2	−3.2
Total spending	100.0	+35.3	100.0

Source: derived from figures in Mental Health Strategies 2006.

helpful to provide some evidence on where additional resources within mental health have gone in the recent past. Using data from the financial mapping returns (converted to real terms), this is shown in Table 20.4.

There has clearly been very substantial variation between service areas in terms of expenditure growth rates over the period shown. Presumably reflecting their priority status, the new specialist teams and secure care enjoyed the fastest growth in spending, and taken together these two areas absorbed over 60% of all the extra resources devoted to adult mental health care, even though they accounted for less than 20% of total spending at the start of the period. At the other end of the spectrum, expenditure on day services actually fell in real terms and a number of other service areas, including acute hospital services and community mental health teams, experienced growth rates in spending that were only around half the growth rate for mental health care as a whole. Looking ahead, some re-balancing of expenditure is implied by the Government's five-year review of the NSF published at the end of 2004 (DH 2004), which identified a number of areas for development over the second half of the planning period, including improved access to psychological therapies and better standards of care in inpatient wards.

Conclusions

The NSF was published in late 1999 and set out a comprehensive prospectus for improving standards in adult mental health care, to be delivered over the first decade of the 21st century. Though not stated explicitly at the time, the resource implications of the new policy were clearly substantial and the evidence presented in this chapter suggests that full implementation of the NSF would require spending on mental health services to more than double in real terms from the level prevailing in the base year of 1999/2000. This was always an ambitious undertaking. Good progress was made over the period 1999/2000 to 2005/06, when an accommodating climate for public spending in general and health care in particular allowed expenditure on mental health services to rise by nearly 50% in real terms.

Looking ahead, the prospects are less favourable and it cannot realistically be expected that spending will grow as rapidly in the second half of the NSF planning period as in the first. Some shortfall in funding is therefore likely and calculations presented here suggest that probable expenditure in 2010/11 will be around 20% below the level required to deliver the NSF in full. This is still a substantial achievement and there is little doubt that better resourcing has led to major improvements in the quality of mental health care since 1999, albeit with some variations in performance both between services and between different parts of the country. The likely shortfall in funding implies a need for continuing debate on priorities. In an increasingly constrained spending environment, what will be the best uses of additional resources in the coming years?

References

Audit Commission 2006 Managing finances in mental health. Audit Commission, London

Boardman J, Parsonage M 2007 Delivering the Government's mental health policies: services, staffing and costs. The Sainsbury Centre for Mental Health, London

Boardman J, Willmott S, Henshaw C 2004 The prevalence of needs for mental health treatment in general practice attenders. British Journal of Psychiatry 185:318–327

Centre for Public Mental Health, Durham University 2006 Adult mental health service mapping: reporting autumn 2004 and spring 2006. (http://www.amhmapping.org.uk/reports/)

Department of Health 1999 National service framework for mental health: modern standards and service models. DH, London

Department of Health 2000 The NHS Plan: a plan for investment, a plan for reform. DH, London

Department of Health 2001a The mental health policy implementation guide. DH, London

Department of Health 2001b Shaping the future NHS: long term planning for hospitals and related services: consultation document on the finding of the national beds inquiry. DH, London

Department of Health 2004 The national service framework for mental health – five years on. DH, London

HM Treasury 2004 Stability and security and opportunity for all: investing for Britain's long-term future: new public spending plans 2005–2008. HM Treasury, London

HM Treasury 2006a Public expenditure statistical analyses 2006. (http://www.hm-treasury.gov.uk/economic_data_and_tools/finance_spending_statistics/pes_function/function.cfm) HM Treasury, London

HM Treasury 2006b Financial statement and budget report. HM Treasury, London

Layard, R, Clark, D, Knapp M, Mayraz G 2006 Implementing the NICE guidelines for depression and anxiety: a cost–benefit analysis. (http://cep.lse.ac.uk/research/mentalhealth/default.asp) Centre for Economic Performance, London School of Economics

Mental Health Strategies 2006 The 2005/06 national survey of investment in mental health services. (http://www.dh.gov.uk/PublicationsAndStatistics/Publications/Publications Statistics/PublicationsStatisticsArticle/fs/en?CONTENT_ID=4134717&chk=1NpN4i) DH, London

New Zealand Mental Health Commission 1998 Blueprint for mental health services in New Zealand: how things need to be. Mental Health Commission, Wellington

New Zealand Mental Health Commission 2005 Annual Report for the year ended 30 June 2005. Mental Health Commission, Wellington

New Zealand Ministry of Health 1994 Looking forward: strategic directions for the mental health services. Ministry of Health, Wellington

New Zealand Ministry of Health 1997 Moving forward: the national mental health plan for more and better services. Ministry of Health, Wellington

NHS Information Centre 2006 NHS hospital and community staff (HCHS): medical and dental England: 1995–2005. (http://www.ic.nhs.uk/pubs/nhsstaff)

NICE 2004a Anxiety: management of anxiety disorder (panic disorder, with or without agoraphobia, and generalised anxiety disorder) in adults in primary, secondary and community care. NICE, London

NICE 2004b Depression: management of depression in primary and secondary care. NICE, London

Wanless D 2002 Securing our future health: taking a long-term view. HM Treasury, London

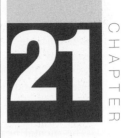

The role of the voluntary sector

A. McCulloch • G. Howland

Introduction

There is a lot of rhetoric about the role of the voluntary sector in mental health but rather less evidence and thoughtful analysis. While we should not promise more than we can deliver, this chapter will attempt to offer a realistic analysis of the current and future roles of the voluntary sector in mental health. In doing so, we will consider the background, including definitions of the voluntary sector and the current policy environment, and the current and future roles of the sector in mental health. We will offer empirical evidence in the form of a survey of leading voluntary sector providers. In particular, we will attempt to assess the sector's potential to support change and to consider how its role needs to change if we are to continue successfully to modernise mental health services.

The title of the chapter begs a number of questions and raises a number of issues including:

- what is the voluntary sector?
- what are its current roles?
- what should be its future roles?
- what realistically can the sector achieve?
- how can this contribution be facilitated?

These are important questions, given the increasingly large volume of services being delivered by the sector, in addition to its historic role in campaigning and pressing for change, as well as meeting gaps in service provision.

What is the voluntary sector?

There are many definitions of the voluntary sector and it has an ancient history. Organised religion is usually seen as the basis of the first voluntary organisations which in some countries have become inextricably entwined with the state.

The specific voluntary provision of mental health services also has a long history. According to one source the first mental hospital was founded in

Damascus in the 8th century (Howells 1975) and run according to Islamic principles. Charities for the relief and support of people with mental health problems and other conditions in England go back at least as far as the Middle Ages (The Bethlem was founded in 1247), and multiplied in Tudor times. Modern mental health charities started to emerge in the 19th Century. Together (previously MACA), for example, is 120 years old, Mind is over 60 years old and the Mental Health Foundation will be 60 in 2009.

The mental health voluntary sector in England has therefore existed for at least 800 years. It has gradually moved away from its religious roots, and state recognition has been increasingly important. Elizabeth I granted a Royal Charter to a range of organisations which still exist today and most major charities have a number of different structural and governance links with the state. But the essence of the voluntary sector must be the 'voluntary' or independent aspect which has its roots in voluntarism and free independent or collective action by citizens (Etzioni 1968).

Van Til (1988) usefully provides a typology of voluntary action and uses the term *voluntarism* to refer to organised voluntary action within society. It is voluntarism with which this chapter is concerned. It is obvious that today's voluntary sector often has a very limited relationship with volunteering. Whilst many voluntary sector agencies use volunteers most are run by paid staff and employ professionals from various disciplines. What typifies these agencies are the following principles (after Anheier 1995):

- they are formally constituted organisations, often companies limited by guarantee with charitable status
- they are private, i.e. separate from the state, albeit often partly state funded
- they are not profit distributing
- they are self governing
- they have some meaningful voluntary input e.g. donations, volunteering.

It is these agencies which this chapter deals with.

Mental health sector

What does it mean to work in the 'mental health sector'? Ultimately all human action has a potential mental health impact; and most major voluntary agencies if effective could have a positive impact on the mental health of populations or sub-populations with which they are concerned (e.g. through providing better lives or meaningful activity). Whilst it is impossible to measure it could be argued that the voluntary sector is intrinsically bound up with public mental health and that participation in corporate voluntarism or individual voluntary action is mentally healthy. However, for the purposes of this chapter we can only examine the role of voluntary agencies which explicitly wish to work on mental health or mental illness as one of their primary aims. These include:

- bespoke mental health service providers
- voluntary organisations dealing with mental health as their main focus
- service providers where mentally ill clients are a major explicit focus of their broader activity (e.g. Turning Point).

The current role of the mental health voluntary sector

In volume terms, the largest role of the voluntary sector in mental health is in the direct provision of services. Other important roles appear to include:

- lobbying and campaigning
- research and development
- information provision
- support for carers and users including advocacy.

It is hard to gauge the relative importance and impact of these different functions. However it is relatively easy to measure the size of the sector in financial terms.

Current Government policy and the voluntary sector

We will now assess how Government policy impacts on the sector. As we have already highlighted, the voluntary sector has been a provider of services for many hundreds of years, but the sector has a much wider role than simply service provision. A role which encompasses research, education, training, campaigning, lobbying for change and developing innovative ideas for often highly distinctive client groups with very specialised needs.

The current Government is particularly keen to promote public sector service provision by the voluntary sector, but this has not been the case with all Governments, and many mental health voluntary sector service providers, while keen to do more for the specific client groups they serve, wish to see mental health service *transformation* rather than simply the *transfer* of existing, often poor quality, mental health services across sectors.

Relationship between Government and the voluntary sector

The relationship between the voluntary sector and national and local Government has fluctuated over time as different initiatives have been brought forward by national Government. For example, the introduction of the NHS in 1948 substantially reduced the provision of general hospital care by local Government and the voluntary sector. By contrast, the introduction of the Community Care reforms in the early 1990s and consequent disinvestment from local authority service provision gave a significant boost to the provision of housing programmes within the mental health voluntary sector.

In 2006, the Government's new emphasis on public service delivery through social enterprise appeared to offer the voluntary sector a key role in mental health service transformation (Hewitt 2006).

Investing in and personalising public services

The current Labour administration has sought to increase substantially, in real terms, expenditure on health services while relating this new investment closely to health service reform. So, for example, the mental health National Service

Framework was introduced to target new mental health service investment towards the introduction of new specialist community teams (e.g. early intervention, crisis intervention/home treatment and assertive outreach teams).

At the start of its second term, the Government began to talk also about moving away from what it described as 'one size fits all public services' towards 'personalised public services' which remained, particularly in the case of health, universally available and free at the point of use, but which utilised a plurality of providers to increase choice. In October 2001, the Prime Minister, Tony Blair said:

> 'In developing greater choice of provider, the private and voluntary sectors can play a role. Contrary to myth no one has ever suggested they are the answer. Or that they should replace public services. But where they can improve public services, nothing should stand in their way.'

Building the voluntary and community sector

The current Government wants to build up what it describes as the Voluntary and Community Sector (VCS) for a number of reasons including:

- voluntary and community organisations help to build a sense of community (i.e. create social capital)
- they unleash the power and the potential of individual and collective action which strengthens our democracy
- they can deliver personalised public services, particularly for those from marginalised and disadvantaged groups
- they are a means through which communities can influence the decisions and actions of those responsible for commissioning and delivering public services (e.g. local government and the NHS).

There is also the suspicion among many in the VCS that the Government also sees the voluntary sector as a 'cut-price alternative' to current state providers. This perspective has been reinforced by initial proposals to establish a national mental health tariff at prices below the cost of service provision, which would require the VCS to make up the difference through 'charitable subsidies'.

Commissioning from the voluntary and community sector

In order to support the VCS in taking on an enhanced role in public service delivery the Government established a cross-cutting review to inform its 2002 Spending Review. This highlighted five key areas of reform and made a number of recommendations to:

- involve the VCS in planning as well as delivery of services
- forge long-term partnerships with the sector

- build the capacity of the sector
- legitimise full cost recovery for the sector
- promote implementation of the Compact (developed jointly by the Sector and the Government in 1998).

In addition, it established the Active Community Directorate in the Home Office to implement the Review's recommendations and initiated the Future-builders fund (essentially, a long-term loan fund of £125 million, made available initially over 3 years) to overcome obstacles and increase the scope and scale of VCS service delivery.

In 2005, the National Audit Office reviewed progress on improving working with the VCS (Third Sector) in their report Working with the Third Sector (June 2005) and found that progress had been patchy. In particular, it noted that a number of funding issues continue to cause difficulty, including late confirmation of funding, little progress on longer term funding and difficulty in achieving full cost recovery. While some Government departments had been pro-active in improving relationships with the VCS, many had not.

Following this report, in July 2005, the Department of Health announced the establishment of a Third Sector Commissioning Task Force to:

- promote a sound commercial relationship between public sector commissioners of services and the Third Sector as providers
- help to remove barriers to entry for all providers
- promote equality of access for all types of Third Sector organisations in the provision of public services.

The Task Force's first report 'Embrace Partnership Now' (Third Sector Task Force 2006) is a statement of 'work in progress' restating what needs to be done to remove barriers to Third Sector participation in service delivery. It makes a series of commitments to further action, and urges commissioners and providers to consider what behavioural changes are needed to make the vision of greater Third Sector service provision a reality. Significantly for our purposes, it includes a guide to commissioning from Third Sector organisations (which the Government defines as including voluntary and community organisations, charities, social enterprises, faith groups, cooperatives and mutuals) and a 'model' block contract for the provision of social care services. These developments will require a change in mindset among NHS Commissioners.

In addition, it will also require changes in the Third Sector. To realise its full potential with an increasingly diverse and challenging market, Third Sector organisations will need to more effectively communicate their unique selling points to commissioners, develop strategies for ensuring the services they deliver are of the highest possible quality and effectiveness, and secure robust and transparent systems of governance (Hewitt 2006).

The work of the Task Force is important and continuing and its initial ideas are already being factored into the Government's latest guidance on health reform and commissioning (DH 2006).

Transfer or transform?

While the Government is increasingly seeking to *transfer* existing services to the VCS, the mental health VCS is increasingly talking about *transforming* public services and making them more relevant to individuals and communities needs and wants.

We do appear to be at the start of a period of major change in mental health primarily because we may be moving from a model based on mental illness to a model based on mental well-being, recovery and social inclusion. Therefore the interventions required to manage this are shifting from traditional medical approaches to care to psychosocial models of individual and community support and development.

This shift in emphasis together with the Government's desire to see the Third Sector play a much larger role in delivery is a major development opportunity for the voluntary sector (the appointments of the Director General for the Third Sector and the Director General for Social Inclusion and the launch of the Third Sector Action Plan have started to put the Government's desires into practice).

Expanding the provider role of the mental health voluntary sector

The provider expertise of the mental health voluntary sector has been built largely on the provision of housing programmes and a range of community support initiatives. While the voluntary sector currently provides some clinical services, and some voluntary sector organisations are keen to provide more, generally the sector has much less experience than the NHS or the private sector in this field.

Clearly, the VCS could either buy in or gradually grow the clinical expertise that would enable it to become a provider of a 'full range' of mental health services but it does not have it 'in house' at the present time. In addition, the sector lacks a whole range of infrastructure skills and resources (e.g. in relation to finance, human resources and IT) which are significant barriers to the type of exponential growth needed to transform public services from the outside. So the dilemma facing Government is to bring together the guaranteed funding, specialist clinical skills and resources of the statutory sector, with the innovation, user and community focus and engagement of the voluntary sector, to personalise public services.

The Government is starting to address this dilemma through an expansion in the role of social enterprise. However, sustained Government intervention is likely to be required, over the next 5–10 years, to shake up existing relationships between the statutory and voluntary sector and transform mental health services through new organisational models of delivery.

Beyond the voluntary sector: transformation through social enterprise?

In May 2006, the Government created the Office of the Third Sector, headed by Ed Miliband, the first Minister for the Third Sector, to seek to address these dilemmas. In his speech to the Third Sector Summit on 22 June 2006 (Miliband 2006) he set out his vision of the hybrid future contribution that the Government wishes the Third Sector to make as:

> 'First, working in partnership with the public sector to deliver services directly to people where the sector is best suited to doing so, particularly in highly specialised areas ... This is not just about delivering existing services in a different way but about doing things which were not previously recognised as an important part of public services, working in partnership with people: so-called co-production of the service.
>
> 'Second, the third sector can innovate so that the public sector can learn the lessons in the services it provides ... The challenge this provides for government is how we can find ways of replicating this successful learning in other public services where the third sector can show the way forward.
>
> 'Third, I believe the third sector has an essential role to play as a source of voice for users ... an essential part of driving up the standards of service ... I want to send a clear and unambiguous message that amid the talk of the increased public service delivery of the third sector, it is important for government not to downgrade this important function that you have.'

For Public Sector and Third Sector organisations intent on working together to deliver service transformation, social enterprise, particularly through the vehicle of community interest companies, appears to offer a key route forward. The new DH Social Enterprise Unit will encourage innovation and entrepreneurialism in health and social care and pave the way for new services which better meet patients and service users' needs and wants. To help with this a Social Enterprise Fund was established from April 2007, to help with set-up costs. This shift towards health and social care delivery through Social Enterprise has also been endorsed by the Opposition.

In conclusion, the building blocks are now in place that will enable the Third Sector providers who want to do so, to play a much larger role in public service delivery in the future. The speed and extent of this major strategic shift will depend now on 'cultural and behavioural change which are, of course, the biggest challenges of them all, and must be recognised and embraced as critical and integral to the success of the reform programme' (Third Sector Task Force 2006).

Our survey of major mental health voluntary organisations

This then is the context within which major voluntary sector organisations in mental health are currently working. In order to understand the organisations' own views on the change process we carried out a survey of key organisations in mid 2006. This part of the chapter reports on the results of that survey.

Methodology

A mixed multiple choice and open ended questionnaire was sent to the Chief Executives of the 19 largest and most influential mental health provider charities in Great Britain. These were selected using a combination of founder membership of the Mental Health Providers Forum and turnover as recorded in the Top 3000 Charities 2006/7 (Caritas Data 2006). The emerging list had 'face validity' as far as the authors were concerned. Fifteen of the charities responded, producing a strong representation of the views of the leading voluntary sector providers in Great Britain including major charities in Scotland and Wales. These are not, of course, representative of smaller and informal groups which may be equally important in delivering services and change. Individual charities were promised anonymity. The issues covered in the survey were:

- current and future roles
- current and future funding sources
- major factors affecting business development
- perception of the environment and market
- views on key issues surrounding the sector
- governance.

The survey results

Roles

Table 21.1 summarises the current roles of the respondents. The organisation which did not consider a major role to be service provision, does provide national support for local service provision. In terms of role development, responses can be summarised as follows:

- No role change envisaged – 3
- Expansion of existing roles – 3
- Increase in lobbying and campaigning – 3
- More research and evaluation or service development consultancy – 2
- More user involvement – 2

Table 21.1

Current roles of the respondents

Roles	Number of charities (15 respondents)
Service provision	14
Lobbying and campaigning	5
Research and development	2
Information provision	5
Support for carers and users and advocacy	8

- More partnership working – 2
- Clearer audit trails/accountability – 2
- Recovery orientation
- More clinical services
- More information provision.

Funding sources

Organisations were asked about their primary funding sources (delivering at least 20% of income) and how these might change over the next three years. Table 21.2 summarises the current key funding sources of the organisations. In terms of changes over the next three years:

- Increased fundraising activity (non-statutory focus) – 5
- No change envisaged – 3
- More contracts (NHS focus) – 2
- Diversification – 1
- More individual purchasing – 1
- Reduction in statutory funding – 1
- More benefit monies – 1
- More restricted income – 1
- Lower donor income – 1
- More partnership monies – 1.

The environment

The respondents were asked about the major factors affecting their businesses (Table 21.3).

The future

They were also asked what major changes they expected to see over the next three years (Table 21.4). Colleagues were then asked to rate various relevant

Table 21.2

Key funding sources	
Funding sources	**Number of charities with this source (15 respondents)**
Statutory sector contracts	13
Other contracts	2
Private donations	2
Institutional grants and donations	2
Consultancy	0
Other	2

Table 21.3

Environmental factors affecting charities	
Major environmental factors	**Number of charities with this response (15 respondents)**
Availability of statutory funding	14
Attitude of statutory partners	9
Public attitudes to the sector	4
Availability of suitable staff	6
Government policy	10
Other	1

Table 21.4

Expected changes over next three years	
Areas of change for the charity	**Number of charities responding (15 respondents)**
Business volume will grow faster than RPI	14
Volume will stay the same	1
Volume will shrink	0
Labour market will improve	3
Labour market will stay the same	7
Labour market will become more adverse	4
Statutory sector will use voluntary organisations and partnership more	10

statements on a 5-point Likert scale (Table 21.5); numbers of charities out of a possible 15 are indicated in each box, full statements are listed in the footnote. One respondent said:

> *'If they are not careful the statutory sector will miss an excellent opportunity of engaging with service providers in the not-for-profit sector. They should start seeing us as part of the solution and not part of the problem.'*

Other open ended responses pointed to the importance of individual budgets and commissioning, and to risk sharing. One respondent felt that regulation was important but was a blunt instrument in managing the market.

Table 21.5

Rating on 5-point Likert scale					
Statement	Strongly agree	Agree	Neither	Disagree	Strongly disagree
The role of the voluntary sector is poorly understood	3	11	0	1	0
The role of the voluntary sector is undervalued	5	9	0	1	0
The voluntary sector is more innovative	3	8	3	0	0
The voluntary sector has a stronger user focus	4	11	0	0	0
My business is ready to expand	4	8	0	1	0
Our independence is threatened	2	3	3	7	0
The statutory sector treats us as an equal partner	0	0	3	8	4

Footnote: The statements organisations were asked to rate on a 5-point Likert scale were as follows:
(a) The role of the voluntary sector is poorly understood by the statutory sector
(b) The role of the voluntary sector is undervalued by the statutory sector
(c) The voluntary sector is more innovative than the statutory sector
(d) The voluntary sector has a stronger customer/user focus than the statutory sector
(e) My business is ready to respond to Government plans to allow our sector to expand
(f) Our independence is threatened by over-reliance on statutory funding
(g) The statutory sector treats us as an equal partner in business relationships

Governance

The charities were asked whether changes to the governance process were planned to respond to the market:

- None planned – 5
- Set up trading arms/subsidiaries – 3
- Recruit new trustees with market relevant knowledge – 2
- Carry out formal review of the governance process – 2
- Involve more users in governance – 2
- Improve performance and information management – 1
- Reflect changes to the governance of the UK – 1.

Respondents indicated in clarification of the final point, that the markets would develop very differently in England, Scotland and Wales – a radical shift towards the voluntary sector was expected only in England.

Discussion of the survey results

The findings of the survey will not surprise many working in the mental health sector, but the results do provide some important pointers to the future. They confirm the evidence that service provision is the leading role for mental health voluntary organisations, followed by support for users and carers, information and campaigning. R&D is relatively poorly developed. It is interesting that three of the organisations consider that campaigning is a key area for expansion and a further two wish to develop research and service development. This suggests that in future more organisations may be seeking to 'complete the policy and research into practice' cycle by actively seeking national change and service transformation. This to some extent fits with the evidence base on change which suggests that innovation requires more than just the provision of excellent services locally but a coordinated strategy involving R&D, communications, policy and leadership. It is also worth noting that three charities underlined their commitment to the expansion of existing roles.

The organisations are overwhelmingly funded by the statutory sector. It is interesting that few other sources of funding hit the 20% level. Only two of the 15 organisations had major levels of private donor funding – this raises key issues about independence which we will consider later. Five organisations were considering increasing their fundraising activity and two their contracting, but given that some respondents and other evidence suggests that the donor market may be difficult over the next five years, this activity might not hugely alter the massive reliance on statutory income within the sector, and for some this will rise.

Views on the environment were particularly interesting or stark. Obviously organisations that rely on statutory funding will consider its availability key (14 out of 15) but 10 also considered Government policy key despite the scepticism in services which sometimes exists about policy impact. Nine also cited attitudes of statutory partners and six the labour market.

In terms of the future, sector leaders clearly believe Government intentions about a shift in resources towards the sector. Fourteen believed their businesses would grow and none believe they will get smaller. Most believe that partnership will move up the agenda. There is a fairly gloomy view about the labour market – 11 out of 15 believe it will get worse or stay the same.

The survey placed a key emphasis on assessing attitudes and beliefs. All but one of the respondents agreed, or strongly agreed, that the role of the voluntary sector is poorly understood by the statutory sector and that it is undervalued. Twelve disagreed or strongly disagreed that the statutory sector treats the voluntary sector as an equal partner. However, most believe that it is more innovative and has a stronger user focus. Again, all but one respondent thought their business was ready to expand. There were mixed views on whether organisation's independence was threatened by changes in funding and policy – five thought it was and seven thought it was not.

Finally, we looked at governance. Perhaps surprisingly quite a few organisations envisaged no change to governance, but perhaps organisations have already addressed the issues arising from becoming large providers. Three intended to set up trading arms and eight intended to improve governance arrangements in various ways.

Analysis of survey results and conclusions

We are fairly clear about the origins and current role of the mental health voluntary sector, but what of the future? It seems to the authors that there are a number of key questions about the future role of the sector which have to be answered:

- Is the sector 'fit for purpose' to meet the challenge of Government policy?
- Can the sector transform services and communities instead of just adding to service volume?
- Related to this is the age old question – is the sector is genuinely innovative?
- What will be the advantages and disadvantages of sector expansion?
- How can a better relationship with the statutory sector be engendered?
- How will the broader environment impact upon change?

The results of the survey show that the sector is optimistic about its ability to grow. This is far from being the same as saying that it will be able to meet all the challenges posed by Government policy statements. For example, only one of the leading providers stated that it wished to take on clinical services. Whilst this may not be necessary or desirable, it is clear that if the vision is to transform services the sector will have to provide different kinds of service and not just the same services under a different label. We know that, for example, some are seeking to do this and are developing services such as expert user and carer programmes, psycho-social interventions and assertive outreach, as well as embryonic holistic 'managed care' programmes. At the moment though the majority of services remain housing and employment based, many of which are frankly unexciting, not necessarily evidence based and not necessarily much different to statutory provision elsewhere. Whilst it is almost certain that the sector can and will grow much of this growth may be a change in volume coupled with transfer of existing services from the statutory sector, rather than the radically new 'personalised services' that the Government is seeking.

As far as innovation itself is concerned, there is much evidence both from our survey and the wider literature that many organisations and opinion formers believe that the voluntary sector is more 'innovative' than the statutory sector. Osborne (1998) provides the most detailed and thoughtful analysis of these issues seen by the authors. His conclusions seem to apply very much to the current situation of the mental health voluntary organisations. He has seven key messages for voluntary organisation leaders:

1. '... it is wrong to perceive innovative capacity as an inherent characteristic of (voluntary organisations).' Innovation – and perhaps subsequently transformation – is only one role of sector.
2. The sector must be clear about the type of innovation being pursued and its managerial implications – transformational change requires strong leadership whereas low level incremental innovation is much easier to achieve.
3. Voluntary organisation structures do not necessarily foster innovation. The survey was disappointing in that radical changes to governance do not seem to be envisaged in the sector, but they may be necessary if transformation is to occur.

4. An outward looking stance amongst all levels of staff was necessary for innovation to be fostered.

5. '... managers ... (must) ... take a deliberate strategic approach to the relationship of their organisation to its environment – in terms of the local community, its key stakeholders and the larger societal environment.'

6. Innovative organisations are more likely to receive statutory funding. This is a controversial but interesting finding to which we will return below.

7. Leadership within the organisations have to be fully aware of the institutional environment and must attempt to be proactive in shaping it. Encouragingly, the survey suggested a number of organisations are attempting to influence the organisational environment more strongly.

Reflecting on the work of writers such as Osborne, our own knowledge of the sector and its history, and the survey, we have developed a 'balance sheet' or SWOT analysis on the possibility of sector expansion (Table 21.6).

One of the key messages from the survey was that voluntary organisations and the statutory sector will have to work harder to understand each other so that they can work together to transform outdated mental health services. This must be a joint and equal responsibility.

Voluntary sector leaders clearly have a key role in talking to the statutory sector and building understanding. Crude and unrealistic messages about the alleged superiority of voluntary sector approaches cause scepticism and cynicism – a more balanced message about strengths, weaknesses and partnership is required.

At the same time, the statutory sector needs to be incentivised and/or required to treat the voluntary sector as an equal partner. The move away from guaranteed block funding for the statutory sector to payment by results may be one way in which this process can be accelerated. Evidence based commissioning, disinvestment from interventions (such as in-patient care) that lack an evidence base, and a requirement to participate with the voluntary sector in joint

Table 21.6

SWOT analysis	
Strengths	**Weaknesses**
Value-led	Governance
Innovation	Quality variable
User and carer involvement/ownership	Management
Diversity	Vulnerability
History	Lack of infrastructure for clinical and
Lack of bureaucracy	professional input
Multidisciplinary team working	Short-term funding/access to capital
Voluntary	HR and IT infrastructure
Opportunities	**Threats**
Policy mood music	Speed of change
Changing zeitgeist in mental health sector towards	Funding pressures
integrated models	Labour market
Emphasis on partnership and social enterprise	Blunt nature of regulation
	Lack of statutory sector understanding/
	support/collaboration

social enterprise companies would all help to facilitate and speed up much needed change.

Whatever the future of New Labour, its debt to Etzioni and other key thinkers on voluntarism is shared by the new leadership of the Conservative party. It is unlikely therefore, in the authors' view that the macro policy environment will shift radically away from emphasising voluntary sector involvement in the reshaping of public services including mental health services. Our voluntary organisations are not perhaps fully ready for the challenge, but they must get there quickly. Improved governance, evidence based commissioning, equal partnerships with statutory sector providers, including through social enterprise and longer-term contracts will all assist this process. However, transformational leadership from voluntary sector managers is likely to be key to ensuring the sector helps create mental health services fit for the century.

Acknowledgements

The authors are grateful to the respondents to the survey for providing full and frank responses. We are also grateful to Alison Frankish for administering the survey and to the Mental Health Foundation for funding the research.

References

Anheier H 1995 Theories of the nonprofit sector. Voluntary and Nonprofit Sector Quarterly 24(1):15–24

Blair A 2001 Prime Minister's speech to public sector workers on Public Service Reform. British Library, London, 16 October

Caritas Data 2006 Top 3000 Charities 2006/7. Caritas, London

Department of Health 2006 Health reform in England: update and commissioning framework. DH, London

Etzioni A 1968 The active society. Collier-Macmillan, New York

Hewitt P 2006 Social enterprise in primary and community care. Social Enterprise Coalition, London

Howells J (ed) 1975 A world history of psychiatry. Baillière Tindall, Edinburgh

Miliband E 2006 Speech to the Third Sector Summit, London, 22 June

Osborne S P 1998 Voluntary organisations and innovation in public services. Routledge, London

Third Sector Commissioning Task Force 2006 No Excuses. Embrace partnership now. Step towards change! Department of Health, London

Van Til J 1988 Mapping the third sector: voluntarism in a changing social economy. Foundation Center, New York

Further related reading

HM Treasury 2002 The role of the voluntary and community sector in service delivery: a cross cutting review. HM Treasury, London

Home Office 1998 The compact on relations between government and the voluntary and community sector. Home Office, London

National Audit Office 2005 Home Office: Working with the Third Sector. National Audit Office, London

22

Mental health legislation

P. Bartlett

The failure of reform

> '[The National Service Framework] will be backed up, in due course, by changes to bring the law on mental illness up to date to reflect modern treatments and care, following the root and branch review conducted by the independent expert group under Professor Genevra Richardson.'
>
> (DH 1999a, p1)

So claimed Frank Dobson, then Health Secretary, in his introduction to the National Service Framework (NSF) for mental health. This optimism was to prove misplaced. The Act that was eventually passed in the summer of 2007 was yet another set of piecemeal amendments to the existing legislation, little more than a fig leaf to disguise the failure of the efforts to achieve reform over the previous nine years. The 'root and branch' review had well and truly withered on the vine.

In substantive terms, the tale of the crumbling of mental health law reform is an account of a demise of ideals also contained in the NSF. It is for others in this volume to discuss whether these values have survived elsewhere, but in the Mental Health Act, there is now only the barest shadow of the optimism and dynamism of the NSF. This is, perhaps, not entirely a surprise. The NSF was designed essentially to provide standards of service that people will use voluntarily. Its ethos is about providing service options; it virtually never mentions the possibility that people might need to be forced to use the services. By comparison, coercion is a traditional part of mental health law: involuntary admission and treatment without consent are two central themes to the discipline. Mental health law as traditionally conceived and the NSF would never be obvious bedfellows. Nonetheless, the divergence in their paths over the last nine years is striking.

The process of reform was commenced in 1998, with the appointment of an expert panel chaired by Professor Genevra Richardson to advise on legislative reform. The Richardson Committee made a serious attempt to take into account the changes in social, political and policy attitudes that had occurred since the previous major law reform in 1959 and the lesser reform in 1983. Its starting premise was that people with mental illness should be treated as far as possible in a fashion analogous to people with physical illnesses – a principle of non-discrimination.

The Committee included a set of principles that were to guide the interpretation of the Act, including the principle of least restrictive alternative, a preference for consensual care, user involvement, respect for diversity, respect and support for carers, and rights to the provision of information. They also adopted an approach of 'reciprocity' – that when compulsion was used on a person, that person had a corresponding right to services. While it stopped short of calling for inclusion of formal standards of service provision in the Mental Health Act itself, users were to be given a right to a needs assessment, with the expectation that at this assessment their concerns about their mental health would be taken seriously. Carers too would have the right to have an individual's mental health needs assessed. The Committee made it clear that their proposals would only be effective if appropriate services were offered, anticipating the proposals of the NSF.

The overall focus by the Richardson Committee on user autonomy was given tangible form in both substantive and procedural recommendations. A more stringent test of the health or public safety benefits required for involuntary admission was proposed for people who had capacity to make decisions than for people who lacked that capacity. Involuntary treatment would be restricted for involuntary in-patients, pending a mandatory independent review seven days following admission. Involuntary treatment in the community would not be permitted without such a review. The review panel would not consider merely whether compulsion was warranted, but would have before it a full treatment plan for the individual, put together by a multidisciplinary team according to a variety of prescribed medical and social criteria. Full tribunal hearings would be available at this stage if requested by the user, and a full tribunal hearing would in any event be mandatory if compulsion were to continue beyond 28 days. A variety of civil rights protections were introduced into those hearings, including a formal right to advocacy (DH 1999c).

There is much here that intersects with the ethos of the NSF, including the involvement of users, the provision of appropriate services, the promotion of independence, non-discrimination in service provision, and the expectation that services would promote independence.

However, this vision for a new Mental Health Act began to be undercut even as the Richardson Committee was being formed. At the initial meeting of the Committee, Paul Boateng, then the Under Secretary of State for Health under whose responsibility the Committee fell, stated (DH 1999c, p142):

> 'But if there is a responsibility on statutory authorities to ensure the delivery of quality services to patients through the application of agreed individual care plans, so there is also, increasingly, a responsibility on individual patients to comply with their programmes of care. Non-compliance can no longer be an option when appropriate care in appropriate settings is in place. I have made it clear to the field that this is not negotiable.'

Consistent with the 1997 Labour Party manifesto, the Government further made it clear that community treatment orders would be part of any reform package. Even at this early stage, the emphasis was changing from autonomy to compulsion.

This trend continued with the publication of the Government's green paper in response to the Richardson Committee. For example, the Government accepted that principles ought to be contained in the new legislation but altered the focus of the list proposed by Richardson to emphasise public safety concerns and the coercive role of the law. Thus it added a specific principle that 'the safety of both the individual patient and the public are of key importance in determining the question of whether compulsory powers should be imposed', and it altered the principle of least restrictive alternative to require that 'where compulsory powers are used, care and treatment should be located in the least restrictive setting consistent with the patient's best interests and safety and the safety of the public'(DH 1999d, p15). It specifically dissented from Richardson's view that autonomy and consensual care should be guiding principles of the legislation (DH 1999d, p16). The Government took the view that capacity was irrelevant to compulsion: compulsion was a matter of protection from risk (DH 1999d, p32). The Government further proposed reducing the procedural safeguards proposed by the Richardson Report.

— At the same time as this process was happening, a parallel programme of law reform was in place relating to personality disorder. The Fallon Committee had been appointed in 1998 jointly by the Department of Health and the Home Office to investigate allegations of mismanagement at Ashworth Special Hospital. Its eventual report did not restrict itself to that institution, but addressed a range of concerns relating to criminals with personality disorder. The Mental Health Act 1983 required that an effective treatment must be available for 'psychopaths' if they were to be held beyond 28 days under that legislation. The Fallon Committee proposed that people with a serious personality disorder making them dangerous to the public ought to be able to be detained whether or not medical treatment was available for that disorder. It further proposed that criminal law should be amended to allow reviewable, indeterminate sentences for these individuals (DH 1999b). The Government largely accepted these proposals, and proposed a new set of procedures to confine people with 'dangerous and serious personality disorder'.

The logic of combining the Richardson and Fallon streams of law reform at the time appeared compelling. Both were, effectively, proposing revision of the existing mental health legislation, and parallel revisions moving in different directions did not seem to anyone to be a sensible approach. The Government responded by publishing a single white paper incorporating both streams of reform in December 2000 (DH/HO 2000). Politically, this was not a success: virtually all commentators, medical and non-medical, roundly condemned the white paper. The perception was that it was a move further towards coercion, turning the psychiatric system into a carceral system for those who might not yet even have committed a crime.

Given the background, this reaction is not a surprise, although some of the criticism was stronger than logic could strictly justify. Much was made, for example, of the Government's decision to do away with the treatability requirement for involuntary psychiatric admission, with no acknowledgement that this requirement applied only to people with a 'psychopathic disorder' or a non-serious 'mental impairment' (to use the terms of the 1983 statute). People who were instead suffering from 'mental illness' – the vast bulk of those involuntarily confined – were subject only to a minimal treatability test, reduced to virtual irrelevance by court decisions. Even the Richardson Committee had not recommended a change to the statutory definition of treatment, suggesting that some people who were largely untreatable could be subject to compulsion under their proposals.

The political climate did have the effect of uniting the opposition, however, and the Mental Health Alliance became an increasingly important political force in opposition to the bill. At its strongest, the Alliance represented roughly 80 organisations across the stakeholder spectrum. The Alliance was a novelty in English/Welsh mental health politics, in that it included both user and service provider organisations on an equal footing, demonstrating how far users could be integrated into broader political coalitions on issues of mental health policy. If this lesson is learned, something significant may have resulted from the reform process. In the early summer of 2007, in the final stages of the reform process, the Alliance did splinter, but significantly, the division was not between users and service providers, nor was it between civil libertarians and paternalists. Instead, it was between psychiatrists and other healthcare professionals on a matter related to professional roles.

In the face of united opposition, the Government's proposals became politically unworkable. Draft bills in 2002 and 2004 were greeted with derision, and the Report of the Joint Scrutiny Committee of the House of Lords and House of Commons on the 2004 bill was highly critical (House of Commons and House of Lords 2005). The Joint Scrutiny Committee stated that the purpose of mental health legislation was to improve services and safeguards for patients and to reduce the stigma of mental disorder. They proposed a capacity-based test for compulsion, and a move away from a focus on protection of the public as the legislative ethos. This can be perceived as an attempt to re-introduce some of the progressive thinking contained in the Richardson Report, and consistent with this view, the Joint Scrutiny Committee went so far as to propose a re-introduction of the separate statutory reform processes relating to mental health legislation and the law relating to dangerous and serious personality disorder.

The Government was unmoved, stating that mental health legislation was about compulsion, not safeguards. It further defended its focus on safety to the public and to users themselves, stating that it was only users and medical and social care professionals who seemed concerned by this focus (DH 2004, p4). If the NSF was to be the carrot, the Mental Health Act was to be the stick, it would seem. Nonetheless, faced with the opposition of the key players, it decided the following year not to proceed with the Bill, and instead to introduce amendments to the Mental Health Act 1983.

The Mental Health Act 2007

The result was the Mental Health Act 2007, which received Royal Assent in July 2007. While the Act is now passed, its terms are not yet in effect, and as of the time of writing (August 2007), it is not yet clear when implementation will occur.

On any meaningful criteria, the 2007 Act must be viewed as a failure of the reform process. Some significant reforms accepted earlier in the process are conspicuously absent from the 2007 Act. There will be no change, for example, to the role of psychiatrists on review tribunals, and principles have been relegated to a non-binding code of practice. The Act's most significant alterations to the existing law are as follows:

- *Categories of Mental Disorder:* The previous definition of mental disorder includes four sub-categories – mental illness, severe mental impairment, mental impairment, and psychopathic disorder. Under some sections of the Act, it was necessary to identify which of these applied to the patient. The government has removed these distinctions, although it still intends learning disability will only be treated as a mental disorder if it results in abnormally aggressive or seriously irresponsible conduct, as in the current Act.

- *Definition of Mental Disorder:* The 1983 definition also provided that nobody would be held to have a mental disorder 'by reason only of promiscuity or other immoral conduct, sexual deviancy or dependence on alcohol or drugs' (Mental Health Act 1983, s. 1(3)). Under the 2007 amendments, only dependence on alcohol or drugs is outside the scope of the definition. The effect of the 1983 provision had been significantly reduced by judicial interpretation (see, e.g., *R v MHRT, ex p Clatworthy* [1985] 3 All ER 699); the 2007 amendments remove the last vestiges of those restrictions. The Government was adamant that homosexuality would not fall within the scope of the definition: it simply was not a mental disorder. On that point, it may well be correct; but it will become much easier to bring other sexual behaviour, including paedophilia and sexual obsessive behaviour, into the realm of mental disorder.

- *Criteria for Detention:* consistent with its removal of the sub-categories of mental disorder, the government proposes to abolish a separate and more stringent treatability test for people with (non-severe) mental impairment and psychopathic disorder. Instead, the availability of appropriate treatment will be required for all compulsory detentions.

- *Nearest Relatives*: the nearest relative of a confined person has a variety of rights relating to discharging a detained person and blocking the detention of a person. The 1983 Act had a hierarchical list defining who will be nearest relative. The 2007 amendments include civil partners on this list at a level equivalent to heterosexual married spouses. The 1983 Act allowed the nearest relative to be replaced by court order, but the detained person had no right to apply for such an order: if he or she wanted a different person to act in that capacity, there was nothing he or she could do. The 2007 amendments allow the confined person to apply for replacement of the nearest relative, and expands the grounds for replacement to include that the individual is 'not suitable to act' as nearest relative. The user will thus still have to show unsuitability, and as such the Act remains a long way from allowing users to choose their own representatives.

- *Community Treatment Orders:* The 2007 Act introduces Community Treatment Orders (CTOs). While treatment by force in the community is not to be allowed, persons subject to CTOs who refuse to take their medication will be able to be compulsorily re-admitted to hospital on an expedited basis and without reference to the full range of requirements for usual civil confinement. A CTO may be imposed only when an individual is already an in-patient in a psychiatric facility, but notwithstanding the attempts of the House of Lords, there is no formal requirement that the individual be a 'revolving door' patient. This is one of the few substantively significant innovations in the 2007 Act. As it will extend the power of the state over users in the community, it is particularly disappointing that CTOs have such a weak evidence base: both the most recent Cochrane study (Kisely et al 2005) and indeed the systemic review commissioned by the Department of Health as part of the reform process (Churchill et al 2007) conclude that there is little evidence that CTOs improve results.

- *ECT*: The 2007 amendments do, for the first time, outlaw the imposition of electro-convulsive therapy onto competent and refusing persons. Further, individuals will be able when competent to refuse ECT, with that refusal continuing to have effect during a subsequent period of incapacity.

- *Advocacy*: The 2007 amendments require the Government to make advocates available for detained persons, persons subject to CTOs and persons subject to guardianship. The precise scope of this service is yet to be determined.

- *Professional Roles:* under the 1984 Act, applications for compulsory detention are made by an approved social worker. Under the Government's proposals, the individual fulfilling this role will no longer need to be a social worker, but might for example be a community mental health nurse. The role will be re-named 'approved mental health professional'. Further, under the current Act, the patient's 'responsible medical officer' must be a registered medical practitioner, almost always a psychiatrist with specific training. The Act will allow other professionals with appropriate experience to fulfil this role. Innocuous though this amendment appears, it is on this point that the Mental Health Alliance fractured. During the legislative process, the government accepted an amendment that required a registered medical practitioner to be involved in extensions to detentions. Psychologists, occupational therapists and mental health nurses broke from the alliance over this point, alleging that it undervalued their disciplines.

- *Bournewood patients*: These are patients who lack the capacity to decide whether they will consent to informal admission to psychiatric and other care facilities. A decision of the European Court of Human Rights in 2004 held that the rights of these patients in England and Wales were insufficiently protected. The 2007 amendments are complex. In essence they apply the terms of the Mental Capacity Act to these individuals, but ensure that some of the determinations required by that Act are made by people who have some independence from the admission in question.

That, it would seem, is to be the summation of nine years of law reform.

Stuck in the old days?

At this stage, it is worth remembering why reform of mental health law really is overdue.

The long hand of history

The first major statutory schemes relating to mental health law arise in the early nineteenth century, with the original County Asylum Act in 1808, a comprehensive re-write of legislation governing private madhouses in 1828, and a string of statutes regulating and clarifying the Royal Prerogative powers. Detention of criminal lunatics was handled as part of the County Asylum Acts, but also from 1860 by its own set of statutes. All four of these statutory schemes were amended in a cut and paste fashion throughout the century, in literally dozens of public acts. The streams were largely independent, however. The County Asylum Acts regulated the publicly funded county asylums, where admissions and discharges were administered by poor law officials and Justices of the Peace. The Madhouse Acts regulated private institutions, including charitable hospitals, and admissions were controlled by the family of the insane person and private medical practitioners. The Royal Prerogative statutes did not concern confinement, but rather decision-making authority over the individual's person and estate. The Lunacy Act of 1890 consolidated these various strands into one statute, but did not consolidate the strands themselves; the paupers who had been under the jurisdiction of the County Asylum Acts continued to be subject to a set of rules quite different from private patients, for example.

The first half of the twentieth century offered two significant alterations. The first was to add yet another strand of legislation, the Mental Deficiency Acts. These provided the basis of the current guardianship provisions of the Mental Health Act; they also provided the legislative framework for some early care in the community, before the Second World War. Second, the Mental Treatment Act of 1930 introduced informal admissions for the first time – perhaps the most significant alteration in mental health law ever. Through this period, the old legislative provisions continued to exist, supplemented by the new.

It is in this legislative context that we must understand the 1959 Mental Health Act. The creation of the National Health Service in 1948 had largely removed the distinction between public and private facilities, with the incorporation of charitable hospitals into the public sector, and the old legislative distinctions appeared to make less and less sense. Where the 1890 Act had left the distinctions largely untouched, but included all legislative strands in one statute, the 1959 Act actually tried to consolidate the divergent strands into one. The solution of the 1959 Act was largely to ram the different processes together. Where compulsory admission up to that time would be in the hands of poor law/social service officials if the patient was poor and the family if the patient was able to afford private care, for example, under the new system all compulsory admissions required both family and social services involvement. Again, a proper re-drafting of the act did not occur; many of the clauses were carried over from previous legislation. This was compounded in the 1983 amendments, as further tweaking occurred. The Mental Health Act 2007 introduces yet another set of cut-and-paste amendments.

The result is that there has not been a proper re-write of the statute since the original statutes were passed at the beginning of the nineteenth century. Clauses from that period are still contained in the Act, often expected to speak in entirely new contexts, and piecemeal amendments have made the Act virtually incomprehensible. This is a fundamental point that the legislators have seemed to miss: if an Act is incomprehensible, it is unlikely to be followed. Sadly, and tangential to the instant discussion, the government draft bills were also largely incomprehensible – almost models of bad drafting.

The first reason that a new Act is necessary, therefore, is the incoherence of the current law.

Developments in policy and practice

The second set of reasons that a new Act is necessary flow from recent changes in social and political thinking regarding mental disability. As noted above, the last major considerations of mental health law were in 1959 and, to a lesser degree, 1983. Both, therefore, pre-date the rise of the disability rights movement and in particular the political rise in importance of non-discrimination based on disability. In current policy and practice relating to care of people with mental disability, it is roundly accepted that the service user has a pivotal role to play in service provision. It is easy to forget how far behind the current Act is in these regards, so some examples are appropriate by way of illustration.

As an obvious example, once a person is detained in a psychiatric facility, his or her views about treatment for his or her mental disorder cease to be relevant for at least three months. Under section 63 of the Mental Health Act, the responsible medical officer (RMO) can simply treat, in a manner that he or she thinks appropriate (unless the treatment is psychosurgery or ECT, which are subject to different rules). It matters not whether the patient has capacity to consent, or what the reasons might be for any refusal. Under the Act, it is not even necessary to tell the person what treatment is being given. There is no appeal or formal challenge available envisaged by the Act to these treatment decisions by the RMO. Since 2002, the courts have held that where an alleged violation of the Human Rights Act is at stake, an application may be made to the courts on that point (see *R (Wilkinson) v Broadmoor* [2001] EWCA Civ 1542), but the courts have never yet found in favour of a patient on one of these applications, preferring to defer to medical discretion. Certainly, the Code of Practice states that patients must be informed of the nature, purpose and likely effects of treatment (para 14.5); but the Code is mere guidance. It does not have the force of law.

Similarly, consider the substantive portion of the current standard for confinement under section 2 of the Act:

2(2) An application for admission for assessment may be made in respect of a patient on the grounds that:

(a) he is suffering from mental disorder of a nature or degree which warrants the detention of the patient in a hospital for assessment (or for assessment followed by medical treatment) for at least a limited period; and

(b) he ought to be so detained in the interests of his own health or safety or with a view to the protection of others.

This is a purely professional decision, couched in highly discretionary language. How serious must the disorder be to 'warrant' detention? What does it mean to say that the individual 'ought' to be detained? Further, the criteria are astonishingly broad. The disorder need not be both of a nature *and* degree warranting detention – either nature *or* degree will suffice (*R v MHRT for South Thames Region, ex p Smith* [1999] COD 148). And clause (b) will be satisfied if *any* of health, safety or protection of others are compromised. What this all seems to mean is that if two doctors and an approved mental health professional (formerly, an approved social worker) think the individual needs admission, he or she is going in: there is no real substantive standard here. Certainly, the person detained may appeal to a review tribunal, but that tribunal is to apply a linguistically identical standard: the problem of lack of clarity and discretion has not disappeared, but merely moved to the tribunal level.

It is appropriate to emphasise that virtually universally, the professionals in question do not restrict themselves to these bare legal minima. Of course medical professionals tell patients in the first three months of detention how they are proposing to treat them; no doubt most would be shocked to discover it was not law but mere good practice to do so. Similarly, of course those in charge of hospital detentions take those decisions seriously and carefully, albeit in the absence of meaningful statutory guidance. That merely emphasises the present point, however: the law is manifestly lagging behind the practice norms taken for granted in the profession. A new statute is required.

These are obvious examples. The more difficult questions involve what the standards and processes involved in such an act might be. When the 1959 and 1983 Acts were passed, there was little doubt that mental disability per se warranted special statutory attention. On its face, that now appears inconsistent with a policy of non-discrimination. The Richardson Committee itself recognised this tension (DH 1999c, p18):

> 'While we received overwhelming support for the principle of patient
> autonomy many respondents pointed both to the contradiction inherent in
> the elevation of non-discrimination in a statute which then permits the
> compulsion of individuals essentially on grounds of mental disorder, and to
> the failure of our Draft Proposals to maintain a consistent approach to
> patient autonomy throughout.'

After defending its view that capacity was relevant to compulsion, it proceeded to consider whether compulsion of a competent person could be justified (DH 1999c, p19):

> 'There was a much larger body of opinion [among those submitting views
> to the Committee] which was prepared to accept the overriding of a capable
> refusal in a health provision on grounds of public safety in certain
> circumstances. The reasons given were in part pragmatic and in part driven
> by principle. Essentially most of those who commented accepted that the
> safety of the public must be allowed to outweigh individual autonomy where
> the risk is sufficiently great and, if the risk is related to the presence of a
> mental disorder for which a health intervention of likely benefit to the
> individual is available, then it is appropriate that such intervention should

be authorised as part of a health provision. Mental disorder unlike most physical health problems may occasionally have wider consequences for the individual's family and carer, and very occasionally for unconnected members of the public affected by the individual's behaviour, acts and omissions. The Committee supports this reasoning and in what follows we seek to describe a framework which adequately reflects it.'

While acknowledging the pragmatic attractiveness of this line of argument, it is difficult to see that this really answers the question about discrimination. Certainly, public safety is a concern; but other groups are statistically more dangerous than people with mental disabilities, and yet are not subject to special legislative treatment involving their preventive detention. Certainly, mental health issues may affect people in the individual's family or others in the community, but how different are these effects from physical conditions that are not subject to intervention?

We still have not really articulated why people with mental disability should be treated differently, if indeed they should. A justification may well exist, but it is not 'obvious' in the way that it seems to have been in 1959 and 1983. The Richardson Committee began to ask appropriate questions as to what a modern Mental Health Act ought to contain and how it ought to be shaped, but that discussion has only begun. As such, perhaps it is useful to think of the current demise of the mental health law reform process not so much as a failure, but as a purchase of time, creating a hiatus in which we can come to articulate our terms with a new legislative universe. The need for a new statute has not gone away; but it is not yet clear what it should say.

Is that all there is?

So how much time do we have? There can be little doubt that the current government will feel little enthusiasm for engaging in a new round of reforms in the foreseeable future; but will it solely be up to them?

Mental health law has been fiercely litigated under the Human Rights Act since that legislation took effect in 2000, and increasingly, mental disability issues are the subject of litigation before the European Court of Human Rights. Many of these cases do not result in a finding of a human rights violation, but some do. In practice, such cases may force the Government's hand, as occurred in the *Bournewood* litigation, noted above.

These cases are not going to stop, and a number of the matters at issue are central to the current mental health legislation. As an obvious example, the European Committee for the Prevention of Torture and Inhuman or Degrading Treatment or Punishment (CPT) has included the following provision in their standards for psychiatric facilities (p57, para 41):

'Patients should, as a matter of principle, be placed in a position to give their free and informed consent to treatment. The admission of a person to a psychiatric establishment on an involuntary basis should not be construed as

authorising treatment without his consent. It follows that every competent patient, whether voluntary or involuntary, should be given the opportunity to refuse treatment or other medical intervention. Any derogation from this fundamental principle should be based upon law and only relate to clearly and strictly defined exceptional circumstances.'

As yet, cases challenging the English approach to treatment of psychiatric patients without consent citing this provision have failed; but the CPT is the Council of Europe body charged with the enforcement of Article 3 of the European Convention on Human Rights and Fundamental Freedoms. The European Court of Human Rights routinely cites the CPT authoritatively in its judgments. It is highly unlikely to say that the CPT simply misunderstands the scope of the Article. The English law is vulnerable, and a successful challenge to the structure of treatment under the Mental Health Act would create a significant difficulty in the administration of the Act.

This is perhaps the clearest point of vulnerability in the current statute, but it is by no means obvious that it is the only one. Mental health law is being routinely challenged under the Human Rights Act. While the success of these applications has been mixed, there is every reason to believe they will continue. The existing legislation was not designed to withstand such challenges, and indeed the passage of the Human Rights Act and the potential vulnerability of the Mental Health Act 1983 to successful challenge thereunder was one of the reasons for the establishment of the Richardson Committee. Those problems have not gone away, and will only increase. Human rights as enforced by the courts are to some degree a moving target: as the standards of human rights discourse increase, evidenced for example by new international treaties and conventions, the scrutiny of the courts also increases.

In this progression, the Mental Health Act 1983 will prove increasingly out of step, and the current band-aid approach can only continue for so long. There is little or no support for the current legal régimes among the major stakeholders. As Lord Patel commented to the House of Lords during the debate surrounding the 2007 Act, 'the Mental Health Act appears to be a set of second-rate provisions, outdated attitudes and the shifty machinations of a Home Office forever seeking unfettered powers of social control' (Hansard, HL, 26 February 2007, col. 1482). It is difficult to see that the statute will be effectively implemented by those that subscribe to that view.

Whether the Government is enthusiastic or not, it seems inevitable that a return to root and branch mental health reform will prove necessary sooner than the Government may wish.

References

Churchill R, Owen G, Singh S, Hothopf M 2007 International experiences of using community treatment orders. (Accessed 5 August 2007: http://www.iop.kcl.ac.uk/news/downloads/Final2CTOReport8March07.pdf) King's College London

Department of Health 1999a Mental Health: National Service Framework. Series no HSC 1999/223 (Available electronically at http://www.dh.gov.uk)

Department of Health 1999b Report of the Committee of Inquiry into the Personality Disorder Unit, Ashworth Special Hospital (Fallon Report). Cm 4194. The Stationery Office, London

Department of Health 1999c Review of the Mental Health Act 1983 (Richardson Committee Report). DH, London

Department of Health 1999d Reform of the Mental Health Act 1983: Proposals for Consultation. (Green Paper) Cm 4480. The Stationery Office, London

Department of Health and Home Office 2000 Reforming the Mental Health Act (White Paper). Cm 5016. The Stationery Office, London

Department of Health 2004 Government Response to the report of the Joint Committee on the draft Mental Health Bill 2004. Cm 6624. (http://www.dh.gov.uk)

European Committee for the Prevention of Torture or Inhuman and Degrading Treatment or Punishment 2002 CPT Standards. CPT/Inf/E (2002) 1, Rev 2004

House of Commons and House of Lords 2005 Report of the Joint Scrutiny Committee on the Mental Health Bill. PP HL (2004-5) 79/HC (2004-5) 95

Kisely S, Campbell L A, Preston N 2005 Compulsory community and involuntary outpatient treatment for people with severe mental disorders (review). The Cochrane Library, vol. 3

23

The National Service Framework for mental health:
never mind the quality, feel the width?

C. Brooker • S. Onyett

Introduction

In concluding remarks to his review of the NSF for mental health, Appleby (2004, p74) stated that:

> 'We are now five years into a 10 year programme of reform. No one would claim that the problems that have affected mental health care for decades have been solved, or that we have yet the services nationally that service users deserve and that staff can feel proud of. We have seen, however, large increases in spending and staff numbers, greatly increased use of modern treatments, over 500 new specialist community teams and the lowest suicide rates on record. It is an exciting, impressive and promising start.'

The preceding chapters in this book have all attempted to grapple with a fair and often independent appraisal of the extent to which such changes have taken place. Chapter 1 underlines the primacy of recovery-orientated approaches in the delivery of modern mental health care. This final chapter, Chapter 23, synthesises the conclusions reached by all the other chapter authors under a number of headings: *inclusion* (Chapters 2–4); *specific service user groupings* (Chapters 5–9); *service components* (Chapters 10–16); *support mechanisms* (Chapters 17–22). Each of these sections is now considered below.

Users/carers

The chapter by Faulkner considers the policy framework for *user involvement* and the different levels at which users can be involved. Engagement with users

CHAPTER 309

The NSF for mental health: never mind the quality, feel the width?

covers a wide spectrum including involvement in: individual care; individual services; organisation-wide; research and development; training and development and finally national policy. There have been marked improvements in levels of such engagement but Faulkner carefully identifies some of the dilemmas that remain. First, the crucial importance of the need to come to a shared understanding about what 'user involvement' means. Second, the need for diversity is often not achieved with many service users being predominantly white and male. Tokenism is still a problem with able and articulate service users being seen as somehow 'unrepresentative' and representation often failing to translate into actual authority when it comes to key decisions.. There is also still more that needs to be done to 'capacity-build' at a grassroots level. Ten years ago, however, the clamour was for service users to be involved, the call now is develop understanding about how this is best done.

Carer involvement is examined by Repper and, unlike user involvement, it is clear that, over the last decade, carer involvement has not been the same success story.

Repper highlights the NSF standard in this area (Standard 6) which gave carers the right to an annual assessment with Local Authorities handed the lead responsibility. Appleby's five year review concluded with respect to Standard 6 that 'we have too little to report on improving the support we offer to carers' – scant progress, indeed. Repper postulates that carer exclusion might well have its roots in theories about the aetiology of mental illness where 'family blame' models predominated in the 1960s and 1970s. However, accepting carers as experts threatens professionals and where the focus of intervention is on the user this can create conflicts of loyalty for staff, especially when confidentiality is taken into account. What is also clear from pioneering work in the field is that professionals often lack the skills necessary to work with families as a whole. Carers themselves want services that include them, that are flexible, accessible and responsive and integrated. Before this occurs professionals need to change their attitudes towards carers in a significant manner. As Repper concludes 'the main difficulty for services and providers seems to lie not in how to work with carers but working with them at all'.

Sayce's chapter charts changes in attitudes to *discrimination* on the basis of mental illness. She shows how attitudes within Government have changed remarkably over the past 20 years, largely as a consequence of lobbying undertaken by both the voluntary sector and professional organisations. The Disability Discrimination Act (1995) has been a major cornerstone of change, enshrining key principles such as the applicability of the concept of long-term disability in relation to mental illness. Not that this legislation has necessarily changed the attitudes of society. A Department of Work & Pensions survey (2001) showed that only 37% of employers would take on someone with a mental illness. Sayce reports a large study of the physical health of people who experience mental health problems commissioned by the Disability Rights Commission (DRC) which showed, unequivocally, that:

'Five year survival rates show lower survival rates for patients with mental health problems for almost all key conditions.'

(Hippisley-Cox 2006)

A new body, the Commission for Equality and Human Rights (CEHR), will replace the DRC and track progress in improving these outcomes. The CEHR will possess formal powers to enforce change within organisations where there is evidence of patterns of discrimination. Sayce concludes by pointing out that it is vital that people with mental health expertise engage with the new commission at this strategic level. However, in mental health practice, services can make a huge difference by: employing vocational workers; supporting people to recognise that they have a DDA case; give helpful advice about who can take on a professional training; and finally, and importantly, raising expectations.

Client groups

The book examines the implications of the NSF for a number of different priority groups using mental health services: those from Black and ethnic minority groups (Chapter 5); women (Chapter 6); those with a dual diagnosis (Chapter 7); people with a personality disorder (Chapter 8); and finally, the users of forensic mental health services (Chapter 9).

Bennett's analysis of the *Black and minority ethnic* (BME) issues implicit in the NSF is highly critical. She presents compelling evidence that people from BME communities continue to experience racial inequalities in mental health care and she notes the lack of any specific NSF target to address the issue. The 'Delivering Race Equality' initiative has only been recently established but already the implementation of its action plan has been criticised for the inadequacy of resources and the lack of central leadership and commitment to the programme. For example, Winterton, a health minister, sent out a letter to Strategic Health Authorities outlining her concern about the progress with DRE programme – only 170 out of 500 community development workers were in post by the target date set for 2006. Bennett also questions the assumption that increasing community workers will impact upon the over-representation of people from BME groups in acute in-patient care.

Appleby's mid-term review acknowledged that the needs of *women* were not being met. The new guidance for commissioners and providers, introduced in 2002, is discussed by Carlisle in her chapter. The guidance was wide-ranging but couched in generalities and without specific targets. More recent policy guidance on commissioning women-only day services (DH 2006) has been forthcoming but there has been no effort as yet to report or evaluate the impact of these strategies and little new resource to implement change.

Dual diagnosis has also become an increasingly significant issue over the past eight years. Appleby (2004) suggests that dual diagnosis will be a priority over the remaining life of the NSF with work in this area highlighting: the need for better collaboration between services; better training for staff; 'intensive' efforts to prevent drug misuse; and the prevention of drug misuse in in-patient units. It is clear that much policy attention has been focused in this area with the development of training materials, competencies, good practice guides and even documents giving advice for carers. This squares uncomfortably, however, with recent research by Kipping in London, which showed that whilst specialist posts were being funded, very few boroughs had strategic plans in place to improve dual diagnosis services and this includes identifying the funding for education and training.

Dent-Brown and his colleagues examine progress with services for people with a *personality disorder* (PD). They argue that the pessimism that, historically, has characterised work with people experiencing PD has significantly reduced. Two major factors explain this paradigm shift: interventions are now more effective; and the original conception of PD as a stable condition has been strongly challenged by recent research. Investment has certainly been made in the field of PD. A national training initiative for education and training, costing £2m, was rolled out through CSIP. The team from Nottingham University that evaluated the project concluded that short-term delivery of training was highlighted at the expense of long-term sustainability. In addition, during 2004/05, 11 pilot sites received a total of £10.9m to provide community-based local PD services. A team has been commissioned to evaluate the services but has yet to report. However there are serious concerns that monies from the DH sent out to PCTs for the continued commissioning of PD services have not been ring-fenced. This coupled with the general lack of resources for education and training, highlighted many times in this book, perhaps tempers the 'therapeutic' optimism alluded to earlier.

The final chapter in this section considers the users of forensic services. Senior and Shaw examine each of the NSF standards in relation to this group. The authors contend that although forensic services per se have not specifically been addressed by the NSF, the NHS Plan, for example, did commit resources to the development of prison in-reach services. These resources are scant, however, with a median of four staff per team. New so-called *integrated* mental health teams in prisons are now being expected to take on the functions of CMHTs and primary care against the backdrop of a very high prevalence of mental health disorder in these settings. The integration of mainstream mental health services with prison mental health services also needs much improvement as the second national survey of prison in-reach amply demonstrates (Brooker et al 2007). Forensic mental health services outwith prisons have never been addressed specifically by the NSF or in its review. Indeed, prisoners apart, no official review of the NSF has made specific mention of the services required by mentally disordered offenders.

Service components

The NSF for mental health, in combination with the National Plan, laid out plans for both new functional service models and improvements to existing provision. Targets, largely quantitative, flowed from these intentions and Appleby (2004) provides a commentary, in his midway five-year review, on the amount of progress achieved in relation to each NSF standard. Seven years into the implementation of the NSF, and from perhaps a more objective stance, our contributors give another perspective.

Assertive outreach is a real success story, suggests Freeman, which is admired throughout the world – ironically perhaps in the USA most of all. He argues that assertive outreach is the notable achievement of the past decade with 263 teams now surpassing the target of 220 teams by 2003. Interestingly, many

AO services predated the implementation of the NSF and were being established as far back as the early 1990s. Freeman does, however, argue that many clinicians would benefit from additional skills training in higher levels of the psychological therapies (a theme that grows and develops in this section). It should be pointed too that no recent national research been commissioned to examine the extent to which, according to PIG guidance, assertive outreach teams are working as envisaged.

McGowan and colleagues appraise the development of teams for *early intervention* (EI) in psychosis – perhaps the latecomer to the party. In terms of the quantitative indices often used to describe successful implementation, EI teams surpassed the number of target teams outlined in the National Plan. However, this chapter digs deeper and questions the extent to which these teams are: confident of future funding; operating 'faithful' models; and offering a wide enough skill mix. A recent separate study (Brabban & Kelly 2008) has surveyed the skills set of EI practitioners and commented that:

> *'The tight Government timescale for the establishment of early intervention*
> *teams neglected to take into account the lack of sufficient experts in the field*
> *able to lead such developments locally (Newstead & Kelly 2003). The rushing*
> *of such service development in order to receive funding may have been a reason*
> *for the lack of appropriately skilled practitioners being recruited to the teams.'*

The survey by Onyett and Linde (Chapter 16) raises perhaps similar concerns in relation to the establishment of *crisis resolution teams* (CRTs). Here, however, even quantitative targets had not been met. The survey reported by Onyett and Linde, undertaken in 2005, established that although the very disparate figures of the number of teams (243 vs 335) against the national target could be partially explained by merging of teams, overall the capacity of teams with respect to staffing was at around 88% of recommended levels. Other difficulties unearthed in the national survey included: specific staff shortfalls (input from social workers, OTs, psychologists and psychiatrists was low); only half of CRT staff agreed that they had been trained to work in CRTs; the key PIG requirement for gatekeeping of hospital admissions was only reported by 68% of teams; and only two-thirds of teams offered a service between 10pm and 8am. When CRTs were asked if they could describe themselves as fully set up only 40% were able to do so. Not surprisingly, younger teams (those less than a year old) were some way off recruiting to the ideal caseload size of 20–30 service users.

In Chapter 13, Boardman poses a critical question that has seemingly been ignored over the life of the NSF 'where do *community mental health teams* sit in the brave new world of service re-design'? He points out that there has been no commissioned research to prospectively evaluate the impact of new functional teams on the work of generic CMHTs. The PIG for CMHTs (last revised in 2002) stated that:

> 'most *patients [sic] will have time limited disorders and be referred back*
> *to their GPs ... when their condition has improved' whilst 'a substantial*
> minority *will remain with the team for ongoing support.'*

Boardman & Parsonage (2006) estimated that in order to provide these functions an extra 11,107 care staff would be required by 2010. CMHTs, despite earlier anxieties, have emerged as the co-coordinators of care and treatment for people with a SMI and a point of access for primary care. However, as practice-based commissioning gains momentum will GPs be less interested in service users with a serious mental illness?

Primary care – often the first port of call for most people with mental health problems – is the specific focus of Ricketts and Ekers in Chapter 15. They note that one creative solution to the high prevalence of mental illness in primary care settings was to cultivate a new role, that of the graduate mental health worker (GMHW). Appleby (2004) is cited, who, in his review, laments the fact that commissioners gave a lower priority to the introduction of GMHWs (than other specialist mental health teams) such that by 2004 only 339 were in place compared to the target figure of 1000. Positive changes in primary care are observed too, including the increasing currency of 'stepped care' and the inclusion of mental health issues in the Quality Outcomes Framework. The fact that probably only 1% of people who need CBT in primary care receive it (Layard et al 2006) has led to the development of community interventions, book prescription schemes, computer-delivered treatments and guided self-help strategies. Despite these advances, record amounts of anti-depressants are prescribed year on year in primary care and the availability of psychological treatments falls gravely below the standard demanded in the NSF, i.e. access to effective interventions 24 hours a day.

Simpson reminds us that the first new NSF-related policy guidance for *acute care* was not forthcoming until 2002. It was an overdue initiative that came on the back of a series of critical reports and research studies coupled with a decline in actual bed numbers from 67,000 in the late 1980s to 13,200 in 2005. The policy itself and further developments such as the design of training materials, investment in research and monies for a capital building programme were all timely. However, the recent context of severe NHS financial funding problems (2005/06) has led to the freezing of vacancies and the cutting of yet more in-patient beds (SCMH 2005). Effective care-planning, including compliance with the requirements of the CPA, remain in Simpson's word 'elusive'. Meanwhile, the service user profile in acute care has become more challenging, with dual diagnosis and treatment resistance common, as, indeed, are offending histories. Whilst there was initially evidence that in-patient environments were becoming safer (suicide rates dropped initially but then rose again), aggressive, antisocial and uninhibited sexual behaviour continue to pose 'daunting questions' for organisations, as do other key blocks and barriers to the maintenance of positive change (Brennan et al 2006).

Service support

Apart from the direct provision of services, there are other significant strands of activity that have supported the implementation of the MHNSF. In this section four are identified as follows: mental health promotion (Chapter 14); research and development (Chapter 17); and education and training (Chapter 19).

Guite and Bywaters (Chapter 14) refer to the decision to include *mental health promotion* (MHP) in the NSF, as Standard 1, as 'brave and inspired' largely because the potential scope of MHP is so all encompassing. The first set of performance targets for MHP included: a local needs assessment; specific action to promote mental health in particular settings; action to reduce discrimination; housing, welfare benefits and housing needs to be written into enhanced care programmes. Whilst the presentation of LITs' local MHP self-assessments paints a mixed picture of progress, the investment in MHP has remained low throughout the period totalling just 0.08% of all mental health investment in 2005/06. In 2001, the Durham Service Mapping programme attempted to identify progress with MHP but respondents found it impossible to provide meaningful data. The authors of this chapter argue that there have been improvements in the field, but that all too often MHP is being led 'by a handful of dedicated persons with virtually no budgets'.

Research and development is examined by Clark and Chilvers and they point out that the MHNSF was one of the first to prescribe future service design drawing on the best available research evidence. That some aspects of this evidence-base were weak was acknowledged, indeed implicit, in research funding priorities over the past decade. The strategic review of mental health research (DH 2002) set this agenda concluding, inter alia, that there were few multi-centre large scale studies, few systematic reviews of evidence, little involvement of users/carers and a lack of funding. By 2004, £9m had been committed to 69 projects all aimed at supporting implementation of the NSF. In addition, in order to facilitate the conduct of large multi-centre RCTS, the Mental Health Research Network (MHRN) was created. However, as the MHRN gained momentum, the National Forensic programme was terminated in 2007. Although the budget of £2m a year was small, this latter programme was crucial in ensuring, for example, that research money was allocated to new areas of mental health care such as offender health care which PCTs became responsible for in April 2006. Although advances have undoubtedly been made mental health research monies still remain proportionally small in comparison to other areas of health care such as cancer and cardiovascular disease. A question mark too hangs over the new generic National Institute for Health Research Programmes (e.g. applied research programmes and regional research for patient benefit schemes) and whether or not mental health can hold onto a fair share of total health research expenditure.

Education and training is addressed by Rushforth and Baguley – both of whom have been closely associated with the NIMHE workforce programme. They suggest that the NSF programme of reform requires:

> '*a radical rethink of core values which embraces the whole system of care, questions traditional clinical practice, workforce skills mix and in particular recognises the role of the service user in redesigning education and training provision which is responsive to user need, evidence based and fit for purpose.*'

The lack of skills in the existing workforce has been highlighted throughout this text and there are several reasons which include the amount of money in

CHAPTER **23** 315

The NSF for mental health: never mind the quality, feel the width?

the system to pay for relevant training and the extent to which traditional educators/trainers have the skills to provide what is necessary. Certainly, studies have questioned the ability of Higher Education Institutions to prepare practitioners, citing some lecturers lack of recent clinical experience – thus they possess little experience of the skills and interventions they are supposed to teach. Some progress has been made in expanding that component of the workforce that is best described as 'non-professionally affiliated'. We have already seen how the target for 1000 GMHWs by 2004 had slipped significantly and that of the 3000 STR workers aimed for by the same date only 1990 were projected to be in place by the summer of 2006.

What is undeniable in the workforce arena is the plethora of training initiatives that have been spawned nationally. The list is a long one but includes: the 10 Essential Shared Capabilities; Mental Health Awareness Training for Prison Officers; an interactive CD-Rom toolkit for GMHWs; distance learning CBT packages (PRAXIS); an audit tool for mental health training; a £2m regional training initiative for personality disorder; CRT specific training; training for the management of violence and aggression; dual diagnosis packages; training for teams; a curriculum for physicians' assistants; nurse prescribing course; and medication management programmes. The evidence is that many of these initiatives, often rolled-out through CSIP, received significant front-loaded investment but became diluted or 'washed-out' very quickly (Repper & Brooker 2002), and were implemented in a highly variable fashion (Brabban et al 2006, Brooker & Sirdifield 2006, Greatbatch et al 2006). The much more difficult exercise of course, within the current education and training commissioning environment, is to invest sustainably in the right levels of training for the most appropriate staff. In 2003, 80% of LITs assessed themselves as either red or amber on the development of local education and training plans – we suspect little has changed, especially given the financial constraints endured by the NHS during the period 2005/06.

Legislation

A strong contrast is revealed in this chapter between government's concern for public protection and the various lobby groups who have consistently objected to the coercive nature of newly proposed legislation. Bartlett argues that it is this debate that has largely stymied progress with legislative reform, leading in 2007 to a much watered down Mental Health Act receiving royal assent in July. Bartlett lists the Act's most significant changes as: categories of mental disorder; definition of mental disorder; criteria for detention; nearest relatives; community treatment orders; ECT; professional roles and Bournewood patients (i.e. those lacking capacity to consent to informal admission). Furthermore, it is argued that English law here is vulnerable through (a) being challenged under the Human Rights Act and (b) the law is arguably at odds with European policy. One successful challenge here would create serious problems with the administration of the act. Interestingly, Bartlett asserts that beside the detail, the nature of the new Mental Health Act (2007) conflicts with the ideals outlined in the NSF.

Costs

In a comprehensive and thorough review Parsonage (Chapter 20) examines the costs of implementing the NSF. He notes that unlike New Zealand, where detailed financial information has been presented regularly as the new national mental health strategy has been implemented, the situation in England has been less coordinated. Although the Wanless Report indicated that delivery of the MHNSF would be equivalent to annual uplift in spending of 8.8% annually, no specific breakdown was given, nor were any assumptions underpinning the estimate outlined. If the information from the Mental Health Strategies analysis of financial mapping returns is robust, spending would need to increase from 2006 by 9.6% per annum until 2010–2011 to fully implement the NSF. The sophisticated analysis undertaken by Parsonage indicates that this is unlikely and that funded capacity for adult mental health care will be 80% of the NSF target level. In this scenario, and despite the achievements related to increases in mental health spending, how will competing priorities for funds from 2007 on be determined?

The voluntary sector

In Chapter 21 McCulloch and Howland provide original data, gleaned from a survey, which examines the contribution that will be made to the modernisation of mental health services. The SWOT analysis that is reported summarises the position well. Opportunities abound both in terms of the current policy emphasis on integrated models and in social enterprise. These openings play well to the strengths of the sector which is always values-led, largely innovative, lacks bureaucracy and embraces diversity. The authors acknowledge the weaknesses of the voluntary sector, often in relation to management and governance. However, as future service providers, there are clearly issues to resolve in relation to ensuring the input of clinical and professional staff. Finally, threats to the third way are seen as the speed of change, the labour market and, importantly, a lack of understanding on the part of the statutory sector. The final message is that, whatever hue any future government might be, there will be no shift away from the role of the voluntary sector in reshaping mental health services in partnership – the sort of partnerships that might well see joint social enterprise companies becoming de riguer.

Summary

Appleby's 5-year review of the implementation of the NSF comments that we suffer from an English inclination towards punishing self-criticism. It is too easy to be cynical about the progress achieved since the historic achievement that the NSF represented. There is a real need to mark and celebrate the very considerable achievements of the wider variety of stakeholder involved. We want to particularly highlight the progress that has been made in user participation, and an increased imperative to focus on the implications of social inequalities (e.g. as arising from race, gender or disability) when developing and providing services.

CHAPTER 317

The NSF for mental health: never mind the quality, feel the width?

However, holding on to and building on that progress and the promises of a better future requires very clear-eyed and candid recognition that mental health service implementation still remains in many places a stunted and frail plant requiring continued attention and nurturing. The use of Local Area Agreements as the vehicle for partnership working, the new environment for commissioning (especially practice-based commissioning), and a potentially more competitive and covert provider environment means that the need for committed leadership, resources and policy attention remains as significant as ever. Even in the area of user participation successive health commission surveys on the views of service users suggest that progress on the ground has stalled. Of particular concern is the need to be constantly developing the next generation of skilled and committed stakeholders in mental health care and particularly practitioners. This remains one of the areas that have been most consistently neglected.

Being the first of the NSFs significantly impacted on the former 'Cinderella' status of mental health care. We have been allowed our place at the ball. However much more needs to be done before we can assume a 'happy ever after' outcome for this particular princess.

References

Appleby L 2004 The National Service Framework – five years on. Department of Health, London

Boardman J, Parsonage M 2006 Delivering the Government's mental health policies: services, staffing and costs. The Sainsbury Centre for Mental Health, London

Brabban A, McGonagle I, Brooker C 2006 The ten essential shared capabilities; a framework for the mental health practice. Journal of Mental Health Workforce Development 1(3):4–14

Brabban A, Kelly M 2008 A national survey of psychosocial intervention training & skills in early intervention services in England. Accepted for publication in the Journal of Mental Health Workforce Development

Brennan G, Flood C, Bowers L 2006 Constraints and blocks to change and improvements on acute psychiatric wards – lessons from the CITY Nurses project. Journal of Psychiatric and Mental Health Nursing 13(5):475–482

Brooker C, Sirdifield S 2006 Mapping the introduction of a mental health awareness in custodial settings self-directed workbook across eight care services improvement partnership patches. Journal of Mental Health Workforce Development 1(4):29–35

Brooker C, Gojkovic D, Shaw J 2007 The second national survey of prison in-reach teams. Final Report to the Department of Health

Department of Health 2002 A strategic review of mental health research. DH, London

Department of Health 2006 Supporting women into the mainstream – commissioning Final Report to the Department of Health (http://www.socialinclusion.org.uk/publications/Womens_Day_Services_Doc.pdf)

Department of Work and Pensions 2001 Recruiting Benefit Claimants: Qualitative research with employers in ONE pilot areas. Research Series Paper No. 150 (prepared by Bunt K, Shury J, Vivian D). DWP, London

Greatbatch D, Lewis P, Owen S, Tolley H, Wilmut J 2006 Evaluation of the Personality Disorder Training Initiative. Final Academic Report to the Department of Health. The Centre for Developing and Evaluating Lifelong Leaning, Nottingham

Hippisley-Cox et al 2006 Cited in Equal Treatment: Closing the Gap. A Formal Investigation into physical health inequalities experienced by people with learning disabilities and/or mental health problems. DRC, London

Layard R, Clark D, Knapp M, Mayraz G 2006 Implementing the NICE guidelines for depression and anxiety: a cost–benefit analysis. (http://cep.lse.ac.uk/research/mentalhealth/default.asp) Centre for Economic Performance, London School of Economics, London

Repper D, Brooker C 2002 Avoiding the Wash Out: Developing the organisational context to increase the uptake of evidence-based practice for psychosis. Northern Centre for Mental Health, York

Sainsbury Centre for Mental Health 2005 The care programme approach – back on track? Sainsbury Centre for Mental Health, London

Index